Law, Liability, and Ethics

for Medical Office Professionals

Third Edition

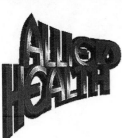

Law, Liability, and Ethics

for Medical Office Professionals

Third Edition

Myrtle Flight, J.D., M.Ed., C.M.A.

Former Assistant Director
Blue Hills Regional Technical School
Adjunct Faculty Massasoit Community College
and Northeastern University
Member of the Massachusetts Bar

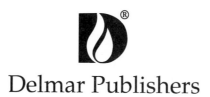

Delmar Publishers

an International Thomson Publishing company I(T)P®

Albany • Bonn • Boston • Cincinnati • Detroit • London • Madrid
Melbourne • Mexico City • New York • Pacific Grove • Paris • San Francisco
Singapore • Tokyo • Toronto • Washington

Cover Design: Scott Keidong
Cover Illustration: Clare Johnson

Delmar Staff:
Administrative Editor: Marlene Pratt
Editorial Assistant: Sarah Holle (Acting Developmental Editor)
Production Coordinator: Barbara A. Bullock
Art and Design Coordinator: Timothy J. Conners

COPYRIGHT © 1998
Delmar is a division of Thomson Learning. The Thomson Learning logo is a registered trademark used herein under license.

Printed in the United States of America
8 9 10 XXX 05 04 03 02

For more information, contact Delmar, 3 Columbia Circle, PO Box 15015, Albany, NY 12212-0515; or find us on the World Wide Web at http://www.delmar.com

Library of Congress Cataloging-in-Publication Data:

Flight, Myrtle, 1935-
      Law, liability, and ethics for medical office professionals / Myrtle
    Flight. —3rd ed.
        p. cm.
        Includes bibliographical references and index.
        ISBN 0-8273-8183-2 (alk. paper)
        1. Allied health professionals—Legal status, laws, etc. — United
    States. 2. Medical professionals—Malpractice—United States.
    3. Medical ethics—United States.   I. Title.
    KF2914.F58   1997   97-9100
    344.73'0411—dc21   CIP

Contents

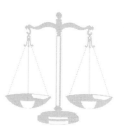

Act (ERISA); Occupational Safety and Health Act (OSHA); Medical Waste; Unions and Health Care Workers; Working Conditions; Collections

Preface

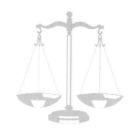

This book is intended to introduce the legal side of the medical office to employees and provide a foundation of law to be used as a guide against which individual behavior may be measured. It is intended to help prevent medical malpractice litigation by exposing the student to legal concepts of standard of care, scope of employment, criminal and civil acts, contract, negligence, and ethical concepts. It is not an exhaustive study of medical law and ethics but one directed toward informing and alerting employees in the health care delivery system of the legal and ethical aspects of their employment.

There are no hypotheticals used as examples in this book. Every case and article quoted is based on real life experiences of plaintiffs and defendants, individuals and institutions. Older cases provide stability to the system and form the foundation for society's expectations. More recent cases reflect current societal issues. A complete list can be found in the bibliography.

To those who enjoy law, reading cases is like eating peanuts. They have one and keep going until they finish the entire package. Cases are used to teach principles of law because the fact patterns are easy to remember— the mere mention of some "bizarre" situation calls to mind the legal concept behind the "story."

Law is dynamic. When there is dramatic change in society, it forces modification of legal concepts. Managed care, a reality in the nineties, represents a change in the way health care is accessed and medicine practiced. This change will force a shift in fact patterns presented to the courts in testimony and will contribute to the modification of existing legal theory in the resulting decisions. An icon is placed next to managed care materials to assist students in identifying the latest "state of the law."

Today, judges and legislators are struggling to determine who should be held legally responsible when a patient in injured. The Kennedy-Kassebaum Bill, known as the Health Insurance Portability and Accountability Act of 1996, presents many questions that will require future judicial determination, as do other acts passed by Congress and state legislatures. These questions will permeate every aspect of managed care. For this reason, managed care issues are integrated into the entire text rather than being isolated in a single chapter.

As we approach a future where provider, payor, and patient may all fall under the same corporate umbrella, legal and ethical issues assume greater importance in balancing the scales of justice.

Acknowledgments

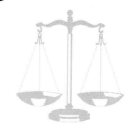

Approximately twenty years ago, the seed for this book was planted by Sister Winifred Kelley at Aquinas Junior College in Milton, Massachusetts. I was struggling to teach medical assistants office procedure with a limited text, while Sister Winifred was struggling to teach medical assistants law and ethics with no text. She was adamant that the students learn about the interaction of law and medicine. With the exception of a few articles in *Medical Economics,* and a couple of drug companies' pamphlets on upcoming medical malpractice crises, there was little material available geared to the medical office assistant.

At the time, Dr. Jules Rubin of Canton, Massachusetts, provided us with his medical periodicals, which we clipped and cut in our search to develop a resource file of relevant case material. A few years later, on a trip to New York, I purchased the book *Medical Malpractice Law,* by Angela Roddy Holder, from a secondhand bookstore; this provided at least one factual pattern for each legal point. At this stage, the complexities of substantive law, coupled with ignorance of procedural matters, yielded nothing but confusion.

The experience of being involved in a labor lawsuit (sex discrimination in promotion) further developed my interest in law, and the professionalism of Alan McDonald, the attorney who successfully represented me in the case, challenged my stereotype of lawyers. I applied and was accepted in 1979 to the New England School of Law evening program, graduated in 1983, passed the Massachusetts Bar in 1984, and have been a sole practitioner since November 5, 1985. While in law school, Professor Jonathan Brant, now Judge Brant, allowed me to independently research the materials fundamental to the chapters on law. My interest in ethics developed at a later date.

Some of the material in the book has been modified from articles written for and published in *The Professional Medical Assistant,* a magazine published by the American Association of Medical Assistants. Other information is abstracted from the newsletter *Legal Issues for Medical Office Personnel* published through my law office in Canton, Massachusetts; the *Journal of the American Medical Association* (JAMA); subscriptions to the *Wall Street Journal, New York Times, The Boston Globe,* and *The Patriot Ledger;* and daily living experiences. The material on medical ethics has been researched primarily in *Hasting Center Reports* and the journals of The American Society of Law, Medicine, and Ethics.

There are many individuals who have helped in one way or another in the writing of this book: Richard Pillard, M.D., whose patience helped me develop the confidence necessary to test my talents; Mary Wade, whose friendship and standards of excellence have reinforced my own striving; my son Curtis and his wife Barbara, my daughter Linda and her husband Peter, who have each contributed in his or her own special way; Lisa Arpino, who has kept the law office functioning throughout the entire life of this project; Mary Lou Stocker, who helped edit the first edition of the manuscript; Susan Arthur, whose excellent secretarial skills and dedication made production of the first manuscript possible; Alice Petrescu, who responded to a cry for help and competently completed the first edition; and Brooke Thompson-Mills, whose skill, endurance, and perseverance resulted in the completion of the second edition, third edition, workbook and instructors manual. The third edition would not have been completed without the assistance, skill, and encouragement of Pat Cully in the developmental phase and the efforts of Debbie Segal, a promising young attorney in my office, in the final stages.

Leslie Boyer, editor at Delmar, inspired me with her calm and reassuring manner to keep moving even when the final effort of completing the first edition seemed more than I could muster. Marion Waldman put forth the impetus for the second edition. And Sarah Holle, "more than a voice over the phone at Delmar," was inspiring and understanding throughout the process of producing the third edition.

Saying thank you to all of the people mentioned seems hardly enough, but I do thank you—each and every one. Because a book is a culmination of life's experiences, there are many unnamed individuals who have contributed to this material. Those I acknowledge here have contributed something special that made a dream become reality. The picture on the book cover is a reproduction of a painting by my sister, Claire Johnson. To Claire I express a special gratitude.

Above all, I acknowledge and am deeply grateful to my husband, Curtis, who supplied moral support and endless patience as I wrote and rewrote this book while trying to adhere to deadlines and the vicissitudes of private practice.

Myrtle R. Flight

I would like to acknowledge the following for providing valuable input in the development of the third edition:

Reviewers

Julie Hosely, R.N., C.M.A.
Carteret Community College
Moorehead City, NC

Karen Berger, M.T. (ASCP), C.L.S. (NCA)
Antonelli Medical & Professional Institution
Pottsdown, PA

Chris Hollander, C.M.A.
Denver Institute of Technology
Denver, CO

Sue Hunt, B.A., M.A., R.N.
Middlesex Community College
Bedford, MA

Charlotte Jensen, B.S., M.P.A.-H.S.A.
Cabrillo College
Aptos, CA

Linda Scarborough, R.N., C.M.A.
Lanier Technical Institute
Oakwood, GA

Brooke Koons, R.N., B.S.N.
Antonelli Medical & Professional Institution
Pottsdown, PA

Chapter 1

From Examining Room
to Courtroom

*The doctor's secretary knowingly misrepresented herself as a nurse, and
practiced medicine by diagnosing and treating a patient. Although the
secretary died before trial, the jury directed a verdict against her estate.*

Stahlin v. Hilton Hotels Corp.
484 F.2d 580 (1973)

OBJECTIVES:

You have just read part of a decision from a medical malpractice lawsuit in which a secretary, the defendant, was found guilty. After reading this
chapter, you should be able to:

1. appreciate the need to understand the law applicable to a medical
   office.
2. recognize that employment in a medical office carries with it legal
   obligations for the patient, employer, employee, and the state.
3. distinguish between the standard of care required of professional and
   nonprofessional personnel by the courts.
4. distinguish between practicing as a multiskilled health care professional and practicing medicine.

BUILDING YOUR LEGAL VOCABULARY

due care	medical malpractice	respondeat superior
layperson	mental incapacity	revoke
liability insurance	procedures manual	standard of care
litigious	reasonable person	vicariously liable

The facts in the following case were not disputed:

CASE STUDY   Mr. Stahlin, a guest at a Hilton Hotel, was dressing for dinner. His foot became tangled in his shorts and he fell backward, striking his head against the wall. A friend called the hotel desk for help. Mrs. Anderson, secretary to the physician on call, went to his room and identified herself as a nurse. She recorded the facts of the injury, examined Stahlin's head and took his temperature, blood pressure, and pulse; and after observing a bottle next to the bed containing pills for a heart condition, told him to stay in bed for twelve hours. The next day at noon his friend admitted him to a hospital where he was diagnosed as having a subdural hematoma. Surgery was immediately performed which left him with residual brain damage. Stahlin sued the hotel for negligence, the doctor and his assistant for malpractice, and won.

Stahlin v. Hilton Hotels Corp.,
484 F.2d 580 (1973)

IMPORTANCE OF LEGAL KNOWLEDGE TO MEDICAL OFFICE PERSONNEL

Today health care workers are caught in the middle of medical malpractice litigation, fraud and abuse regulations, employment hearings and managed care mergers. On one side, there are **litigious** patients, aggrieved relatives, and aggressive attorneys. On the other side, there are defendant physicians and other health care professionals, as well as hospitals, nursing homes, laboratories, and health maintenance organizations. The public expects miracles from modern medicine, politicians are increasingly involved in regulating medical care, and medical malpractice **liability insurance** is becoming increasingly expensive. Each case in this book will demonstrate that when one is involved in the delivery of health care to the public, one risks potential legal danger.

You cannot learn to avoid lawsuits for yourself or your employer, or handle your own job confidently, until you understand the nature and scope of the problem you face. That is the purpose of this text—to provide you with the basics of law so that you will recognize situations that may lead to a **medical malpractice** action against you or your employer. Understanding the ingredients of a medical malpractice action will allow you to practice preventative procedures and to recognize when you need an attorney.

Personal Protection

It is important to protect yourself from needless litigation and loss of reputation, personal wealth, or earning power by understanding basic principles of the law. This text does not guarantee that you will be able to do this after reading it, but you will be more sensitive to situations that are potential trouble spots, and you will develop thought patterns that can help you avoid legal pitfalls. For example:

A young woman, nineteen years of age, who had just completed an accredited medical assisting course, found her first job with a specialist in internal medicine. Seventy-five to one hundred individuals walked daily by her desk to meet with the doctor. Approximately twenty-five were scheduled in her appointment manual.

One afternoon the police came, and she was arrested along with the doctor. The doctor was indicted on several counts of illegal narcotic distribution, and she was indicted as a conspirator. Her salary stopped. The profession for which she had trained was no longer a potential source of employment, and she was faced with the reality of having to defend herself in a court of law.

The case took three years to go through the legal system. The doctor was convicted of twenty counts of illegal distribution of narcotics; the charges against her were dismissed without trial. She was never proven innocent or guilty.

Now she is twenty-two years of age, tainted by her employment record, and unable to find a job in a doctor's office or any other health care facility in the area. Potential employers will not hire her for fear that she might have been involved in illegal narcotics distribution, for fear that their office might therefore become suspect of the same by her presence.

(Author's Experience)

The above anecdote is an example of criminal law. You have now read examples of medical malpractice and criminal law. Later in this text, you will be introduced to concepts of employment law. As an informed employee, you must be aware of your contractual agreement with an employer, along with issues of discrimination, sexual harassment, and, in some situations, union membership and collective bargaining. In addition, you must remember that you work in a field that is regulated by state medical practice acts and other federal and state legislation.

Patient Protection

Patients trust that they are being treated by qualified personnel. Licensure laws can be interpreted as serving patients' interests by defining the education and experience required to perform certain procedures. A license indicates that the holder has the basic minimum qualifications required by the state for that occupation. License requirements also control employers by setting standards for hiring that ultimately protect the public. Licenses are granted by licensing boards that also have the power to **revoke** the licenses. The grounds for revocation include unprofessional conduct, substance abuse, fraud in connection with examination or application for a license, alcoholism, conviction of a **felony,** and **mental incapacity.**

Often employees of a health care agency are closer to the patients and more sensitive to their needs than are physicians. The requirements of privacy and respect for the confidential relationship between physician and patient must be met: privacy and confidentiality have ethical as well as legal bases. Permission to touch and the right to perform certain procedures are interwoven with state medical practice acts.

Many patients refer to everyone who works in a physician's office as a nurse, regardless of whether the individual is a registered nurse, licensed practical nurse, nurses' aide, medical technician, medical assistants, secretary, or receptionist. A medical office assistant who wears a white uniform, particularly with a cap, appears to represent a nurse. Today, many unlicensed personnel are assuming and performing tasks formerly done by the office nurse. These unlicensed employees may have been trained through a variety of disciplines. The conduct of a person who represents a nurse and purports to act as a nurse is judged by the same standard of care as though the individual were a properly licensed nurse.

It is not uncommon for unqualified individuals to forge, steal, or otherwise make use of a legitimate license without the knowledge of the owner, as in the following:

An R.N. who was preparing to move to Florida had a stroke and was admitted to a facility where she died a short time after admission. An aide who was working in the facility noticed that all the papers of the deceased nurse were in good order and ready to be sent to Florida, so she forwarded them for processing and received a license in the deceased nurse's name. She then moved to Florida with the license and impersonated the R.N. She might have gotten by with it except for one mistake; she was caught passing a bad check and sent to jail.

The prison psychologist who tested her doubted that she was educated as an R.N. Alerted to this suspicion, the Florida licensing board discovered that there had been a number of reports of incompetence on her record though her credentials appeared to be in order. After reviewing the records, a representative of the board visited the "registered nurse" in jail and was surprised to find that she was considerably younger than the records indicated. Confirmation of the birth and death dates in the deceased nurse's home state proved that the license the aide held was obtained by **fraud.**

Isler, Charlotte, "Six Mistakes That Could Land You in Jail,"
RN, p. 66 (February 1979)
Copyright © 1979 Medical Economics Company, Inc.,
Oradell, NJ. Reprinted with permission.

In addition to protecting the patient, the law also operates to protect the public as a whole. Certain health matters must be reported by physicians in every state: births and deaths; venereal and other communicable disease; injuries resulting from violence such as stab and gunshot wounds; child and elder abuse; blindness; immunological proceedings; requests for plastic surgery to change a person's fingerprints; and cases of industrial poisoning.

Physician Protection

Physicians are **vicariously liable** for the behavior of their employees while the employees are working within the scope of their employment. In the employment setting, this is known as **respondeat superior**—"Let the master answer." It is sometimes difficult to decide whether an employee is acting within the scope of employment. The test used is whether the behavior serves the interest of the employer or furthers the employer's business. For example, a physician tells a medical assistant to give a patient an injection of penicillin and asks the nurse to prepare the syringe. The doctor leaves the examining room. The nurse, without being directed to do so, gives the patient the injection but neglects to tell the patient what is being injected or ask if the patient is allergic to penicillin. The patient suffers a severe allergic reaction. The physician is vicariously liable under the doctrine of respondeat superior for the **negligence** of the nurse if the patient is injured and sues.

DUTY OF THE PHYSICIAN

Once it has been established that there is a doctor-patient relationship, the doctor has a duty to the patient to diagnose and treat the patient's injury with **due care.** Due care assumes that the doctor possesses the qualifications and training to provide competent medical care for the patient. Office personnel extend the physician's effectiveness; therefore, the duty of due care requires the doctor to provide competent office personnel. Although the following case is old, it is still recognized law:

CASE STUDY   A physician permitted his servant to give treatments to his patients during his absence. The physician tried to avoid liability on the grounds that the servant acted independently during his absence. The court stated "that a physician who tells a patient that an office assistant will give treatments during his absence is in effect assuring . . . that the patient may safely receive the treatment from the office assistant."

Mullins v. Duvall,
104 S.E. 513 (Ga. 1920)

Due care includes the responsibility of hiring personnel who are qualified to carry out the tasks assigned by the physician. In another case, the court found negligence on the part of the physician on the grounds that he left the treatment of the patient largely to the office assistant, whose medical training and experience were almost nonexistent. The patient had a severely injured thumb that required thirty-seven stitches, and he returned for treatment on seventeen different occasions. The condition of the thumb became worse. "A girl who merely graduated from high school and had worked in a hospital as a nurses' aide for about two years was permitted by the physician to treat the patient in at least twelve out of seventeen visits. She removed the stitches, squeezed pus out of his thumb, prescribed pills, injected penicillin, removed bandages and reapplied bandages to his hand, and even advised the patient as to the treatment to be followed" (*Delaney v. Rosenthal*, 196 N.E.2d 878 (Mass. 1964)). The judge determined that in allowing his patient to be treated by the assistant, the doctor breached his duty to the patient. The breach resulted in injury. Due to the procedures performed, plus the level of education and training of the assistant, the responsibility fell on the employing physician.

In a medical office, each employee has a duty to care for the patient. Each job requires special qualifications because specific tasks are to be performed. These qualifications and tasks should be documented in a **procedures manual.** As long as the employee stays within the parameters of a job description, the standards for the position will most likely be enforced. Once the employee performs a procedure not included in the job description, standards of professionals who usually perform that procedure will most likely be upheld.

STANDARD OF CARE

The practice of medicine includes various activities ranging from the routine and repetitive to those requiring advanced training, skill, and judgment. On one hand, it is wasteful and inefficient to require years of college, medical school, internship, and residency to qualify a person to perform routine duties that can be learned in a few months of specialized technical training. On the other hand, even the most routine procedure may be critically important and result in a crisis requiring the skill and judgment of a highly trained professional to save the patient. People in different positions may be held to different standards of care, as is shown in the following:

CASE STUDY   Kyle Crowe, a twenty-two-month-old baby, awakened ill and was taken to the office of Dr. Provost, a physician, at about 9:30 in the morning. There he was examined by the doctor. The diagnosis was nasopharyngitis, an infection of the tonsils and throat. He received an injection of four hundred thousand units of penicillin as well as a prescription for Cosa-Terrabon, an antibiotic to be given by the mother.

At about 11:30, the child became critically ill and was rushed back to the doctor's office. The physician had left the office and the nurse tried to contact him on the phone. He called back a few minutes after noon. The nurse informed him that the mother thought that the child was much worse, had had a convulsion, and was running a high temperature. The nurse informed the doctor that she thought the child was about the same as when the doctor saw him earlier in the day. Upon this assurance, Dr. Provost decided he would have lunch and then return to the office.

The office receptionist returned from her lunch and the nurse left the office for her lunch. A very few minutes after the nurse left, the child's condition became worse and he vomited while lying on his back on a treatment table. The receptionist called the physician at approximately 12:30 p.m. and told him the child's condition was worse. The child died within a few minutes after vomiting and prior to the return of the physician and the nurse.

The case turned on whether the receptionist, after the child vomited, would have known to use her finger, or a bulb syringe, to extract the vomitus; and whether she would have known not to have the patient in an upright position but to have turned the child on his side or stomach. The court determined that the receptionist was not required to have knowledge of, or perform, these lifesaving procedures. The verdict went against the nurse and the doctor employer. Charges were not pressed against the receptionist.

Crowe v. Provost,
374 S.W.2d 645 (Tenn. 1963)

In the preceding case, the doctor and the nurse were held to a higher **standard of care** than the receptionist. It was determined that the doctor and nurse were professionals who had special knowledge and skill that members of the public as a whole do not possess. The receptionist was viewed as a layperson. The distinction between professional and **layperson** is very important for employees working in health care. To be classified as a professional, an individual must have an independent basis of professional knowledge from which to make an independent decision.

CASE STUDY   Once a person attempts to treat another's individual illness or to perform a medical procedure, the standard of care required may be the same standard of skill and knowledge as a physician. For example, a student, who had some previous experience in drawing blood and had received permission from his professor, drew blood from other students in the professor's office. Due to the student's lack of experience taking vital signs and administering first aid, one of the students from whom blood was taken fainted and fell, knocking out six front teeth. The injured student sued. The court determined that "the withdrawal of blood is a medical function, and that it was the duty of the professor to provide the same standard of care as a physician, including having a place to lie down, and knowledge of what to do if someone fainted, as would a physician drawing blood."

Butler v. Louisiana State Board of Education,
331 So. 2d 192 (La. 1976)

PARAMETERS OF RESPONSIBILITY IN THE MEDICAL OFFICE

The Norman Rockwell painting of the family doctor at his roll-top desk writing notes of the day's activities in the ledger depicts an era in office management that has disappeared. In those days, when the medical office workload increased, physicians relied on their wives, other doctors' wives, daughters, and friends to handle office business. As office procedures became more sophisticated and complex, the modern office staff came into being. In most situations, registered nurses, licensed technicians, and professional secretaries share office responsibilities. In other practices, a "hybrid" health care professional known as a medical assistant serves as a combination nurse-secretary-technician. The scope of knowledge required and the amount of responsibility carried by this employee are extensive.

Medical office personnel are the link between the patient and the doctor when arranging office visits, laboratory tests, therapeutic appointments, and hospital admissions. They are crucial in the development of good relations between physician and patient. It is important that members of the office staff understand the legal issues involved in practicing medicine and the importance of good staff-patient relations. Good staff-patient interactions minimize the nonmedical and nonlegal variables involved in malpractice and may prevent a legitimate complaint from developing into a full-blown lawsuit.

Medical Assistants

Although the professional status of medical assistants has grown during the past few years, many state laws and regulations, including medical practice acts and nursing practice acts, either do not acknowledge the existence of the medical assisting profession or do not authorize the delegation of administrative and clinical duties to medical assistants.

As a member of society, one is expected to carry out interpersonal relationships in a responsible manner that will not cause harm. This is known legally as holding an individual to a **reasonable person** standard. A medical assistant is a health care professional. The requirements of a professional relationship differ from those of a personal relationship. As a practitioner in the medical office, greater responsibility is encountered, demanding more of the practitioner than what is demanded under the reasonable person standard. Violation of this professional standard of care is the basis of medical malpractice lawsuits.

For medical assistants, the standard of care that is required is difficult to predict. For registered nurses and other members of the office staff, professional guidelines for accepted practices are more clearly defined. When a physician allows a medical assistant to perform certain functions, the delegation of responsibility is based on the premise that the assistant can perform the functions as well as the doctor, or as well as the nurse if the procedure is usually performed by a nurse. It also follows that the assistant may be held to the same standard of care as the doctor or nurse.

In a 1986 case, *Riff v. Morgan Pharmacy,* it was held that each member of the health care team "has a duty to be, to a limited extent, his brother's keeper." The plaintiff was given a prescription for Cafergot suppositories with instructions for using the medication (one every four hours), but neither the prescribing physician nor the dispensing pharmacist added the admonition that no more than two should be used per headache and that no more than five should be used per week. The warning was included in the product's package literature and was well known to health professionals. The plaintiff, who did not read the product's literature, used the medication as directed and suffered toxic effects.

CASE STUDY   Fallibility is a condition of human existence. Doctors, like other mortals, will from time to time err through ignorance or inadvertence. An error in the practice of medicine can be fatal; and so it is reasonable that the medical community including physicians, pharmacists, anesthesiologists, nurses, and support staff have established professional standards which require vigilance not only with respect to primary functions, but also regarding the acts and omissions of the other professionals and support personnel in the health care team.

Riff v. Morgan Pharmacy,
508 A.2d 1247 (Pa. 1986)

PRACTICING MEDICINE

The practice of medicine is generally held to mean diagnosis, treatment, and/or prescription for prevention or cure of any human disease, ailment, injury, deformity, or physical or mental condition. To practice medicine, one must have a license. Traditionally, only physicians could practice medicine. With the emergence of new health care providers such as nurse practitioners and physicians' assistants, there has been a trend toward allowing individuals other than medical doctors to practice medicine. Permission to practice medicine today is not a *carte blanche* to perform any procedure, to provide each treatment, or to prescribe every drug. Each individual who practices medicine is held to professional and/or statutory guidelines and accepted standards of care. In the case of *Stahlin v. Hilton,* a medical secretary was convicted of practicing medicine without a license. The following is another example:

CASE STUDY   MacMahon was a college graduate with a background in food chemistry, biology, and physiology and the proprietor of a food store in New Jersey. He sold "certain trade-name package products."

One witness testified that on her first visit to the food store she told MacMahon that she had distress in her stomach and pressure around her heart. He told her it came from eating improper foods and advised her not to eat starches or meats but to eat plenty of fruits and vegetables. He gave her a package of Sorbex.

On another visit she told MacMahon that she had a pain under both ears and down the side of her neck. He told her that her glands were not functioning properly and that she needed iron. He gave her a bottle of Seatabs and told her to take one to four tablets daily.

On the third visit she informed MacMahon that she had an irritation around the waistline and an itch. He informed her that she had an acid condition; that she should not use any common table salt; that she should eat lots of fruit, vegetables, and lemons. He gave her a package of Vegebroth and told her to use it twice a day.

The Supreme Court of New Jersey upheld MacMahon's conviction stating that "Whether or not the substances he sold and prescribed are to be classed as medicines or not makes no difference. Clearly MacMahon attempted to diagnose the physical condition of the witness and to ascribe a cause for its existence and prescribe for such condition."

Pinkus v. MacMahon,
129 N.J. 367, 29 A.2d 885 (1943)

A medical assistant is neither licensed nor certified to practice medicine and cannot decide the course of treatment for a patient on behalf of a physician. It is best for the assistant not to discuss the patient's symptoms with the patient but to listen only, making a memorandum for the physician of the complaints listed. If a patient makes the statement, "I'm not happy with my care," the medical assistant should not hide the information from the physician nor attempt to handle the complaint alone. If the patient is not cooperating with the treatment prescribed by the physician, the medical assistant should make a note informing the doctor and attach it to the front of the record. Medical assistants are the first contact with a patient, and often the last, and are therefore in a key position to influence the physician-patient relationship.

Because it is unlawful for the medical assistant to practice medicine, it is unlawful to diagnose over the telephone or during an office visit. Even though the assistant knows that a particular illness is prevalent and that the physician will prescribe an over-the-counter drug, to decide the course of treatment for a patient is practicing medicine. It is similarly illegal to take an X-ray of an obviously broken arm without a physician's directive.

In dealing with medication, it is unlawful for a medical assistant to dispense drugs. A prescription is an order given for a specific person directly from a physician to a pharmacist. This order may be given by telephone or by written instruction on a prescription blank signed by the physician. Each order should bear the name and address of the patient, the name and quantity of the drug or drugs prescribed, directions for use, and the date of issue. The Los Angeles County Medical Society sent the following directive to its doctors:

> When you ask your office assistant to instruct or refill a prescription, you are placing both the assistant and yourself in jeopardy. The physician's aide who directs a pharmacist to fill or refill a prescription becomes guilty of the practice of medicine without a license. A physician who directs his assistant to do this places his license in jeopardy by assisting an unlicensed person to practice medicine. The conclusion of this directive is that when you want a pharmacist to fill or refill a prescription, let the pharmacist hear the doctor's voice, or better, have written orders on a regular prescription blank.
>
> Roche Laboratories Medico-Legal Seminar,
> Los Angeles, CA

SUMMARY

Understanding of the law that applies to a medical office is important for employees in order to protect themselves, their employer, and the patient. Because medicine is becoming an occupation closely regulated by state and federal law, it is necessary for employees to be aware of statutes and regulations that influence the procedures they are permitted to perform. Medical assistants are professionals working in the delivery of health care and are held to a higher standard of care than laypersons who do not have special knowledge and training. Other professionals working in medical offices are held to the standard of care established by their licensing organizations at the state level and by registration boards at the national or state level. Certification means that the individual has attained the levels of education and training necessary to meet minimum qualifications required by the certifying agency.

Part of being a health care professional includes knowing the parameters within which one is allowed to practice. Most office employees are not licensed to practice medicine and must carry out their responsibilities without making decisions outside their area of expertise.

SUGGESTED ACTIVITY

Observe a medical assistant at work for one hour and document the number of times that person borders on practicing medicine.

STUDY QUESTIONS

1. Give three reasons why it is important for a medical assistant to be knowledgeable of the law.
2. Discuss: A mistake you make in a medical office may affect your entire future.
3. Research the medical practice acts in your state that affect medical assistants. You can do this using the index of your state laws and looking up the appropriate statute. Most public libraries carry these books. Internet access may also be available.
4. List four representations a receptionist wearing white might make to a patient.
5. How does respondeat superior work in a medical office?
6. List seven questionable procedures performed by a medical assistant in the case of *Delaney v. Rosenthal*.
7. Distinguish between a charge of negligence and one of malpractice with regard to medical assistants.
8. Why is it difficult to set a national standard of care for medical assistants?
9. Check each citation in this chapter and identify the book, volume, and page number where the case may be found. Then go to a law library or your local library and look up one case. Copy and read the entire decision.
10. A procedures manual tells who can do what procedure and the accepted practice for performing a particular task. Draft a procedure for keeping the reception area clean and free of out-of-date periodicals.
11. Give an example of a medical assistant practicing medicine.
12. Write a brief memo informing a physician that a patient told you he did not agree with the doctor's diagnosis.

CASES FOR DISCUSSION

1. Dr. Finch, a California doctor, was accused of murdering his wife. The physician was found guilty and sentenced to jail, where he was a model prisoner and received early parole. Residents in a small town in another state were looking for a physician and, upon Dr. Finch's parole from prison, asked him to practice there. Dr. Finch accepted the offer, passed the state medical examination, and worked as an X-ray technician while waiting for the paperwork to be completed by the Board of Medical Examiners. The board refused Dr. Finch a license to practice, stating that conviction of murder was sufficient to justify permanent revocation. The physician appealed. Should the court agree with the Board of Medical Examiners?
2. The plaintiff is a licensed physician and a board-certified family practitioner. A controversy between the physician and the hospital began when the head nurse and the night supervisor in obstetrics expressed

concern to the hospital administration about the plaintiff's delivery techniques. Another physician wrote to the hospital's chief of staff, transmitting the nurses' complaints and requesting an investigation according to the hospital's bylaws. As grounds for the request, the second physician listed incompetence in the performance of deliveries and care of the newborn, unauthorized use of experimental drugs, falsification of medical records, improper conduction of labor, and the performance of procedures exceeding granted privileges. An investigation was conducted within the hospital by one committee, followed by a hearing by a second committee to determine whether the doctor should be allowed practice privileges. The hospital refused the physician privileges. The physician appealed, taking the case to court. What should the appeals court find?

3. A woman was admitted to the hospital, where her blood was incorrectly typed as Rh positive. During the surgery she was given a transfusion of Rh positive blood. Following recovery from surgery, the patient became pregnant and subsequently gave birth to a stillborn child. Who should be responsible for the error—the hospital, the doctor, or the technician?

4. On a particular day, two individuals with the same name were admitted to the hospital. Their blood samples were mixed up; the first patient received the transfusion intended for the second and died. The trial court held that the physician was not responsible. The case was appealed. How should the appeals court decide?

5. A patient was seriously ill at his home several miles from the doctor's office. The only people available to take care of him were his wife, his daughter, and the wife of a neighbor. None of these women were nurses. Because of the lack of training of his caretakers, the condition of the patient deteriorated. Should the physician be found negligent in this situation?

6. The plaintiff was suffering from emphysema and went to see Dr. Phillips, who treated him by removing one of the carotid bodies from his neck. The patient sued Dr. Phillips, alleging injuries from this surgery, which was not a medically accepted method of treatment for emphysema. At trial, Dr. Phillips testified he utilized this surgery between 1,200 and 1,500 times and that 75% of his patients were helped to some extent. Three physicians who testified for the plaintiff stated that carotid surgery is an unaccepted method of treatment for emphysema. Should a physician who uses a form of treatment that is not accepted by at least a respectable minority of the medical profession be subject to liability for harm caused thereby to the patient?

7. A psychiatrist discharged from the hospital a patient who had received electroshock treatment. Prior to the discharge, the psychiatrist did not see the patient. The physician also ordered a prescription for a heavy sedative to be taken at home. He did not warn either the patient or the patient's wife about the drug. The patient went home, was confused and sedated, and set himself on fire with a cigarette. The injuries

suffered from the fire were critical. Should the court determine that the psychiatrist was responsible for the patient's injuries?

8. Ella Hicks, a licensed cosmetician, wanted to offer ear piercing as a service to her customers. She filed a petition with the Arkansas State Medical Board requesting a declaratory ruling that the piercing of ears was not within the definition of the practice of medicine or surgery. After a hearing, the board decided that ear piercing was encompassed in the phrase "the practice of medicine" as defined in the Arkansas statutes. The cosmetician took the case to appeal. Should the appeals court define ear piercing as practicing medicine?

Chapter 2

Functioning Within the Legal System

"The only thing we have to fear is fear itself."

Franklin Delano Roosevelt
First Inaugural Address (March 4, 1933)

OBJECTIVES:

The possibility of having to defend oneself in court brings a knot in the stomach, a sense of self-doubt, and nightmares to all but the most hardened criminal. Fear of the unknown, the knowledge that even your most noble act may be made to look shabby and questionable under cross-examination, affects your ability to deal with the situation. Knowledge is the best antidote. After reading this chapter, you should be able to:

1. differentiate between the origins of statutory, common, and administrative law.
2. identify the steps necessary for the passage of federal and state legislation.
3. distinguish between the appellate paths of the federal judicial system and the state judicial system.
4. identify three administrative law agencies involved in the regulation of the medical office.
5. identify the parties to a lawsuit.
6. explain the importance of a legal citation in legal research.
7. understand basic procedures in trials of medical malpractice cases.
8. identify the stages of an appeal.
9. demonstrate techniques that aid in being a good witness.

BUILDING YOUR LEGAL VOCABULARY

aggressive	cross-examination	negotiate
appeal	damages	negotiation
assertiveness	decision	perjury
bench trial	deposition	preponderance of evidence
beyond a reasonable doubt	direct examination	pretrial conference
burden of proof	disposition	preventive medicine
cert. denied	district attorney	psychological
common law	documentation	substantive law
confidentiality	incident report	testimony
constitutional right	interrogatory	witness
contingency	judgment	writ of certiorari
credibility	motion	

STATUTORY LAW

Under the Constitution of the United States and the various state constitutions, the federal and state governments are given the power to pass laws to govern the people. While federal law is uniform throughout the country, state laws vary. Included among the powers of state legislatures is the authority to delegate certain types of regulations to cities, towns, and counties, as well as to various agencies and commissions. On the federal level, the creation of the Social Security Administration and Federal Tax Bureau (IRS) are examples of statutory law. Medical practice acts and licensing are regulations set by state statutes.

Medical practice acts and health care licensing regulations directly affect medical office personnel. In addition, some states have nursing practice acts, while others do not. As health care becomes increasingly specialized, emerging professions find themselves embroiled in "turf wars." As economics become an increasing concern, cross-training among professionals becomes a necessity.

In order to survive in the medical office arena, medical assistants recently have been filing bills and lobbying in state legislatures to define and protect their right to practice. Others identifying themselves as multiskilled health care professionals are interested in the same issues. The legislative process is similar in each state and requires moving parties to make the original ideas leading to development of law.

ADMINISTRATIVE LAW

Legislative statutes require enforcement. In order to enable government to exercise its authority and enforce the law, the legislature delegates authority to administrative agencies. Administrative agencies make rules having the force of law and adjudicate disputes involving the application of those rules

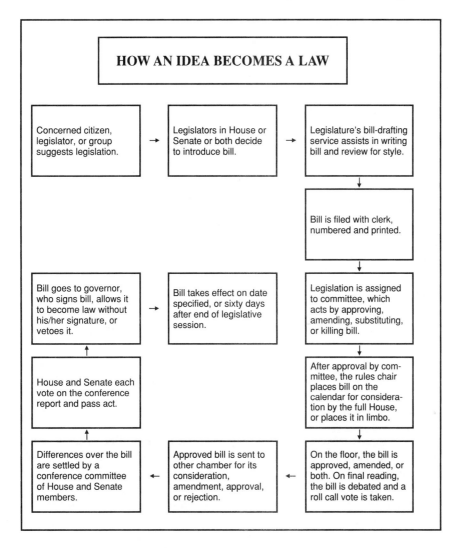

HOW AN IDEA BECOMES A LAW

Concerned citizen, legislator, or group suggests legislation. → Legislators in House or Senate or both decide to introduce bill. → Legislature's bill-drafting service assists in writing bill and review for style.

Bill is filed with clerk, numbered and printed.

Bill goes to governor, who signs bill, allows it to become law without his/her signature, or vetoes it. Bill takes effect on date specified, or sixty days after end of legislative session. Legislation is assigned to committee, which acts by approving, amending, substituting, or killing bill.

House and Senate each vote on the conference report and pass act. After approval by committee, the rules chair places bill on the calendar for consideration by the full House, or places it in limbo.

Differences over the bill are settled by a conference committee of House and Senate members. Approved bill is sent to other chamber for its consideration, amendment, approval, or rejection. On the floor, the bill is approved, amended, or both. On final reading, the bill is debated and a roll call vote is taken.

to particular parties under certain circumstances. In carrying out their responsibilities, agencies usually perform one or more of the following functions: (1) rule making, (2) adjudication, (3) prosecution, (4) advising, (5) supervision, and (6) investigation.

Administrative law is any law concerning the powers and procedures of administrative agencies. It usually does not include the **substantive law** put out by the agencies, which is better classified as tax law, labor law, social security law, and so on.

COMMON LAW

Common law is distinguished from law enacted by legislatures, or statutory law, in that it is made up of a body of principles and rules that are common to the entire population. Common law, which originated in England and is of Anglo-Saxon descent, is a body of law accumulated over the centuries. Judges wishing to be fair in the administration of justice have decided cases by looking to the past and basing their decisions on similar past decisions whenever the facts are the same. This has given rise to the principle of stare decisis, which translates as "let the decision stand." Stare decisis gives stability to the court system, yet allows for flexibility whenever there is a new fact pattern. Common law is distinct from equity law, which is based on the changing principles of ethics, morals, and conscience.

Common law is separated into criminal and civil law. There are statutory crimes as well as common law crimes. Of interest to medical office personnel is medical malpractice, which falls under the category of civil law, in the section on tort, subsection negligence, subsection medical malpractice.

MEDICAL MALPRACTICE

It is estimated by malpractice attorneys that approximately ten percent of the malpractice lawsuits that are filed actually go to court. It is also estimated that of those that go to court, only ten percent follow through to a final **judgment.** The remainder of cases are settled out of court. Settling out of court may take place anytime prior to judgment.

Malpractice cases follow the same procedures as other civil litigations, and pass through the following phases.

Phase I

The first phase is the time period in which the alleged negligence occurs. The patient becomes aware that he or she has been injured or that something is not quite right, and the doctor or other professional perceives that there may be trouble. Insurance companies require the filing of **incident reports,** which do not admit fault, at the earliest possible time. Sometimes professionals deny there is a problem and fail to file an incident report. Sometimes they try to shift the burden of guilt onto the patient. Anger becomes a major problem. The patient is angry, the relatives are angry, and the doctor becomes angry. Professionals would do well to remember the cliche, "If you are rude you will be sued." If the physician is unable to smooth over the incident, a medical assistant or other member of the office staff may be able to dissipate the anger and head off litigation by practicing **preventive medicine.**

The practice of preventive medicine assumes the positive qualities associated with **assertiveness** in today's society and discards the negative aspects of **aggressive** behavior. It has been shown that Americans prefer to stay with a trusted regular doctor. Office personnel can work to make this happen by improving the relationship between the physician and patient. In a book by R. M. McGraw, *Ferment in Medicine,* the following **psychological** factors are found to be at the root of many malpractice cases: "the need to be noticed, the need to be thought worth something, and the need to be loved." Recent studies of quality control experts reaffirm the importance of the doctor-patient relationship. There is a high correlation between satisfaction with health care and the development of a trusting relationship between the professional and the patient. A professional office staff can complement the physician in all these areas. Many times a patient is more comfortable and finds it less intimidating to ask questions of a medical assistant or medical secretary.

Phase II

Once the patient seeks the advice of an attorney concerning the harm allegedly done, the second phase is entered.

The first thing an experienced medical malpractice attorney will do is attempt to obtain a copy of the medical records. This may be done by asking the patient to obtain personal records or by having the client sign a statement releasing the physician from the contract of **confidentiality** with the patient. The attorney then forwards the release to the physician and requests the records. Often physicians charge for releasing records.

The lawyer has one or more physicians review the records and may have an independent physician examine the patient. Then, taking all this information into consideration, the attorney decides whether to take the case. Often malpractice cases are taken on a **contingency** basis, which means that the lawyer will not be paid until the case is completed. If the attorney loses, there is no fee or payment.

During the second phase, the insurance company, the doctor, and the attorney for the patient may **negotiate** a settlement. If the **negotiations** break down, the patient's attorney files a complaint. Once a complaint is filed, the patient becomes the plaintiff and the doctor becomes the defendant. Both sides now conduct formal "discovery," which consists of **depositions, interrogatories, motions,** and (often) further negotiation.

The end of the second phase of the lawsuit comes when a **pretrial conference** is held. Medical malpractice cases are usually presented before a tribunal or other type of hearing to determine whether the case has merit before it enters the trial phase. Even if the plaintiff loses at the hearing, there are built-in procedures to protect the plaintiff's **constitutional right** to take the dispute to trial. (See the chart of The Civil Case Process in the appendix.)

Phase III

A trial is a means of settling a dispute between two parties before a judge or a jury. The plaintiff presents the facts of the case as he or she sees them, and the defendant has the opportunity to present the facts of the case as he or she sees them. The jury determines which set of facts appear to be correct. The judge controls the trial and makes decisions about the law being tested by the opposing parties. Rarely is a trial as dramatic and colorful as those portrayed on television and in the movies. The attorneys are just people trying to make a living by presenting their clients' cases. The judge is trying to offer both parties a fair hearing, as well as keep cases moving through the court. The **witnesses** are ordinary people interested in telling their story. The members of the jury are trying to listen and make a fair decision. In **bench trials,** the judge serves as both judge and jury, ruling on the law as well as the facts. Once the **decision** comes down, **disposition** is pronounced, and **damages,** if any, are awarded, the lawsuit goes into Phase IV.

Phase IV

Either side has the right to appeal the decision. Usually the party losing pursues an appeal. The following chart indicates the route of **appeal** for most medical malpractice cases tried in the state court system:

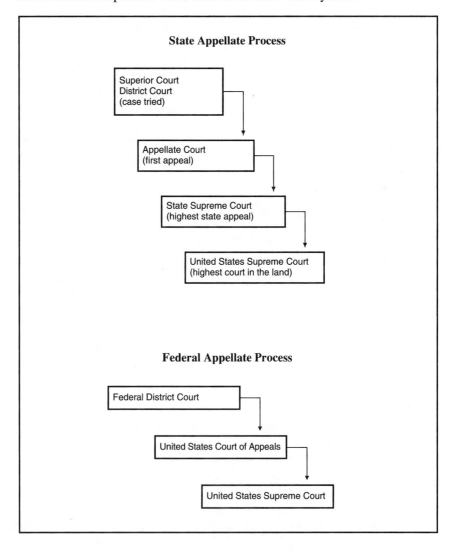

Generally, a decision can be appealed only on matters of law. This means that the legal principles of the lower court's decision are challenged, not the facts of the case. Not every case that is appealed goes to the United States Supreme Court. From cases tried in the state court system, only those concerning conflicts between state constitutional law and the Constitution of the United States can be appealed to the United States Supreme Court, with certain defined exceptions.

When you review the citations of Supreme Court cases, some will be marked **"cert. denied."** This means that the Supreme Court received a **writ of certiorari** from the party appealing the decision and refused to hear the case, letting the state law stand. According to *Black's Law Dictionary,* a writ of certiorari is an order by the appellate court that is used when the court has discretion on whether to hear an appeal.

PREPARING YOUR CASE FOR COURT

Most cases are won outside the courtroom. The preparation of the attorney and the witnesses is crucial to winning a lawsuit. When considering your **testimony,** look at both sides and see where you fit into the total picture before you get to the hearing. Try to anticipate what defense the other side will offer to your remarks. Try to be objective about your strong points and weak arguments.

- Pay attention. Trials sometimes become very boring, and it is hard to follow what is happening. If you are testifying or going to be testifying, it is important to recognize that the judge and jury are looking at you, trying to determine whether you are a credible witness. The way you behave is being observed at all times. If you are attending a deposition, everything you say is being recorded and can be used against you at trial to test your **credibility.** If you feel tired while you are testifying, you may ask for a recess. Do not daydream and mentally remove yourself from the situation. It is important that you concentrate on what is happening.
- Behave in a professional manner. The people who are listening to you testify do not know you. The way you look and present yourself is very important when assessing your credibility. Respond clearly and in your own language to the questions. Sit up straight and do not chew gum, tap your fingers, or twirl your thumbs or hair. Dress in a manner consistent with the competent employee you are portraying.
- Answer the question. When someone asks you a question, do not give flippant, offhand responses. Do not make a joke or answer quickly in an attempt to get the whole thing over with. Think about what you are saying, and if you are given something to read, make certain that you read it thoroughly. In addition, if you do not know an answer, say so; do not fabricate something.
- Cooperate with your attorney. If your attorney objects to a question, do not answer anyway because you think it will not hurt you. When an

attorney objects to a question, he or she may be telling you how to handle the subject matter. Confer privately with your attorney during a recess about any disagreements or questions.

- Honesty is the best policy. Remember, you are testifying under oath, and any false statement may ruin the total credibility of your story. Lying under oath is **perjury.** If the opposing attorney asks you if you have discussed the case with anyone, the answer is yes. Of course you have discussed the matter with someone else, particularly your attorney. Many times a perfectly credible and true story is totally lost to the judge or jury when a client swears he or she never discussed it with anyone before the trial.

Criminal and civil procedures are covered in volumes of material and take at least two semesters to study in law school and years to perfect in the courtroom. The purpose of this book is not to cover the matter extensively but to give you some idea of how you will fit into the picture if you must testify in a lawsuit.

THE ART OF EXAMINATION

The method used to present the facts to the judge and the jury is adversarial. This means that both the plaintiff and the defendant try to win their case by interviewing their own witnesses and cross-examining witnesses from the opposing side. Asking questions in an attempt to reveal certain information is an artistic endeavor. A witness should be prepared for both **direct examination** and **cross-examination,** which require different questioning techniques by the attorney and responses from the witness.

The following is an excerpt from *Fatal Dosage,* a book written by Gary Provost concerning the true story of a nurse on trial for murder. The defendant in this case is on trial for knowingly giving an overdose of morphine to a terminally ill patient. The **district attorney** is prosecuting the case for the Commonwealth of Massachusetts. Attorney Pat Piscitelli is defending the nurse, Anne Capute. In addition to giving an example of the techniques of **direct** and **cross-examination,** this section was chosen to show the importance of medical record **documentation** and the extent to which an individual may be required to testify to support a medical record. Mrs. Costello, Anne Capute's supervisor, is testifying about record-keeping practices at the hospital. The district attorney, Mr. Pina, in the direct examination, is trying to emphasize the number of times and the amount of morphine injected into the patient:

MR. PINA: What did you discuss about that notation, 10:15 on Saturday night?

MRS. COSTELLO: We discussed Anne's understanding. Again we discussed Anne's understanding of the presence of apnea.

MR. PINA: What did she say?

MRS. COSTELLO: She indicated to me, as I previously testified, her under-standing of apnea.

MR. PINA: Was what?

MRS. COSTELLO: Absence of respiration.

MR. PINA: Did you discuss anything else about the 10:15 notation?

MRS. COSTELLO: I don't remember specifically that we did.

MR. PINA: What did you discuss next?

MRS. COSTELLO: We discussed the "11:15 morphine sulfate, forty-five mil-ligrams, s.c., in right arm, nail beds are bluish, extremities warm, apnea ten to fif-teen seconds in duration. Not responding. Condition very poor. Valium ten mil-ligrams, IM times two at 6 p.m., and 9:45."

MR. PINA: Would you tell us what that discussion was?

MRS. COSTELLO: I asked Anne to describe to me the effects of that dose, forty-five milligrams, on the patient . . . and Anne stated to me that it would kill her. "My God, it would be enough to kill an elephant." After this discussion Anne acknowledged to me, "I must have killed her."

Provost, Gary, Fatal Dosage,
pp. 196, 197 (1986)

In this direct examination, the questions to the witness (Mrs. Costello) are open-ended and she is able to answer freely and in her own words. The work of the plaintiff (in this case, the district attorney) is to get the facts of the case into the record and prove the elements of the case. In a criminal case, the **burden of proof** is **beyond a reasonable doubt.** What follows is the cross-examination of Mrs. Costello by Attorney Pat Piscitelli. He is try-ing to discredit Mrs. Costello's testimony and the hospital's procedure for documenting medication.

The hospital's procedure for documenting medication had been criticized. Its procedure for the narration of nurses' notes had been criticized. Nursing care poli-cies were often in conflict with other policies. One physician did not write progress notes until after the patient had been discharged. Another was using a rubber sig-nature stamp on case histories and physicals.

ATTY. PISCITELLI: Was there a deficiency noted that telephone and verbal orders were not used sparingly and were not initialed by the physician as soon as possible?

MRS. COSTELLO: That's correct.

ATTY. PISCITELLI: Was there also a deficiency to the effect that there was no listing of nurses qualified to administer intravenous medication?

MRS. COSTELLO: That's correct.

ATTY. PISCITELLI: Was there a deficiency concerning the policy of reporting adverse effects of drugs?

MRS. COSTELLO: That's correct.

ATTY. PISCITELLI: Was it also noted that 696 records were not completed and filed within fifteen days?

MRS. COSTELLO: Yes.

> The assault continued. Pat pulled out volumes of nurses' notes showing that all the minor mistakes Anne had made were being made almost daily by dozens of nurses.
>
> Pat showed no mercy. He pointed out four and five mistakes at a time. Before long it grew into hundreds, hundreds of stupid little mistakes of the type that Anne had been criticized for. And Costello, as emotionless as a computer, was helpless. All she could do was sit there and say that Pat was correct.
>
> Provost, Gary, *Fatal Dosage,*
> pp. 200–202 (1986)

The answers given by Mrs. Costello are short, controlled by Attorney Piscitelli as he works both to discredit the record keeping of the hospital and to build sympathy for his client, Anne Capute, by showing that everyone makes mistakes. That is the job of the defense attorney.

SUMMARY

Only a small percentage of the malpractice suits initiated by allegedly injured plaintiffs actually end in court. Each lawsuit that does end in court follows certain phases of development. From the time the alleged negligence occurs to the time the case actually goes to trial, both sides are involved in discovery, which is a form of legal investigation. The outcome of the investigation may be to decide that there is no case, to settle, or to take the matter to a judge or a judge and jury. Once a case has been tried, the matter may be appealed by either side.

It is important that an individual who is a party or a witness in a trial undertake extensive preparation. Time should be spent with counsel preparing the questions and answers that the attorney will ask, as well as anticipating those of the other side. Attention also must be paid to the dress and demeanor of the witness.

SUGGESTED ACTIVITY

The movie entitled *The Verdict,* with Paul Newman, is an excellent portrayal of a medical malpractice cause of action. It accurately demonstrates legal procedures, the problems of the legal profession, the agony of the plaintiff, the role of the judge, the effect of politics on the court, and an example of a "real-life witness" who is involved in a malpractice action in a position similar to that of a medical assistant. The movie can be purchased or rented from a local video store.

STUDY QUESTIONS

1. Comment on the statement, "We are undergoing a malpractice crisis where every case of a doctor's misjudgment goes to court."
2. Incident reports are an important part of the defense of a case. An incident report should be clear, concise, and truly objective. Practice your skills in writing such a report by observing something that happens in your school, office, or home. Document the incident in such a manner that it is truly an objective report.
3. Distinguish between assertive behavior and aggressive behavior.
4. Negotiation is an art and a part of everyday life. Be aware of an incident you have negotiated within the past week. Document the original differences between the parties, the steps that led to a solution, and the final agreement. Review the feelings you had about the experience. Practice negotiating the following situations with your classmates:
    *   a child wants to stay with his or her mother and not come with you to the examining room;
    *   an elderly patient refuses to remove clothing for an electrocardiogram;
    *   you want a raise but your employer says the company does not have the money; and
    *   your employer's daughter calls and wants to speak to her mother right away. This is the fourth call within an hour and your boss does not wish to speak with her daughter again. You wish to remain on speaking terms with the child and obey your employer's wishes.
5. Divide the class into groups of three. Cut out an article from the morning paper, preferably one with medical involvement, and prepare to role-play the parts of witness, plaintiff's attorney, and defendant's attorney. Practice being a credible witness, forming and answering direct examination questions, and forming and answering cross-examination questions. This will give you some idea of how it feels to be a witness and how to answer the different types of questions.
6. Trace a case through the appellate process in your home state.
7. Watch one of the several court programs on television and rate the witnesses as excellent, adequate, or poor on the following items:
    *   the attention span of the witness;
    *   whether the manner of the witness matched the part that was being played;
    *   whether the witness answered the questions directed to him or her; and
    *   whether the witness was cooperative.
8. Watch the movie *The Verdict* and apply the above rating to the witnesses.
9. Search the local telephone book for the names of administrative agencies with offices in your area.

Chapter 3

Intent Makes the Difference

"Anne, do you know the effects of that dosage on a patient?" asked the supervisor. "My God, it would be enough to kill an elephant," responded Anne. "Why did you give her all this medication, Anne?"

"I wanted to keep her comfortable."

Provost, Gary, *Fatal Dosage,*
pp. 196, 197 (1986)

OBJECTIVES:

Above is a conversation that took place at Morton Hospital in Taunton, Massachusetts, when a nursing supervisor first interviewed a nurse later accused of willfully and intentionally killing her patient. The interview was reconstructed in Chapter 2. The facts in this case were not disputed. Approximately a year and a half after the incident, the nurse, Anne Capute, heard the foreperson of the jury bring back the verdict of "not guilty." After reading this chapter you should be able to:

1. understand the reasoning behind the jury's decision.
2. identify other behavior that is classified as criminal.
3. distinguish between criminal and civil causes of action.
4. differentiate between a felony and a misdemeanor.
5. define negligence.

BUILDING YOUR LEGAL VOCABULARY

aggression	cited	deterrence
arson	civil	district court
assault	conspiracy	domestic violence
battery	criminal	euthanasia
burglary	defendant	felony

fiduciary	misdemeanor	robbery
first-degree murder	murder	self-defense
fraud	negligence	sodomy
indictment	plaintiff	statutory
intentional	rape	strict liability
larceny	reformation	superior court
malice	respectable minority	theft
manslaughter	restraint	tort
mayhem	retribution	wanton

DIVISION BETWEEN CRIMINAL AND CIVIL LAW

There are two major divisions of law: **criminal** and **civil.** In the preceding criminal case, the **plaintiff** is the state and the **defendant** is the nurse. The case is **cited** as *Commonwealth [People or State] v. Anne Capute.* A crime is defined as the performance of an act forbidden by law or the omission of an act required by law. In either case, the defendant is punished by society. Crimes are divided into felonies and misdemeanors. A **felony** is a crime punishable by death or imprisonment in the state penitentiary. A **misdemeanor** is a crime punishable by imprisonment in a house of correction or jail for less than one year or a fine. Legislators write and vote on law that determines whether an act is a crime and, if so, whether it is a felony or misdemeanor. These laws are found in the general laws of the state, and such crimes are known as **statutory** crimes. In addition, some crimes are felonies under common law: **murder, manslaughter, rape, sodomy, robbery, larceny, arson, burglary,** and **mayhem.**

Criminal cases are crimes against the state. Civil cases are crimes against the person. The same act may give rise to both criminal and civil causes of action. For example, in **assault** and **battery,** the state tries a defendant for the crime of assault and battery, and a guilty defendant is punished by the state. The purposes of punishment are **reformation, restraint, retribution,** and **deterrence.** The injured party then attempts to collect damages by trying the civil case of assault and battery, and the guilty defendant usually has to pay money damages for harm to the person. The chart of The Criminal Case Process in the appendix describes the route of most criminal cases tried in the state court system.

The most common civil claim in medical law is an action in **tort.** Tort liability is based on one of the following grounds: **intentional, negligence,** or **strict liability.** Intentional torts may be actions toward property or a person. Negligence may be the result of the performance of an act on a patient without using due care or the failure to do something that is required. Negligence is the charge when something just happens—when there was no intent, the outcome was not expected, but the patient was injured. Strict liability is imposed upon a seller for physical harm caused to a user or consumer when a product is in a defective and unreasonably dangerous condition.

In medical malpractice cases when a patient is injured, the intent of the medical professional involved is critical. In order to have a criminal act, the person injuring the patient must have had intent to harm, and the elements of the crime must be present. This differs from an intentional tort where the person inflicting injury had only the desire to act **aggressively** toward the patient. Negligence results in civil injury without intent. "I didn't mean to do it" is often the first comment by the defendant.

CRIMINAL CAUSES OF ACTION INVOLVING HEALTH CARE PERSONNEL

Misdemeanors and Felonies Distinguished

On May 18, 1990, Dr. Gerald Einaugler visited his patient, Alida Lamour, seventy-eight years of age, in a nursing home, mistook a dialysis catheter in her abdomen for a feeding tube, and ordered feeding solution pumped through it. Six days later the patient died, and the doctor was in difficulty. In the past, in a matter such as this, the physician usually would have been considered negligent and would have faced civil suit. In this situation, Dr. Einaugler was criminally prosecuted.

In July 1993, the doctor was convicted of two misdemeanors—reckless endangerment and willful violation of the health laws—and was sentenced to fifty-two weekends at Rikers Island. A doctor's medical judgment had never before been subject to criminal prosecution in New York, and rarely has it been in other states across the country. The attorney general stated that the prosecution of the doctor had nothing to do with punishing him for bad judgment but had to do with the doctor's "willful failure" to care for his patient by transferring her from the nursing home to a hospital as soon as the mistake was discovered.

The American Medical Association (AMA) had concerns that were expressed by Dr. James S. Todd, Executive Vice President:

> "He made a clinical judgment." He used his best judgment as to what to do. Our concern is that mistakes of judgment should not be liable to criminal prosecution. Traditionally, errors in judgment are handled through peer review and malpractice. Society has been poorly served by this decision."
>
> Nossiter, Adam, "A Mistake, a Rare
> Prosecution, and a Doctor Is Headed for Jail,"
> *New York Times*, p. A1 (March 16, 1995)

A misdemeanor is an offense classified lower than a felony and generally punishable by a fine or imprisonment otherwise than in a penitentiary. A felony is defined as a crime of graver or more serious nature than those designated as misdemeanors. Under federal law and many state statutes, it is any offense punishable by death or imprisonment for a term exceeding one year. The crimes discussed in the following text are classified as felonies.

Robbery

Law and medicine interact in many different ways. An individual is guilty of robbery if, while carrying out **theft,** the victim is physically injured or has been threatened and put in fear of bodily injury. For example:

A female receptionist for a North Main Street doctor was cut on the thigh and robbed by an intruder who wanted drugs, reported police. The receptionist, identified as a middle-aged woman, was alone when the intruder entered the office armed with a knife. "He said he wanted the drugs and she told him there were no drugs there," stated the detective.

When he tried to tie her up, he put the knife against her leg and either she moved or he pushed too hard and she received a small puncture wound. He took some syringes before taking the receptionist's jewelry and the money.

The Patriot Ledger,
Quincy, Massachusetts

Murder

"An LPN was sentenced to life in prison in April after pleading guilty to murdering three nursing home residents in St. Petersburg, FL. Authorities are sure Brian Rosenfield killed others; from 1980 to 1990, he was fired from 14 nursing homes for drug use and cruelty to patients. His career ended only when an aide saw him pouring a brown liquid, identified in an autopsy as Mellaril, down a patient's feeding tube. The bodies of five patients who died under Rosenfeld's care were exhumed and traces of Mellaril were found in two of them."

"Headlines," *American Journal of Nursing,*
p. 9 (August 1992)

In Milwaukee, a case involving a medical laboratory that has been accused of misreading Pap smears of two women is testing the question on appeals of whether a corporation can be charged with murder. The matter was brought into the courts after the deaths of the two women were reviewed by an inquest jury. The jury recommended criminal charges against the physician in charge of the lab and a lab technician as well as the lab itself. The physician and technician agreed to practice restrictions. The AMA stated that this was the first case in which a medical lab had been charged with a crime because of an error. Usually charges involving the misreading of a Pap smear are tried as malpractice cases.

Attempted Murder

An attempt to commit a crime is itself a crime. Anyone who attempts to commit a crime by doing any act toward its commission but fails in its perpetration or is intercepted or prevented in its perpetration shall be punished. To prove that a defendant is guilty of an attempt, three things must be proven beyond a reasonable doubt: that the defendant had a specific intent to commit that particular crime; that the defendant took an overt act toward committing that crime, which was part of carrying out the crime, and came reasonably close to actually carrying out the crime; and that the defendant's act did not result in a complete crime.

"Security cameras in the Vanderbilt University Medical Center parking garage spotted Dr. Ray Mettetal on August 22 in a wig, false beard and shoes with lifts. He was seized by the campus police, who became suspicious because of his shabby disguise, and he has been held without bail since then. When he was arrested, a large syringe that investigators said contained a lethal solution of salt water and boric acid was found in the pocket of his padded trench coat.

"Dr. Mettetal, the police said, was bent on revenge; he was out to kill the department chairman whose refusal to write him a letter of recommendation more than ten years ago destroyed his dream of becoming a brain surgeon. The doctor, 44, faces up to 25 years in prison on an attempted murder charge. The man who the police said was his target, Dr. George Allen, Chairman of Vanderbilt's neurosurgery department, was never harmed."

"Doctor Accused of Trying to Murder Ex-Boss,"
New York Times, p. 28 (September 3, 1996)

Robbery is an example of the kind of crime that is usually handled in **district court.** At the other extreme is murder, a crime that would be tried in **superior court.** The trial of Claus von Bulow for the attempted murder of his wife involved the testimony of numerous medical professionals, received national attention, and had an international flavor. Of interest to medical office personnel is the role of the von Bulow medical record that led toward his **indictment.**

For the first week of the von Bulow investigation they simply sat in Reise's office and read and reread all of the medical records. If the question of foul play could be answered, the answer would lie in these medical records and, with the help of doctors and medical authorities, they would have to piece it together from the lab slips, test results, doctors orders and nurses notes.

As Reise and Mirand pored over the records with the patience and persistence of scholars deciphering hieroglyphics, certain things began to emerge. Reise came to suspect that the key words were "the history on this woman is very limited and was obtained from the patient's husband."

The history that Claus von Bulow originally gave at the time of the first coma contained statements that his wife had been using barbiturates and that she took a large quantity of alcohol the evening before her coma. Yet, Reise noted, the very next page of the medical record contained results from blood tests done when Martha von Bulow arrived at the hospital, December 27, 1979, which showed no barbiturates or alcohol. Reise remarked, "Right off the bat that didn't make sense to me."

From the record Reise and Mirand came to believe that von Bulow had deliberately misled the doctors who treated his wife. They concluded that he was trying to paint her as a druggie and an alcoholic as a part of von Bulow's calculated strategy to divert doctors from the true cause of his wife's sudden illnesses. At least on the basis of the medical evidence, they had the makings of a case.

Dumanoski, Dianne,
"The von Bulow Case: Trek Through Medical Records,"
The Boston Globe (March 22, 1982)

An act done with intent to kill the victim constitutes murder. Claus von Bulow was on trial for attempting to murder. He was convicted in the first trial and acquitted in the second. The state must prove guilt "beyond a reasonable doubt" in a criminal case. Medical evidence presented in the second trial convinced the jury that they could not determine "beyond a reasonable doubt" that he had attempted to kill his wife. Anne Capute, the nurse who injected "enough [morphine] to kill an elephant," was also tried for murder. In her case, the question was not whether her acts killed the patient but whether she had performed the acts with the intent to kill. In the element of intent, the jury could not find her guilty beyond a reasonable doubt.

Mercy killing differs from the Capute case in that there is intent to kill. Mercy killing is known as **euthanasia.** According to *Black's Law Dictionary,* euthanasia is the act or practice of painlessly putting to death persons suffering from incurable and distressing disease as an act of mercy. It presents legal and ethical problems within the walls of a health care facility as well as without, as shown in the following example, "Florida Man, 75, Gets Life for Mercy Killing of Ailing Wife." The newspaper article reported:

A seventy-five-year-old man was convicted of murder in the "mercy killing" of his wife of fifty-one years to end her suffering from Alzheimer's disease. The judge immediately sentenced Gilbert to life in prison, with a twenty-five-year mandatory term. The state had waived the death penalty, making the life sentence the only possible punishment for **first-degree murder.**

Gilbert had testified that he shot his wife, Emily, seventy-three, twice in the head out of compassion. He called police and surrendered after the shooting. Mrs. Gilbert, killed in the couple's condominium apartment, was senile from brain degeneration caused by Alzheimer's disease and suffered from osteoporosis, a painful bone disintegration. Witnesses testified that she longed for and begged for death.

The prosecutor had urged jurors to ignore pleas for compassion, saying the shooting was premeditated, cold-blooded murder. The defense lawyer begged jurors to ignore laws and set legal precedent with an acquittal.

Pave, Marvin,
The Boston Globe (May 10, 1985)

The issue of euthanasia is a difficult one for society and the courts. For example, six months prior to the above case, a Massachusetts court ruled in the opposite for a defendant in a similar case:

The Andersons, a couple who lived near Long Pond in Centerville, had been married for fifty-two years, but a stroke followed by two operations left the wife, Olive, an invalid. She was paralyzed on one side, could not talk and was incontinent after her second operation. Ten days after her return home from therapy following brain surgery, Anderson, a retired chef, placed a plastic bag over his wife's head and sealed it with duct tape. He then called his daughter, Shirley, who called police.

Anderson made no attempt to cover up his crime. When the Barnstable Police arrived, the tape and bag were still on his wife's face. Anderson pleaded guilty to first-degree manslaughter and was sentenced by the judge to one year on probation.

The Boston Globe (October 31, 1985)

Manslaughter

Manslaughter is defined as the unlawful killing of another without **malice.** In order for there to be conviction for manslaughter, it is necessary to prove that there is **wanton** or reckless conduct. Every physician makes errors in judgment at some point in his or her career, but an error in judgment is not necessarily wanton or reckless conduct. A misdiagnosed condition or error in treatment, as long as a practice is accepted by a **respectable minority** of the medical profession, may result in civil liability. Even if the patient dies, it should not result in criminal liability. Manslaughter is the charge even when a physician does not practice in good faith, uses a form of treatment not accepted by at least a respectable minority of the medical profession, or practices under the influence of drugs or alcohol, causing death to a patient. In the following case, a physician was convicted by the trial court of manslaughter for the death of a fetus during an abortion. The case was appealed to the Supreme Judicial Court of Massachusetts, where the decision of the trial court was reversed.

CASE STUDY   A few days before September 30, 1973, a seventeen-year-old unmarried woman appeared with her mother at the outpatient clinic at Boston City Hospital requesting an abortion. The chief of the outpatient OBS/GYN services interviewed the patient and advised her about alternatives to abortion, which she did not accept. He then inquired about her last menstrual period. She placed it at a date that would indicate she was seventeen weeks pregnant. After physical examination the physician concluded that the gestational age was twenty weeks. He then advised and approved abortion by the saline method (a common method in use for abortions in the second trimester), and referred the patient to Dr. Edelin, the surgeon who would carry out the procedure.

A physician and a medical student in pre-abortion examinations placed the age of the fetus at twenty-four weeks. Another doctor placed it at twenty-one to twenty-two weeks. It was acknowledged that viability of a fetus may occur in twenty-four weeks. This was evidence that the defendant was aware, in advance of the abortion, that he could be dealing with a viable fetus.

Hysterotomy was the method of abortion chosen by the defendant. The defendant's supposed act, which constituted manslaughter, was waiting three to five minutes after he manually separated the placenta from the uterine wall and before he removed the fetus from the abdominal cavity of the mother. The Commonwealth argued that upon the detachment of the placenta, the fetus became a "person" within the manslaughter statute and was killed by a wanton and reckless act of Dr. Edelin before its delivery from the mother's body. The defense contended that there could be manslaughter only when a fetus was born alive completely outside the mother's body and was homicidally destroyed by acts committed at that stage.

Only when a fetus had been born alive outside its mother could it become a "person" within the meaning of the manslaughter statute. Thus, to be convicted of the crime, Dr. Edelin must be found—by reckless or wanton acts—to have "caused the death of a person who had been alive outside the body of his or her mother . . . Dr. Edelin's conduct from start to finish, both prenatal and postnatal, did not provide a basis for submission to a jury of the issue of 'recklessness' or the like . . . Of course manslaughter could not be supported by proof merely of a mistake of judgment . . . there is nothing to impeach the defendant's good faith judgment that the particular fetus was nonviable, and nothing to suggest that belief was grievously unreasonable by medical standards. . . ."

Commonwealth v. Edelin,
3 Mass. Adv. 2795, 359 N.E.2d 4 (1976)

Covering up a death at a nursing home is another perspective of an intentional tort.

Employees at a rest home in this town near Charlotte tried to cover up the death of a resident who had wandered away and frozen to death by dragging her body inside, dressing it in a nightgown and placing it in her bed, the authorities say. On the basis of the account given by the staff at the home, a doctor signed a death certificate saying the 77-year-old woman, Ellie Wall, had died in her sleep of natural causes.

But an anonymous tip to the Cleveland County Sheriff, Dan Crawford, prompted an autopsy, and the office of the state's Medical Examiner determined on Wednesday that Ms. Wall died of exposure last weekend; when temperatures dropped into the 20's. Employees found her body last Sunday morning in a drainage ditch, clad only in underwear. Sheriff Crawford said. "She did not die peacefully in her sleep," he said. "If we hadn't gotten that call, she would have been buried and no one would have known the difference."

The District Attorney is deciding whether to file charges that could include those of criminal neglect and manslaughter.

"Coverup Seen in Death at Rest Home,"
New York Times, p. 33 (February 5, 1995)

Conspiracy

A **conspiracy** is defined as a confederacy between two or more persons formed for the purpose of committing, by their joint efforts, some unlawful or criminal act, or some act that is lawful in itself but becomes unlawful when done by the concerted action of the conspirators. A conspiracy is a separate crime. To prove a defendant guilty of the crime of conspiracy, three things must be proven beyond a reasonable doubt: that the defendant joined in an agreement or plan with one or more other persons; that the purpose of the agreement was to do something unlawful; and that the defendant joined the conspiracy knowing of the unlawful plan and intending to help carry it out. Following is a conspiracy to smuggle drugs into this country:

Federal agents who arrested a self-described doctor in Brooklyn last week on drug charges said the man's apartment—filled with cots, enema supplies and laxatives—was a refuge for smugglers who swallow drug-filled condoms. "The couriers would come from the airport, stay there till they excreted the condoms, then they would go on their way," Michael Nestor, head of the United States Customs Service Investigations Unit on Long Island, said on Friday. "It was a clearinghouse for the swallowers. . . . Mr. Florian, the man who lived in the apartment, told authorities that he was a doctor from Colombia.

"A Clinic Stopover for Smugglers of Drugs
Is Found After Arrest," *New York Times*

Larceny

Whoever steals the property of another shall be guilty of larceny. Stealing is the wrongful taking of the personal property of another with the intent to permanently deprive that person of such property. In order to prove the defendant guilty of larceny, three things must be proven beyond a reasonable doubt: that the defendant took and carried away the property; that the property was owned or possessed by someone other than the defendant; and that the defendant took the property with the intent to permanently deprive that person of the property.

A private nurse whose accusations brought about an investigation into the death of the tobacco heiress Doris Duke has pleaded guilty to stealing valuables from six wealthy patients. Tammy Payette, 28, faces a maximum of 11 years in prison when she is sentenced on December 14, 1995. . . . In January, 1995, Ms. Payette said that Miss Duke, 80, had died of an overdose of morphine prescribed by her doctor, Charles F. Kivowitz, and other drugs rather than natural causes on October 28, 1993. She blamed people who stood to benefit from the $1.2 billion Duke estate.

Ms. Payette will have to make restitution for the valuables, including pearl necklaces and sterling silver corn holders, that disappeared from the homes of patients. . . . In her plea, Ms. Payette admitted to stealing from six patients but not from Miss Duke, although she agreed to make restitution to the Duke estate for two pearl necklaces and jade eagles that are still missing.

"Doris Duke's Nurse Enters a Guilty Plea,"
New York Times, p. 40 (October 15, 1995)

Abuse

Three types of abuse may involve medical office personnel with criminal investigating agencies: child abuse, elder abuse, and domestic violence.

Child Abuse

In 1985, more than 1.9 million children were reported to the authorities as suspected victims of child abuse and neglect. This is more than twelve times the estimated 150,000 children reported in 1963.

Besharov, Douglas J., "Child Abuse and Neglect . . ."
Family Law Quarterly, XXII(1):8 (Spring 1988)

In a study issued on September 18, 1996, by the Department of Health and Human Services, the number of abused and neglected children rose to 2.1 million in 1993—up 98% from 1.42 million in 1986. The number of seriously injured children nearly quadrupled from 141,700 in 1986 to 565,000 in 1993.

Legislative Response   Responding to the concerns of the public, Congress passed the Federal Child Abuse Prevention and Treatment Act (42 U.S.C. § 510) which requires the reporting of instances of physical and mental "injury . . . under circumstances which indicate that the child's health or welfare is harmed or threatened." In addition, every state legislature has legislated child abuse a crime, and physicians have been listed in the statutes as mandated reporters.

Supporting this role for the physician, Susan Black, M.D., President of the Massachusetts Academy of Family Physicians, comments:

> [P]hysicians in a community are well known for handling families in crises. . . . The physician knows where the power is in the house: she or he knows who's got the authority, who's got the love, and who's got some personal issues that may prevent the victim from regaining health. Family physicians also have tremendous credibility in a court . . . and are often the only professional that family members are willing to talk with.

Reporters   Teachers, nurses, and other licensed health care providers are also identified as mandated reporters under state statutes. At times, mandated reporting may cause personal conflict to the physician and other members of the health care team who have been caring for an entire family. But the child, not the parent, is the patient, and it is universally held that confidentiality in the physician-patient relationship does not exist when parents abuse children. At the same time, it is important for reporters to maintain interpersonal relationships with the family in spite of the possibility of being expected to produce evidence against them. In private life, anyone—family, neighbor, or concerned adult—may file a child abuse complaint with a protective agency. In the physician's office within the scope of employment, unless listed as a mandated reporter, personnel should file a complaint only when delegated that task by the doctor.

> Premature return of a child to abusive parents could result in death, serious injury, or life-long psychological trauma. Conversely, inappropriate removal or separation from the parents could result in a future of disrupted foster placements, broken relationships, poor self-esteem, and crippling psychological damage.
>
> Haralambie, Ann M.
> "Special Problems in Custody and Abuse Cases,"
> *Family Advocate* 10(3):15 (Winter 1988)

Failure by a physician to report child abuse is a matter being addressed by medical societies across the country. It is also being addressed by district attorneys:

Dr. Fred S. Berlin, director of a clinic at Baltimore's Johns Hopkins Hospital which treats pedophiles, child molesters and rapists became the center of controversy in Maryland when a new law went into effect mandating that suspected child abuse and neglect be reported by all health-care professionals, including those treating sex offenders. On the day the law went into effect, Dr. Berlin issued a memorandum to patients and prospective patients warning them of the state's new reporting requirement and suggesting a way around it. The memo recommended that people who molested a child consult a lawyer, who could refer them to the clinic for evaluation. That way, the memo said, the disclosure of an incident would be protected by attorney-client privilege.

Berlin's maneuver prompted . . . a request for an opinion from the Maryland attorney general. In an opinion issued February 8, 1990, Attorney General Joseph Curran, Jr. concluded that cases of suspected child abuse or neglect must be reported even if the person relating the information was referred to an attorney, unless the mental health provider is participating in the preparation of a defense to a criminal proceeding that has already been initiated. . . .

The problem of non-reporting by mandating reporters is not limited to those who treat sex offenders. . . . An estimated 60 percent of the cases of suspected child abuse and neglect known to mandated reporters, including physicians, social workers, teachers, probation officers, and mental health workers, were not reported to the CPS during 1986.

"Doctor Tries to Sidestep Child Abuse Reporting Laws,"
National District Attorneys Association Bulletin 9(1) (January/February 1990)

Filing a Complaint   Procedures for reporting suspected child abuse begin by telephoning the Child Protective Unit. Be prepared to give the following information:

1. The name(s), address, present whereabouts, date of birth or estimate of age and sex of the reported child(ren) and of any other children in the household.
2. The names, addresses, and telephone numbers of the child's parents or other persons responsible for the child's care.
3. The principle language spoken by the child and the child's caretaker.
4. Your name, address, telephone number, profession, and relationship to the child. (Nonmandated reporters may request anonymity.)
5. The full nature and extent of the child's injuries, abuse, or neglect.
6. Any indication of prior injuries, abuse, or neglect.
7. An assessment of the risk of further harm to the child, and if a risk exists, whether it is imminent.
8. If the above information was given to you by a third party, the identity of that person, unless anonymity is requested.
9. The circumstances under which you first became aware of the child's alleged injuries, abuse, or neglect.
10. The action taken if any, to treat, shelter, or assist the child.

National Center for Child Abuse and Neglect Specialized Training

Child protective agencies screen the complaint after a report has been filed. Agency social workers determine whether the child is "at risk," monitor care for the child at home or in foster placement, escort the complaint through the legal system, and establish criteria to achieve the goal of the child's return home. The substantiation, or confirmation, of abuse is critical to the well-being of the child and family. Nationwide, about forty percent of all reports are substantiated.

Premature return of a child to abusive parents could result in death, serious injury, or life-long psychological trauma. Conversely, inappropriate removal or separation from the parents could result in a future of disrupted foster placements, broken relationships, poor self-esteem, and crippling psychological damage.

Haralambie, Ann M.,
Special Problems in Custody and Abuse Cases,"
Family Advocate 10(3):15 (Winter 1988)

The agency also decides whether to refer the complaint to the district attorney, who is the prosecuting arm of the state. Once the case is referred to the district attorney, the matter becomes criminal, and the penalty for the abuser may be jail.

Legal Process   Cases that reach the courts are known as petitions for care and protection. Many attorneys are involved in care and protection proceedings. When the petition is presented in court, the child is identified by the attorney representing the protective agency. Additional attorneys are appointed for the child, the parents (often individually), and possibly the grandparents, as well as a court investigator and/or guardian ad litem. The guardian ad litem serves in the best interest of the child while the attorney appointed for the child advocates for the position of the child. The court investigator serves as an extension of the court and investigates the family's history: educational, economic, medical, and psychological. The attorneys for the other members of the family represent and advocate only in their clients' interests.

The Medical Record   In any court procedure, evidence must be offered to the trier of fact in an effort to convict or defend the defendant. In child abuse cases, the medical record often holds critical information that is used in determining whether a child is returned to the parents. Physical examinations document the physical injuries, psychological examinations document the extent of mental abuse and the effect of the family dynamics on the child, and therapists' progress notes are critical in determining whether or not the family is motivated to change to meet the standards set by society.

Confidentiality   Every attorney wants, but is not necessarily entitled to, every medical report. Access to medical records is protected by doctor-patient confidentiality statutes, and the patient holds the privilege to withhold or release the records. Usually parents hold the right to exercise the doctor-patient confidentiality privilege for their children, but when the family is involved in a child abuse investigation, the doctor-patient privilege is held by the protective agency, and permission for release of information about the child must be received from the agency. The parents still maintain the right to withhold or release their own medical records.

Sections of the medical record may cover the issue of fault. Usually the physcian will ask a child, "How did this happen?" following which the doctor will document the answer. It is common practice for an emergency room staff to separate caretaker from child upon arrival at the hospital in order to interview each person individually. The staff then compares notes before making the determination whether the child is "at risk" and whether it is necessary to place the child in emergency protective custody. This information becomes part of the medical record but may not be given as much weight as documented injuries because of the lack of experience of the interviewers in ascertaining truth.

Behavioral Indicators of Child Abuse   Children who are abused physically or emotionally display certain types of behavior. Many of these are common to all children at one time or another, but when they are present in sufficient number and strength to characterize a child's overall manner, they may indicate abuse.

Overly compliant, passive, undemanding behaviors aimed at maintaining a low profile, avoiding any possible confrontation with a parent that could lead to abuse.

Extremely aggressive, demanding, and rageful behaviors, sometimes hyperactive, caused by the child's repeated frustrations at not getting basic needs met.

Role-reversed "parental" behavior, or extremely dependent behavior. Abusive parents have been unable to satisfy certain of their own needs appropriately and so turn to their children for fulfillment, which can produce two opposite sets of behavior in children.

Lags in development. Children who are forced to siphon off energy, normally channeled towards growth, into protecting themselves from abusive parents may fall behind the norm for their age in toilet training, motor skills, socialization, and language development.

Physical Indicators of Child Abuse

- Bruises and welts
- Burns
- Lacerations and abrasions
- Skeletal injuries
- Head injuries
- Internal injuries caused by blows to midline of abdomen

Elder Abuse

> Thirty-two million Americans are 65 years of age or older and make up 13 percent of the population. They account for 44 percent of all days spent in the hospital, 40 percent of all visits to internists, and a third of the nation's health-care expenditures. Persons over 85 years of age have increased in number from 1.4 million in 1970 to 3.3 million in 1990, and will likely top 6 million by the year 2010.
>
> Lewin, Tamar, "As Elderly Population Grows,
> So Does the Need for Doctors,"
> *New York Times,* pp. 1, A16 (May 31, 1991)

As the population of the United States grows older and lives longer, opportunities for elder abuse increase.

Definition   Elder abuse is defined by the California Welfare and Institution Code § 1561(g) (1986) as physical abuse, neglect, intimidation, cruel punishment, **fiduciary** abuse, abandonment, or other treatment with resulting physical harm or pain or mental suffering, or the deprivation by a care custodian of goods or services which are necessary to avoid physical harm or mental suffering.

Types of Abuse   Elder abuse is divided into five classifications:

> 1. 'passive neglect,' wherein a well-intentioned caretaker simply is incapable of meeting the elder's needs;
> 2. 'active neglect,' wherein the caretaker maliciously overmedicates or under-medicates and withholds basic life necessities;
> 3. 'psychological abuse,' including profanity and intimidating verbal conduct;
> 4. 'financial abuse,' wherein a caretaker squanders the patients funds or refuses to make expenditures essential to the medical or general well-being of the patient; and
> 5. 'physical abuse,' which ranges from sexual improprieties to battery, and offends the dignity of the patient.
>
> Palinecsar and Cobb, "The Physicians Role in Detecting and Reporting Elder Abuse."
> *Journal of Legal Medicine* 3:413–41 (1982)

We will deal specifically with four of these subjects.

1. Passive Neglect

Esther, approximately eighty-five years of age, brings her sister, Martha, into the medical office for a visit with the doctor. For the past several weeks, Martha has not been eating well, has been vomiting a bit, and appears generally run down. The medication that the physician prescribed six months ago has been depleted, and no one has renewed the prescription. Martha's clothes are ruffled, her hair is stringy, and she appears unkempt, as does Esther. Prior to this time, Esther has been able to adequately take care of Martha but apparently can no longer do so. Martha is an example of a passively neglected elder.

2. **Active Neglect**

    The case of Anne Capute (described in Chapter 2) at Morton Hospital in Taunton, Massachusetts, could be interpreted as a matter of active neglect.

3. **Financial Abuse**

    Other dimensions of abuse involve money. For example: "You won't believe what happened," reiterated a distraught woman. "My husband's aunt was at home. Sure, she was a bit confused but not ready for a nursing home. Last Friday, Almeida and her daughter, cousins of the aunt, arrived and the next day Auntie was in the hospital. Three days later she was admitted to a nursing home. This morning, the post-man stopped and asked if anyone had been to see Auntie lately. He was just there and water was trickling out the front door.

    "I went to the home, let myself in, and found water everywhere. Someone had left the water faucet on in the second-floor bathtub. Two days later, all of auntie's bank accounts were depleted and the cousins were off to their home, 1500 miles away."

    This is known as "rape of the estate." A relative arrives on the scene, usually at the death of the aged person, takes every article in sight and leaves before the sun comes up, never to be seen again. In this case, the relatives could not wait for the aunt to die. As part of their plan, they implicated a physician in the hospital and nursing home admission process. The court unknowingly cooperated and issued a temporary guardianship to the cousins. The abusive relatives left a legal entanglement that survived the death of the aunt and enriched the pockets of several attorneys. This type of abuse can be identified as financial on the part of the cousins and as passive neglect on the part of the physician.

4. **Physical Abuse**

    The following involves physical abuse and is viewed from the perspective of the employee abuser. "I've been fired," she cried over the telephone, "and it's so unfair. This patient . . .he hit me . . . he kicked me . . . I was only protecting myself. It wasn't my fault his leg got broken. I want to sue. . . ."

    Joanne had been taking care of an elderly patient in a local nursing home. He was a difficult patient, cantankerous at times, verbally abusive, and lately physically abusive. Joanne was getting him ready for bed at night and he "kicked" her. She stated that she grabbed his foot while he was in bed and pushed against it toward his body with her body to protect herself. She heard a "snap," then a "scream" from the patient, and then remembered nothing but confusion. The next day Joanne was called into the supervisor's office and fired for elder abuse.

The abuse was physical in nature. Joanne caused the breaking of the man's leg. This incident took place in Massachusetts where the law requires the reporting of each incident of elder abuse. Joanne was worried, when she talked with her lawyer, that she would not be employable as a nurses' aide ever again and that her sole skill for maintaining herself financially would be taken from her because of this "accident." In fact, that is what happened. Her attorney contacted the state registry of abusers and found that Joanne had been reported two previous times for abusing residents in nursing homes. The registry board would not give her another chance.

Legislation   Procedures for handling elder abuse vary in each state.

In seventeen states, reporting laws specifically cover abused elders, generally those sixty years or older; twenty-one states include the protection of the elderly with that of disabled adults eighteen years and older. Only a tiny minority—Colorado, Wisconsin, Iowa and Wyoming—have "voluntary reporting" laws; that is, they state abuse "may be reported" instead of mandating that it "shall be reported." Nine states have no "in home" adult-abuse reporting law: Indiana, Kansas, Maryland, Mississippi, New Jersey, New York, North Dakota, Pennsylvania, and South Dakota.

Thobaben, M., and Anderson, L.,
"Reporting Elder Abuse: Its the Law,"
American Journal of Nursing 85(4):371–74 (April 1985)

Check your general laws to determine procedures for handling elder abuse cases in your state.

Penalties for Failure to Report Abuse   Nurses can lose their license to practice, be fined from $25 to $1,000, be imprisoned from ten days to six months, and encounter civil liability for damages, for failure to report abuse. Medical assistants fall under the heading of health care providers and, as such, may or may not be penalized, depending on the reading of the state statute.

In Alabama, a nurse who, on a home visit, sees signs that an elder has been abused and does not report it can be found guilty of a misdemeanor and fined up to $500 or jailed. In California, the same nurse, although still guilty of a misdemeanor, could be fined up to $l,000. In Maine, the nurse would be subject to licensing penalties. In many other states, there is no provision for any penalty.

Thobaben, M., and Anderson, L.,
"Reporting Elder Abuse: It's the Law,"
American Journal of Nursing 85(4):371–74 (April 1985)

Domestic Violence

According to *Black's Law Dictionary,* violence is the unjust and unwarranted exercise of force, usually accompanied by vehemence, outrange, or fury.

Domestic violence is not simply one partner hitting another. A man who brutally beats his wife or intimate partner is committing domestic violence. A man who threatens to harm his wife or intimate partner is also committing domestic violence.

Domestic violence exists in a context where an intimate partner uses threatening, manipulative, aggressive, violent, or otherwise coercive behavior to maintain power and control over his victim. A batterer may abuse a victim by tightly controlling her behavior: forbidding her to have contact with friends and family who might support her; stalking her to prevent even casual social contacts; preventing her from working or, if she does work, acting in ways that make it difficult, if not impossible, to keep her job; and controlling financial assets so the victim cannot access them. Finally, the batterer may further attempt to maintain his power over the victim by threatening to hurt or kill her if she tries to leave or divorce him; he may also threaten to take or hurt the children if the victim does not comply with his demands.

Valente, Roberta L., "Addressing Domestic Violence:
The Role of the Family Law Practitioner,"
Family Law Quarterly 29(1):187–96

In 1994, the Violence Against Women Act (VAWA) was passed by Congress as an act incorporated into the Crime Bill (Pub. L. No. 103-322, Title IV, 108 Stat. 1902-55). The VAWA provided $1.6 billion to confront the national problem of gender-based violence. The VAWA recognizes that there is no place—home, street, or school—where women are spared the fear of crime. Under Title I, Safe Homes for Women, the bill addresses the right of women to be free from domestic violence specifically through the interstate enforcement of protection orders. Prior to the passing of the VAWA, the majority of states did not give full faith and credit to protection orders issued in other states. According to *Black's Law Dictionary,* the full faith and credit clause of the United States Constitution (Article IV, § 1) provides that the various states must recognize, with some exceptions, legislative acts, public records, and judicial decisions of the other states within the United States. Without full faith and credit statutes, a state may only protect victims of domestic violence within its boundaries, limiting the protection afforded victims if they leave the state issuing the protective order.

The passing of the VAWA offered women two avenues of protection from domestic violence: the state courts and the federal courts. The original petition for protection against domestic violence is filed in the state courts and through the state court system. The federal courts enter when there is an interstate violation of a protection order and the matter becomes a federal offense, as is shown in the following:

> In January of 1995, the U.S. Attorney for the Southern District of West Virginia charged a man in the first federal domestic violence case. Christopher Bailey was indicted on January 4, 1995, by a grand jury for interstate domestic violence and federal kidnaping after bringing his unconscious wife to a Kentucky hospital. Bailey faces up to life imprisonment and $500,000 in fines. The FBI has been involved in the investigation and has alleged that Christopher Bailey seriously injured his wife in their home in West Virginia and then traveled through West Virginia, Kentucky and Ohio for six days with his wife sometimes tied up in the trunk. Because the federal domestic violence law is untested, Bailey is also charged with federal kidnapping since that crime is "tried and true."
>
> Klein, Catherine F., "Full Faith and Credit
> Interstate Enforcement of Protection Orders Under
> the Violence Against Women Act of 1994,"
> *Family Law Quarterly* 29(2):253–72

The magnitude of the problems rooted in and affected by domestic violence is evidenced not only in the media time allowed for the O.J. Simpson matter but in the facts that follow:

> Four million American women who are married or living with someone as a couple were physically abused in the last year. 20 million were verbally or emotionally abused by their partner.
>
> 95 percent of assaults on spouses or ex-spouses are committed by men against women.
>
> Pregnancy is a risk factor for battering. Several studies indicate that 8 to 20 percent of pregnant women in the public and private clinics have been abused.
>
> 48 percent of all incidents of domestic violence against women discovered in the National Crime Survey were not reported to the police.
>
> Of women who were physically abused by their partners, 92 percent did not discuss these incidents with their physicians; 57 percent did not discuss the incidents with anyone.
>
> In one study in which physicians treated battered women in an emergency department, staff did not discuss the abuse with 40 percent of the patients.
>
> In a study of 476 women seen by a family practice clinic in the Midwest, 22.7 percent had been physically assaulted by their partners within the last year. The lifetime rate of physical abuse was 38.8 percent. However, only six women said they had been asked about domestic violence by their physicians.
>
> A study of a major metropolitan emergency department that had a protocol for domestic violence showed that the emergency department personnel failed to obtain a psychosocial history, ask about abuse, or address a women's safety in 92 percent of the domestic violence cases.
>
> In a survey of 100 senior executives in Fortune 1,000 companies, 57 percent believe domestic violence is a major social problem; 40 percent are personally aware of employees in their company who have been affected by domestic

Doctor's offices, emergency rooms, and ambulatory care clinics offer victims of domestic violence an opportunity to receive help not only in the treatment of current wounds but in the prevention of future incidents. The AMA has made physician assistance in the reduction of domestic violence a priority in the nineties.

Fraud

"Just the facts, ma'am," intoned Sergeant Friday of *Dragnet* fame as he investigated crime over the airwaves in the forties. Today the same line is heard when a fraud squad investigates persons suspected of illegal billing and other crimes of deceit in the health care industry.

Health care **fraud** is the fastest growing criminal enterprise in America—costing government and private insurance plans at least $44 billion per year, according to FBI Director Louis Freeh, in a speech he gave to Congress on March 21, 1995. One Government Accounting Office study put the figure at $100 billion. "Scam artists are bilking the system of billions, driving up the cost of health care for all Americans," said Senator William Cohen from Maine. To prove his point, Cohen showed a six-pack of a flavored "milk supplement"—in chocolate, strawberry, and vanilla—that scam artists peddled at South Florida condominiums and senior citizen centers to get Medicare numbers. These numbers were then used to bill the government for undelivered services and drugs totaling an estimated $14 million.

The high cost of fraudulent claims has given rise to fraud squads. The government is also looking at health care providers. Hospitals, laboratories, health maintenance organizations (HMOs), and doctors' offices are being targeted for investigation.

Fraud includes billing for services that have not been provided. A mental health center in Roosevelt, Long Island, New York, billed the state for thousands of individual psychotherapy sessions that it did not provide or that were shorter than claimed, defrauding Medicaid out of $200,000, according to state prosecutors.

1990 to December 1993 falsely indicating that therapists had provided individual psychotherapy session in excess of 30 minutes to dozens of Medicaid recipients when, in fact, the visits were far shorter, were for less expensive group sessions, or never occurred at all. . . . The indictment also alleged that to conceal the fraud, the defendants "doctored" patients' medical records to make it appear that individual therapy sessions over 30 minutes had been provided.

Officials said that under applicable Medicaid regulations, [the clinic] is reimbursed $30 for each individual therapy session lasting 15 to 29 minutes and $60 for a session lasting more than 30 minutes. . . . All four defendants surrendered to the police and pleaded not guilty. If convicted of all counts, they could each face up to 23 years in prison.

"Four at a Clinic Are Accused of Medicaid Fraud,"
New York Times, p. B2 (February 8, 1995)

No state is immune from mental health fraud claims. In Massachusetts, a federal jury rejected an insanity defense and convicted a Newton psychiatrist, Richard Skodnek, of fraudulently billing Medicare and private insurers $500,000 for patients he never treated. The doctor was accused of routinely making up diagnoses for patients' relatives he had never seen and billing insurers for nonexistent sessions.

Former patients . . . worried about the fallout from the doctor's fraudulent scheme. "My children had never even laid eyes on the man," said one woman whose two teen-agers Skodnek falsely claimed to have treated for severe depression. "To think that somewhere in a big computer there's a psychiatric diagnosis of my kids. It's not fair and it's not right." The woman fears the phony diagnoses could hurt their chances of getting insurance or jobs when they are older.

Investigators say it would be difficult, if not impossible, to track down all the phony diagnoses by Skodnek that found their way into insurance databases. And the 126 criminal charges Skodnek was convicted of were limited to a period investigators knew he was on vacation, which made them easier to trace.

Rakowsky, Judy, "Newton Psychiatrist Found Guilty of Fraud,"
The Boston Globe, P. 24 (August 3, 1995)

"We treat it as a felony," says Jim Garcia, director of Aetna Life Insurance Company's fraud squad, which is one of the largest. Between 1982 and 1984, Aetna identified $20 million in fraudulent billings. The company pays out $7 billion in medical claims a year. Although performing unnecessary surgery may not be a crime, using the U.S. mail to bill for it is. . . . Fraud investigators are quick to state that most doctors and other providers are honest in their billing.

Mills, David, "Insurers Use Police Tactics
to Snare Doctors Who File False Claims,"
The Wall Street Journal (1984)

Fraud squads are not the only ones interested in the honesty of and concerned about fraud in the billing practices of practitioners. Health insurance executives, in a recent article in the *New York Times,* accused doctors of regularly writing erroneous diagnoses for patients who then collect for non-compensable care. Dr. Paul Parker, in an article in *Medical Economics,* related his experience while having his teeth cleaned by a dental hygienist:

> As I opened wide in a dental chair not long ago, my hygienist set me straight about her favorite OBG specialist: "He's a doll. Chronic cervicitis. Vaginitis. Dysmenorrhea. I don't even have to ask, and he puts down a diagnosis. . . . "
> "Don't you know that putting down a false diagnosis is illegal?" I responded. "Maybe," she said. "But it's not such a big deal." She smiled slyly. "Dentists do it, too."

Prosecution is likely to occur when a health provider systematically overbills for nonexistent procedures and laboratory tests and benefits by it. Some allegations go beyond simple bogus billing and enter areas such as "up-coding" (*i.e.,* using a billing code involving a different and high grade service), "unbundling" services normally tied together (in effect double billing), or claims of "substandard" or "medically unnecessary" service.

> In a busy doctor's office, a blood-drawing technician [phlebotomist] from an outside laboratory lends a hand answering the phones, filing records or taking patients' vital signs when the regular nurses are swamped. Common courtesy? No. . . . Such pitching in constitutes an illegal kickback to the physicians. The government also put clinical laboratories on notice that if they put computers or fax machines in doctors' offices, the machines must be used exclusively for the laboratory work, not the physicians' other business. And the labs and the physicians may be breaking the law if they run tests free for physicians, their families and employees, or if they provide free pickup and disposal of needles and other biohazardous waste unrelated to the collection of specimens for the outside laboratory. . . .
>
> "U.S. Warns Doctors, Labs About Kickbacks,"
> *The Patriot Ledger,* p. 3 (October 14, 1994)

But fudging medical claims can backfire:

> It may seem like a little thing to put down a diagnosis for flu, fatigue or a minor infection to enable you to claim medical benefits for routine office visits not covered by your plan. One could argue it's just a matter of semantics to say you're getting psychotherapy for "depression," when it's really marriage counseling you're after, another service not covered by many plans. Lots of time, doctors

themselves bend the truth, thinking they're doing their patients a favor . . . but "these phantom maladies pile up in your records over the years, making you look like a much bigger health risk than you really are" . . . says Bob Tedoldi, president of the National Association of Life Underwriters. "When the insurer obtains your medical records and finds a series of things wrong with you, it might conclude you have chronic problems and deny you life insurance."

Schultz, Ellen E., "Fudging Medical Claims Can Backfire,"
The Wall Street Journal, p. C1 (June 29, 1995)

Procedures Fraud

Fraud in medicine also involves situations other than billing. In March of 1985, two Brooklyn doctors, a husband-and-wife team, were charged with a medical scam in which they offered to perform abortions on women who were not pregnant.

The scheme was uncovered by two female investigators who posed as patients and paid seventy-five dollars apiece for pregnancy tests. The doctors repeatedly represented that the women were pregnant and suggested they undergo surgery for the purpose of aborting the fetus. The investigators were not pregnant.

A similar scam was uncovered by New York City's Department of Consumer Affairs as early as 1974, just four years after the legalization of abortions:

An investigator, posing as a patient, went to several clinics with a sample of a man's urine. One clinic told her that she was pregnant and offered to perform an abortion after testing the male urine. One abortion referral service told the investigator that no test was needed. It offered to set up an appointment for a quick abortion for a fee of $150. Another abortion clinic was closed after a sixteen-year-old girl paid for what was supposed to be an abortion and gave birth six months later.

Capeci, Jerry, "Docs Nabbed in Abortion Scheme,"
The Boston Herald (March 8, 1985)

Delegation of Duties

Health care delivery by proxy is another area that sets the trap for Medicaid and Medicare billings. Even though a paraprofessional can legally perform a given service under the terms of a state's medical practice act, it does not mean that Medicare will pay for the service. For example, a medical assistant who administers an injection while the physician is out of the office may not be covered.

This is an area that has particular significance for medical assistants. In Massachusetts, for example, new Blue Cross/Blue Shield regulations have been promulgated as follows:

Rule 2. To be eligible to receive payment for services from Blue Shield, a participating provider must personally perform those services. Blue Shield will, however, pay a participating provider for services which are performed by his/her assistant who has been approved by and registered with Blue Shield in accordance with this Rule.

Generally, Blue Shield will pay a participating provider for services performed by an assistant: (a) who is a salaried employee of that provider and who works a certain number of regular hours per week for that provider, regardless of the number of patients seen; (b) who is registered, licensed or qualified under Massachusetts law to perform such services; (c) who performs the services under the direct, personal and continuous supervision of a Blue Shield participating provider who practices in the same or related field. . . .

'Direct, personal and continuous supervision' under this Rule means that the participating provider must perform or participate in an initial examination or evaluation of the patient and actively participate in the continuing management of the patient's treatment. While the provider need not be in the room where the assistant renders his or her services, that provider must be on the same premises and immediately available to provide personal assistance and direction. Availability by telephone or other electronic communication does not constitute direct, personal and continuous supervision. The participating provider must also document his/her supervision of assistants in the clinical record of the patient.

The regulations are new, and at this time there are no certain answers to questions about the status of medical assistants and clinical procedures.

Forgiving Copayments

In the May 1, 1989, issue of *Medical Economics,* doctors were warned that "declining to collect deductibles and copayments from patients" may cause problems with Medicare and private insurance companies. "Forgiving copayments and not telling the insurance company you are doing it is not innocent oversight: it's actually fraud." Insurance companies reason that "if a physician says his fee is $100 but he's willing to take no more than the insurance company's reimbursement of $80 then he is actually charging $80. . . . The reimbursement should be 80 percent of the $80, or $64. The difference, $16 in this example, constitutes an overpayment to the doctor."

Kickbacks

The Medicare-Medicaid Antifraud and Abuse Amendments contain a provision that makes it illegal for a person or institution to make or receive payment of any kind in return for obtaining or introducing the referral of Medicaid or Medicare patients. Criminal penalties will be imposed on anyone who knowingly and willfully solicits or receives any kickback, bribe, or rebate in return for referring a patient to a physician, physical therapist, pharmacy, and so on, or for referring to a patient any item or service that may be paid for in full or in part by Medicare or Medicaid.

For example, Felix M. Balasco, a practicing cardiologist in Cranston, Rhode Island, implanted 733 permanent pacemakers in Medicare patients from 1975 through 1980. He continued to implant another 160 pacemakers during the next two years even though he knew he was being watched. "Apparently not content with Medicare's $1,000 per implant payment, he accepted more than $238,000 in kickbacks from two pacemaker companies. Balasco was convicted in federal court of fraud, conspiracy, and extortion." (Crane, Mark, "Why Did It Take So Long to Nail This Crooked Doctor?" *Medical Economics,* pp. 54–64.)

Because many referral opportunities occur in a physician's office, knowledge of anti-kickback provisions of the Medicare/Medicaid Amendments is important. In a situation involving respiratory therapists, the Health-Care Financing Administration (HCFA) stated that "antifraud and abuse laws can be violated if durable medical equipment suppliers pay 'finders' and/or 'referral fees' to respiratory therapists who refer discharged hospital patients to them, even if in addition to making these referrals the therapists set up the equipment in the patient's homes and teach the patients how to use the equipment."

Medicare Part B Intermediary Letter No. 84-9,
"Payments to Respiratory Therapists by Durable Medical
Equipment Suppliers and the Illegal Remuneration Provisions
of the Social Security Act" (September 1984)

Penalties

The government no longer needs to show intent—only that the physician knew or should have known that the charges were improper.

For every claim that Medicare finds was not provided as reported, the physician may be fined $2,000 in civil penalties and held liable for as much as double the amount claimed for each item or service. There is also the possibility of criminal prosecution and sanctions involving suspension from the program. Sanctions have a serious impact to a physician who has built a practice at least in part on income from Medicare patients.

Informants

An investigation is usually triggered by a tip. Tips come from Medicare carriers, peer review organizations, state licensing boards, whistleblowing physicians, ex-staff members, and patients. Investigators make their case through beneficiary or patient interviews, documentation within the medical record, and interviews of other physicians and nurses. Some cases are easy, as in the following: "We had an ophthalmologist who had his machine repossessed for nonpayment by the manufacturer, and for a year after that he was still billing Medicare for procedures performed by the machine. He pleaded guilty and is serving time."

Medical assistants may be considered co-conspirators with the physician in fraud. The gist of a conspiracy is to agree to disobey or disregard the law. Two types of intent must be proven: intent to agree and intent to commit the substantive offense. When an assistant bills for a physician and consents to mark the insurance form in any manner that does not reflect the true situation, the assistant may be found guilty of conspiring to commit fraud. A defendant, of course, may be guilty of participation in a criminal conspiracy without actually profiting from or having any financial stake in it.

Health Insurance Portability and Accountability Act of 1996

On August 21, 1996, President Clinton signed into law the Health Insurance Portability and Accountability Act (the Act) of 1996, also known as the Kassebaum-Kennedy Health Insurance Reform Bill. Included in the Act is a provision requiring every health plan and provider to maintain "reasonable and appropriate" safeguards to ensure the confidentiality of health information. The safeguards are intended to protect the disclosure of "individually identifiable information" that refers to any information that (1) identifies the individual; (2) relates to the individual's physical or mental health—past, present, or future—or payment for health care; or (3) is created or received by a health plan, provider, or employer.

Any health plan provider, or other person, who knowingly obtains or discloses "individually identifiable information" in violation of the Act is subjected to a fine of $50,000 and a year in prison. If the information is obtained or disclosed through false pretenses, the fine increases to $100,000 and five years in prison. If such information is obtained or disclosed with the intent to sell, transfer, or use it for commercial advantage, personal gain, or malicious harm, the fine becomes $250,000 and ten years in prison.

Individuals and organizations may request the United States Health and Human Services (HHS) Inspector General to issue fraud alerts to inform the public that certain practices are considered suspect or of concern to the Medicare and Medicaid programs. As a requirement of the Act, the HHS, in consultation with the attorney general, will issue advisory opinions, within sixty days of request, to determine whether these activities are prohibited by fraud and abuse provisions.

These decisions will attempt to address unsettled areas of past law, whether a waiver of coverage or deductibles or the transfer of items or services for free or for less than market value is "remuneration," and other matters of similar concern. Such waivers will be legal only when they are not used to solicit patients, are not routinely waived by the provider, and are waived only because of a patient's financial need.

Under the Act, health care fraud is made an independent federal crime and includes knowing and willful schemes to defraud any health care benefits program, not just Medicaid and Medicare. Penalties include fines and up to ten years in prison, which may become twenty years if the crime results in serious bodily injury, and life imprisonment if the crime results in death.

The Act establishes the Medicare Integrity program for private investigations and audits, encourages individuals to report fraud, and allows for rewarding individuals who report fraud. In addition, the Act requires HHS to establish a national data bank to record information about providers and suppliers that have committed health care abuse.

Embezzlement

Embezzlement occurs in the medical office when the assistant handling the payments from patients takes the money and uses it for his or her own purposes. In order to have embezzlement, (1) there must be a relationship, such as employment, between the individual who embezzles and the owner of the money; (2) the money must come into the hands of the embezzler because of the relationship; and (3) there must be an intent to fraudulently misappropriate the money.

Physicians are usually embezzled by long-term employees whom they trust and allow a wide berth in the handling of their money. The experience of having this trusted employee steal money often embitters doctors and, once burnt, they never trust again.

Illegal Sales of Drugs

In a New York Veteran's Affairs (VA) Hospital, twelve employees and seventeen patients were charged with the sale or possession of illegal drugs: crack cocaine and heroin. In order to be found guilty of this offense, the substance in question has to be a controlled substance; the individual being charged has to have a perceptible amount of the substance on their person or have distributed some perceptible amount of that substance with the intent to distribute it to another person or persons; and the individual must have done so knowingly or intentionally:

United States marshals and agents from the Department of Veterans Affairs burst into a first-floor cafeteria at the hospital with their guns drawn . . . and arrested several members of two loose-knit drug rings along with a hospital police sergeant who was charged with accepting bribes to allow the drug sales to continue.

Investigators said they believed that two rings operated largely independently of each other, with the employees among them a mailroom clerk, a laborer and two housekeeping aides [who were] smuggling packets of heroin and cocaine into the hospital and selling them to other employees. . . . The other ring consisted mostly of outpatients in the hospital's drug rehabilitation program, who either hoarded or stole bottles of methadone and sold them to other patients in the program, who are usually given carefully controlled doses. . . . Each suspect charged with selling drugs could face up to 20 years in prison.

Kennedy, Randy, "20 Arrested in Drug
Dealing in a Brooklyn V.A. Hospital,"
New York Times, p. B3 (September 14, 1995)

One of the defenses available to the defendants in the above case charges the investigators with illegal search and seizure.

Search and Seizure

The Fourth Amendment of the United States Constitution protects an individual against unreasonable searches of person, house, office, or vehicle and unreasonable seizure of person, papers, and effects. The amendment further provides that no warrant shall issue except upon probable cause supported by oath or affirmation and, particularly, a description of the place to be searched and the persons or things to be seized. It is generally accepted that police may not enter a person's home without a search warrant. In the following case, the defendant attempted to extend the expectations of privacy in his home to his hospital room:

CASE STUDY

On October 18, 1977, at approximately eleven at night, the defendant was stopped, identified, and searched by a Sacramento police officer on the corner of Sixth and T streets. At the time, the defendant, although male, was dressed in women's clothing and carrying a handbag. The officer observed that he was carrying certain matchbooks, a sharp steak knife (six or seven inches long), and a broken crescent wrench. After a warrant check on the defendant proved negative, he was given a certain green card and released. Defendant walked in the direction of nearby Southside Park.

Sometime between 12:15 and 12:45 on the morning of October 19, defendant was seen with an unidentified male in the doorway of the women's restroom in Southside Park. About 8:45 that morning the Sacramento police homicide department was summoned to the scene, where a dead male had been found.

The autopsy revealed the victim had been dead from six hours prior to 10:00 a.m. and it could have been as long as 16 hours. It also revealed the victim had been stabbed . . . the wounds were made by a knife or knife-like instrument. The coroner opined to police officers that the killing had homosexual overtones.

On October 19, the defendant readmitted himself to Sutter Hospital. On readmission, two nurses had observed blood on his shoes and stockings. While in his hospital room, an officer observed a pair of shoes in an open closet with what appeared to be a great deal of caked blood on them. On the way to the station, the defendant requested permission to return to his apartment for his purse and a check. When the officer opened the defendant's purse to check for weapons, he observed blood on the purse and inside a three-by-five green card similar to the one given to defendant by the officer making the stop the previous night. The purse and its contents were seized as evidence. The defendant attempted to suppress this evidence by claiming that his Fourth Amendment rights had been violated.

The contents of the purse were not suppressed because the searching of the purse occurred during a pre-arrest search, which is necessary for the safety of the officers. The question of expectation of privacy and violation of the Fourth Amendment focused on the officer's view of the blood caked boots in the hospital room. The court determined that no Fourth Amendment violation occurs when a nurse permits an officer to enter a patient's hospital room for purposes unrelated to a search, the patient does not object to the visit, and the officer then sees evidence in plain view.

People v. Brown,
88 Cal. App. 3d 283, 151 Cal. Rptr. 749 (1979)

Individuals who are arrested for driving while intoxicated are asked to take Breathalyzer tests and provide blood samples for laboratory analysis. The United States Supreme Court has upheld the admissibility of blood tests by a physician using standard medical procedures where the blood was taken from a conscious person who did not consent but who offered no physical resistance. Other incidents of search and seizure are found in medical treatment situations. For example:

CASE STUDY
A gun battle between the police and three armed men occurred following the robbery of a supermarket. One policeman and one robber were killed; another robber was shot but escaped. A few weeks later, the police picked up an individual they suspected was the robber who got away. He was taken to the hospital, where X-rays indicated metallic fragments in his buttocks. The police obtained a search warrant, and a surgeon removed the metal while the suspect was under local anesthesia. The metal fragments were identified as parts of police bullets and used as evidence against the defendant. He was convicted of the policeman's murder. He appealed the

conviction and the Indiana Supreme Court held that such an extensive intrusion into his body had constituted a sufficiently unreasonable violation of his constitutional rights to require reversal of his conviction.

Adams v. State of Indiana,
229 N.E.2d 834 (Ind. 1973)

Rape

According to *Black's Law Dictionary,* rape is unlawful sexual intercourse with a female without her consent. Matters dealing with rape occur when a victim seeks treatment in medical facilities following a rape and when a patient is raped by personnel providing medical care within the facility. The following case is unique and deals with the issues.

CASE STUDY   The defendant physician was consulted by a twenty-year-old woman for a physical examination. Halfway through the examination he suggested stopping by her apartment to finish. He suggested that she be in bed and have her nightgown on when he came later. During the completion of the examination in her apartment, which took place several hours after her office appointment, he asked if she had trouble sleeping. She replied, "yes" and he gave her an injection, following which she lost consciousness. She awakened while the physician was sexually molesting her. She was afraid that if he knew she was awake he would have seriously harmed her. The phone rang and when she sat up to answer it the physician told her she "had had a bad dream" and left.

The woman reported the incident to the police who determined that she should keep further appointments with the doctor and tell them if he suggested the same procedure. At her next appointment, the doctor again suggested stopping by the patient's apartment. The police arranged to have a closed-circuit television camera concealed in a shoe box in her apartment. When the physician arrived, two policemen, a policewoman, an assistant court medical examiner, and a neighbor watched the television monitor from a neighboring apartment. The physician followed the same routine and as the doctor proceeded to remove her clothing from the waist down, the police entered the apartment and found her unconscious on her back on the couch with the physician on top of her. The physician was charged with attempted rape, assault with intent to rape, assault and battery, and assault. He was sentenced to five years imprisonment.

Avery v. Maryland,
292 A.2d 728 (Md. 1972)

The doctor-patient relationship is determined to be a fiduciary relationship, which means that the doctor is held to the highest standard of trust. According to *Black's Law Dictionary,* the term *fiduciary* refers to a duty to act for someone else's benefit. It is the highest standard of duty implied by law. Such relationships arise whenever confidence is reposed on one side and domination and influence result on the other. While rape is a crime whenever it is committed, it is a particularly heinous one when committed by a doctor in the doctor-patient relationship. Patients must be able to trust doctors. Public policy demands that patients be protected from abuse of power and breach of trust. This policy is intended to cover all persons involved in the care of the ill, children, and the elderly.

CIVIL CAUSES OF ACTION—INTENTIONAL TORTS

Civil law covers all except criminal actions. Most cases in medical malpractice law fall within the civil law of torts. *A tort is a private wrong or injury, other than breach of contract, for which the court will provide a remedy. In order to have an action in tort, there must exist a legal duty between the plaintiff and the defendant, a breach of that duty, and injury as a result of the breach.* Tort liability is classified as intentional, negligent, or liability without fault. For a tort to be intentional, the defendant must intend to commit the act. An intentional tort differs from negligence. In negligence, injury to the patient occurs because the defendant fails to exercise the degree of care required in doing what is otherwise permissible.

Intentional Torts

The importance of intentional torts for the patient or plaintiff lies in the ability of the victims to receive damages for injury. In a criminal case of assault and battery, for example, the victim may get back money, if robbed, but cannot sue for emotional distress, pain and suffering, diminished employability, and so on. This is processed in the courts by the plaintiff filing two complaints: one criminal and the other civil. The criminal complaint functions to punish the perpetrator. The civil complaint functions to make the victim whole. This is an equitable remedy under which a person is restored to their original position prior to the loss or injury.

Intentional torts against the person include assault, battery, intentional infliction of emotional distress, false imprisonment, invasion of privacy, and defamation of character. Defenses available to defendants include privilege, consent, self-defense, the defense of others, and error.

Assault and Battery

Assault is defined as any willful attempt or threat to injure another person with the apparent ability to do so. Battery is nonconsensual touching. A physician may be charged with assault and battery because of failure to obtain informed consent to treatment. Occasionally the charge of battery is filed against a health care provider who has acted in anger. For example:

CASE STUDY   An injury occurred to a four-year-old child that required sutures. When the patient returned with her mother to have the sutures removed the defendant suggested that the child should lie on the examining table and the mother was directed to hold her down. The child began to cry and tried to sit up. This behavior hindered the doctor in removing the sutures and he spanked her quite hard. The bruises remained visible on the child's buttocks for approximately three weeks. The mother immediately removed the child from the doctor's office and took the child to another physician who removed the sutures without incident. The mother then sued the physician for assault and battery and the jury returned a verdict in her favor.

Burton v. Leftwich,
123 So. 2d 766 (La. 1960)

Any time one person is touched by another without permission, there is the possibility of a claim for assault and battery. In the following situation, the parents were not allowed to recover damages when the doctor slapped their child. The doctor acted in **self-defense,** without malice, and the blow was not severe.

CASE STUDY   A twenty-three-month old child was taken to the emergency room of the hospital by her mother for treatment of a lacerated tongue. A second-year medical student attempted to examine the child's mouth and she clamped her teeth on the defendant's left middle finger and bit hard enough to cause blood to spurt from the finger, which was enclosed in a rubber glove. The defendant shouted to the child to open her mouth but she retained her grip on the finger. He twice unsuccessfully attempted to extricate his finger by forcing a tongue depressor into her mouth. He then slapped the child on the cheek with his hand. This caused her to open her mouth and release the finger. A doctor who immediately treated the finger testified that "the wound was deep enough to have touched the bone."

Mattocks v. Bell,
194 A.2d 307 (D.C. 1963)

Invasion of Privacy

The United States Supreme Court has recognized that privacy is a constitutional right. Independence in making certain kinds of important decisions is a privacy interest. For example, Roe v. Wade, a case decided by the

Supreme Court in 1973, determined that a woman's decision to have an abortion was a right of privacy.

CASE STUDY   This right of privacy, whether it be founded in the Fourteenth Amendment's concept of personal liberty and restrictions upon state action . . . or in the Ninth Amendment's reservation of rights to the people, is broad enough to encompass a woman's decision whether or not to terminate her pregnancy.

Roe v. Wade,
410 U.S. 113, 93 S. Ct 705, 35 L.Ed.2d 147 (1973)

The individual's right to expect privacy in situations of medical care must be respected by medical assistants and other health care deliverers. It has been established for many years that the admission of nonessential persons during treatment without the consent of the patient constitutes a violation of the right of privacy. The following is a case heard in 1881 that is still law today:

CASE STUDY   A doctor was called to the home of a woman in labor to deliver her baby. He took a friend with him who was not a physician. The friend was present throughout the delivery and held the woman's hand while she was experiencing labor pains. The doctor did not tell the patient that his friend was not another physician. The patient sued for violation of her right to privacy and the court held that she had a legal right to privacy at the time that her child was born.

De May v. Roberts,
9 N.W. 146 (Mich. 1881)

In the following case, the court held that a medical office staff was guilty of violating a patient's family's privacy by continuing to contact the family:

CASE STUDY   A female patient was hospitalized and died during the period of hospitalization. Approximately one month after her death, a notice was sent to her by her family physician's office with an appointment for her periodic check-up. Her husband wrote to the physician explaining that she had died and that he and his children found the notice upsetting. Shortly thereafter, he filed a wrongful death action against the family physician, apparently for failure to diagnose her illness. Two additional check-up letters were received, the second being addressed to her daughter. The family sued for invasion of privacy and harassment. The court was of the opinion that sending two more letters after being informed that a malpractice suit had been filed against the physician was an invasion of privacy.

McCormack v. Haley,
307 N.E.2d 34 (Ohio 1973)

False Imprisonment

The tort of false imprisonment is defined as intentionally confining a person without the legal right to do so or without their consent. Examples of false imprisonment are found where patients have been kept in a hospital for failing to pay their bills or have been committed to a mental hospital when there was no probable cause to commit, as in the following case:

CASE STUDY

A seventy-nine-year-old woman was tricked into going into a mental hospital by being told that she was going into a regular hospital for treatment. She signed herself in, but as soon as she found out where she was, she tried to sign herself out. She was denied the right to leave. In spite of her age and physical infirmities, she climbed out a second floor window, ran to a telephone, and called her lawyer. Within an hour he had a court order releasing her. The hospital did not raise the argument that she was incompetent. They did not ask for a civil commitment. The court found that the patient had been falsely imprisoned and did not accept the hospital's defense that the patient must try to escape or is assumed to consent.

Geddes v. Daughters of Charity,
348 F.2d 144 (1965)

False Claims Act

The Department of Justice civil fraud section follows provisions of the False Claims Act (FCA), 31 U.S.C. § 3729, to recover funds in the health care area. The government need prove only a deliberate, *i.e.* reckless but not intentional, false claim and may obtain a fine or penalty of $5,000 to $10,000 per claim plus multiple damages. The most difficult aspect of the FCA is to determine the "knowledge" standard, or what one must "know" to be held liable under the act.

The FCA defines "knowing" and "knowingly" to mean that a person "(1) has actual knowledge of the information; (2) acts in deliberate ignorance of the truth or falsity of the information; or (3) acts in reckless disregard of the truth or falsity of the information" (31 U.S.C. § 3729(b)). There is "no proof of specific intent to defraud" requirement. The importance of the FCA for medical office personnel is involved with billing procedures.

On occasion, busy providers may not "know" that the claims submitted on their behalf do not reflect services that were furnished. If those claims were submitted pursuant to haphazard office procedures that were not tailored toward ascertaining the truthfulness of the claims, the provider may be subject to FCA liability.

The clearest recent FCA case involving the imposition of liability stemming from "sloppy" office procedures is *United States v. Krizek* (859 F. Supp. 5, 13–14 (D.D.C. 1994)). There the court found that a physician had submitted claims without supervision. Specifically, the staff would consider that the doctor had furnished a 50-minute psychotherapy session unless they were told otherwise. Such an approximation resulted in the physician, on occasion, billing for more than twenty hours of services within a twenty-four hour period. While the physician claimed that he was at worst merely "negligent" and emphasized the "Ma and Pa" nature of his small practice, the court nonetheless imposed liability ruling that the physician failed utterly in supervising his agents in their submissions of claims on his behalf. As a result of his failure to supervise, [the physician] received reimbursement for services which he did not provide. These were not "mistakes" nor merely negligent conduct. Under the statutory definition of "knowing" conduct, the Court is compelled to conclude that the defendants acted with reckless disregard as to the truth or falsity of the submissions. As such, they will be deemed to have violated the False Claims Act.

Salcido, Robert, "Application of the False Claims Act
'Knowledge' Standard: What One Must 'Know' to Be Held Liable
Under the Act," *The ABA Forum on Health Law* 8(6):1, 6 (Mid-Winter 1996)

Defamation of Character

Violation of a patient's right to privacy may result in the charge of defamation of character being filed against a health care employee. Defamation of character occurs when one person communicates to a second person about a third in such a manner that the reputation of the person about whom the discussion was held is harmed. Letters or broadcast defamation are termed libel, while spoken defamation is slander. Charges against physicians for defamation of character are closely interwoven with charges of invasion of privacy or disclosure of confidential information. The following is a case against a nurse for slander:

CASE STUDY   A woman who was employed by a caterer had a condition which brought about false positive Wasserman tests. She did not have and had never had syphilis. There was no diagnosis of syphilis by the physician treating the woman. The doctor's nurse attended a social affair which was catered by the patient's employer. The nurse told the hostess that the employee was being treated by the physician for syphilis. This information affected the patient's employment and the employer's business. The court held that there was a good cause of action for slander against the nurse.

Schlesser v. Keck,
271 P.2d 588 (1954)

Public versus private interest is a consideration of the court in the above case. In 1920, there was no cure for syphilis and it was a dreaded contagious disease. The courts determined that public interest outweighed private interest.

CASE STUDY   Mr. Simonsen visited Dr. Swensen with symptoms that were compatible with syphilis. The doctor diagnosed plaintiff Simonsen's case as syphilis before obtaining the results of lab tests. He told Simonsen to move out of his hotel, where he was a resident, until a definite diagnosis could be made, in order to prevent the spread of the disease.

The next day after the visit, the doctor learned that the plaintiff was still at the hotel. He called the owner of the hotel and informed him that Mr. Simonsen had a contagious disease. The owner forced Simonsen to move. The Wasserman test came back negative and Simonsen sued Dr. Swensen. The court determined that under these circumstances, the doctor had a duty to disclose this information.

Simonsen v. Swensen,
177 N.W. 831 (Neb. 1920)

Today a similar situation exists with the disease AIDS, which is a contagious disease for which there is no cure. The courts are faced with the same problem in the 1990s that they faced in 1920.

Privacy, in a different context, is illustrated in the following matter:

CASE STUDY   A clerk in a store became ill at work and reported to the store nurse. The nurse diagnosed her problem as venereal disease and reported this to the woman's supervisor. Subsequently the woman was fired from the job. It was later determined, without any question, that the diagnosis was wrong. The court held that the clerk could not recover damages because the nurse had made a good faith mistake and she had a legal duty to report the diagnosis to her employer.

Cochran v. Sears Roebuck,
34 S.E.2d 296 (Ga. 1945)

Intentional Infliction of Emotional Distress

The intentional infliction of emotional distress is sometimes referred to as the tort of "outrageous conduct." This term distinguishes it from insults, indignities, threats, or annoyances. It is a tort that is usually tried before a jury because conviction depends upon whether an average member of the community would consider the conduct outrageous. Use your own judgment in the following case:

CASE STUDY   The plaintiff, her ten-month-old daughter, Marla, and her mother-in-law, Christine Rockhill, were injured in an automobile accident the evening of December 16, 1967. The plaintiff and her mother-in-law suffered cuts and bruises; Marla was rendered unconscious. The plaintiff's husband, a Navy-trained medical technologist who was also a passenger in the car, testified that immediately after the accident Marla was completely lifeless, and he thought she was dead. He tried unsuccessfully to rouse her; she did not respond at all, even to pinches on the arms and legs.

A passing motorist took them to Junction City and arranged for them to be seen by the defendant, Dr. Pollard. They met Dr. Pollard at his Junction City office shortly before nine o'clock in the evening.

Both the plaintiff and Christine Rockhill testified that the defendant was rude to them from the moment they met him. The plaintiff testified: "And the first thing, he looked at us, and he had a real mean look on his face, and this is what he said. He said, 'My God, women, what are you doing out on a night like this?' . . . and my mother-in-law tried to explain to him why we were on the road and her and I both pleaded to him."

Without making any examination, the defendant told them there was nothing wrong with any of them. Marla was still unconscious at this time. According to the plaintiff, "She was very lifeless. I was saying her name, and she would not respond at all. Her eyelids were a light blue. She was clammy, very cold. In fact, I thought she was dead at the time." Christine Rockhill also testified that Marla appeared lifeless, and was noticeably blue around the eyes. Nevertheless, the plaintiff testified that she had to ask the defendant several times to examine the child. When he finally agreed to do so, the plaintiff took her to the examining room and removed her clothes. "He took a stethoscope and laid it on her heart, and that was all he did then, and then he took a knee hammer and put it on her knees, but there wasn't any response at all and that is what his examination consisted of." While plaintiff was dressing the child after this examination, Marla suddenly vomited a considerable amount. Without any further examination of the child or of the vomited material, the doctor told plaintiff that there was nothing wrong, and that the vomiting had been caused by overfeeding.

The physician never examined the plaintiff or her mother-in-law or suggested that they get treatment for themselves elsewhere, although it was obvious that they were injured. Both were limping. Plaintiff was bleeding from cuts on her face and inside her mouth, and had visible bruises on her mouth and her knee . . . The defendant's attention was limited to directing Christine Rockhill to "Get in there and clean yourself up. You are a mess."

When Christine Rockhill suggested that her brother would pick them up at the defendant's office, the defendant said, "My God, woman, I can't stay here until somebody comes and gets you." Although the temperature was below freezing and Marla's clothing and blanket were wet with vomit, he told them to wait outside by a nearby street light while someone came from Springfield to get them.

Rockhill v. Pollard,
259 Or. 54, 485 P.2d 28 (1971)

The court ruled that a jury could reasonably conclude that the physician recklessly failed to perform his duty toward the three plaintiffs.

SUMMARY

When an individual who is working in a medical office breaks a law, intent makes the difference as to whether the behavior is labeled criminal or civil, intentional or negligent. If a patient is injured from an act performed with premeditation and malice, it is determined that the defendant is a criminal. If the patient is injured because of an aggressive act by the defendant carried through without premeditation or malice, the defendant is accused of an intentional tort. If the patient's injury simply happened, the defendant is alleged negligent.

Statutes are laws made by legislatures defining which acts are criminal felonies or misdemeanors and which acts are civil torts. In addition, there are common law crimes: murder, manslaughter, rape, fraud, sodomy, robbery, larceny, arson, burglary, and mayhem.

Most cases in medical malpractice fall within the civil law of torts. Civil actions differ from criminal actions in that one party is asking the court for damages because of an injury committed by the second party. These are private claims rather than claims filed against an individual by the state. Torts include the intentional torts of assault and battery, false imprisonment, invasion of privacy, defamation of character, intentional infliction of emotional distress, and negligence. The defenses available to defendants accused of intentionally injuring patients include privilege, consent, self-defense, the defense of others, and error.

SUGGESTED ACTIVITIES

Visit the local district court. Make arrangements with the clerk of the court before attending and request an interview with one of the judges about philosophy concerning criminals and criminal activity. Try to get to court early to see arraignments, trials, and dispositions. While in the court, keep your eyes on the lawyers and clients in the hall. This is where most of the court's business is carried out. When the lawyers come before the judge, an agreement has usually been reached. Defendants in a district court who are indigent are usually represented by public defenders or local bar advocates. Ask the clerk of court to arrange for a judge to spend some time with the class. Prepare questions in advance and write them down.

STUDY QUESTIONS

1. Criminal law makes the headlines every day in the local paper. Search the morning or evening paper and "clip and save" the criminal actions that are reported. After reading the accounts of the crime, determine whether a medical office may be involved in any aspect of the case and how.
2. Write in two lines the major distinction between criminal and civil law.
3. List and define the purposes of punishment.
4. Murder is a crime. How does murder differ from euthanasia? Do the courts treat the two differently?
5. How is the medical office affected by statutes and regulations on child and elder abuse?
6. How can a medical assistant be unwittingly brought into a criminal action against a doctor for fraudulent billing to Medicare or some other third-party insurer?
7. The laws of search and seizure are important for clinical and administrative medical personnel. Give an example of an application of the law in both instances.
8. List six intentional torts.
9. Invasion of the right of privacy is a constitutional issue. Describe procedures you might take to protect the privacy of a rape victim's identity from a newspaper reporter who follow the ambulance that takes her to the local hospital.
10. A patient who has not paid a bill has come to the emergency room for medical treatment. While there, a medical assistant notices a large amount of money in her pocketbook. The medical assistant tells the security guard. The guard stands at the patient's room and refuses to let her leave until she pays some money toward her bill. Can the patient file charges against the hospital? If so, what will the proper complaint read?

CASES FOR DISCUSSION

1. On a cold, windy afternoon in January, Fumiko Kimura walked slowly across the beach in Santa Monica, clutched her two young children to her, and then, facing her native Japan, waded into the sea. Rescuers spotted the submerged bodies too late to save Kazutaka, four, and Yuri, six months, who gave a tiny gasp for breath and then died. But Kimura survived, consumed with anguish and resentment at herself and those who saved her. "They must have been Caucasians," she thought, "otherwise they would have let me die."

     Kimura was an excellent mother and a dutiful wife to her tradition-minded husband who struggled to support his family as part owner of a small San Fernando Valley restaurant. . . . Even when he returned home in the wee hours, Kimura would be waiting up to bathe his feet—not knowing until ten days before her suicide attempt that her husband . . . as often as not, was returning from the mistress he had been keeping in an apartment for the last three years. Kimura was devastated by the news. To Kimura's Japanese way of thinking, which she continued to cling to after more than twelve years in the United States, she had failed . . . at life itself. She couldn't eat or sleep and talked of suicide with a neighbor. . . . "This was the only honorable way out for a woman like Mrs. Kimura," explains Professor Mamoru Iga, a Japanese-born sociologist. "Like most Japanese, her life was regulated by custom, not law." Should she be prosecuted for murder?

     Reese, Michael, "A Tragedy in Santa Monica,"
Newsweek, p. 10 (May 6, 1985)

2. In most states, physicians are mandated to report child abuse. Following are four hypothetical cases concerning child abuse. Determine whether you would report any of these cases as child abuse:

     - The dirty house case: Mr. and Mrs. Jones and their two preschool children, John and Mary, live in a decrepit house with three large dogs and a number of cats. Mr. Jones works as a laborer. Mrs. Jones is not employed outside the house and does nothing inside either. There is trash all over the house and many cockroaches. The dogs go freely in and out, and the cats use the piles of old newspapers as litter boxes. The smell is horrible. John and Mary are extremely dirty at all times. They seem to eat junk food a lot. They have no toys and play with various odds and ends. However, aside from runny noses, they appear to be healthy and developing normally.

     - The massage parlor case: Sharleen, age 7, lives with her mother, Barbara, in a small apartment over the men-only massage parlor where Barbara works from 4:00 P.M. until midnight. Drinks are served in the waiting room of the massage parlor, and it is possible that there is some drug use on the premises as well.

There are pornographic magazines available and soft-porn programs on the television sets. Some of the videotapes may have been made on the premises. Sharleen spends her after-school time at the massage parlor, sometimes coloring or playing with her own toys, sometimes helping to straighten up the waiting room, and sometimes just going around talking to people. She stays there until Barbara takes her up and puts her to bed, usually around nine o'clock at night.

- The truant case: Bobby, age eight, skipped school several times. A neighbor told his father about it, but when his father confronted the boy, Bobby lied, saying he had gone to school every day. The father viewed these as serious offenses on Bobby's part and he punished Bobby by beating him with a leather strap hard enough to leave marks on the back of Bobby's legs.
- The suicidal child: Margaret, age 14, took a large overdose of medication and then called the hospital. Due to prompt action, she survived. The hospital requested that she have a psychiatric evaluation before her discharge. Margaret's parents refused initially, but when they were threatened with court action, they capitulated. Margaret's evaluation was that she was of normal intelligence but showed signs of "depression, hostility, and impulsiveness." A foster home placement and individual therapy were recommended. Margaret's parents refused to follow the recommendations.

(Hypothetical cases taken from material used at the MCLE/NELI Child Abuse and Neglect Program, Boston College Seminar, October 25, 1984.)

3.   A woman went to the doctor with severe stomach pains. She was examined by a surgeon who, she stated, told her that her spleen was "hanging by a thread" from her collar bone. The surgeon recommended surgery to "build up ligaments" in her spleen. Following the operation, the surgeon informed her husband that it had been necessary to remove the spleen. The pathology report revealed no evidence of any disease in the spleen. The woman and her husband brought a cause of action against the surgeon for fraud. Should the court rule in their favor?

4.   Charles Venner swallowed twenty-four or twenty-five balloons of hashish oil in Morocco, flew to New York, passed five balloons, went on to Baltimore, and was brought by friends to the emergency room of Sinai Hospital "euphoric, disoriented, and lethargic, but responding to verbal orders." While under observation, he passed in bedpans the remainder of the balloons, one broken. The hospital staff saved the balloons and turned them over to the Baltimore police without a warrant. Should the police require a search warrant to use the balloons as evidence in a cause of action for possession of an illegal substance with the intent to distribute?

5. A patient went to a plastic surgeon to have repairs made on his nose. The surgeon took pictures before and after the operation. These were published without the patient's consent in a medical journal article entitled "The Saddlenose." The patient sued the plastic surgeon stating that the pictures were being used to advertise the surgeon's work. Should the patient win?

6. Parents took their thirteen-year-old daughter to the family physician for treatment of a foot infection. He advised the parents that she should stay at home in bed and that they should ask the school for a home teacher. The form the physician signed that went to the superintendent of the school incorrectly stated that the girl was pregnant. The child's parents requested that the physician change the report, but he told them that he had checked his files and found nothing that would indicate that he had made such a report. He also told them that if they brought the report to his office, he would do what he could to correct any error if he had made one. The school would not release the report. The parents continually called the physician. The office nurse told the parents to stop bothering the doctor about the matter and that he would not call the school. The father brought charges against the doctor for libel. Do you think the physician had a defense that would convince a jury?

Chapter 4

Your Words May Form a Contract

Telephone Conversation:
Medical Assistant: "Good morning. Doctor's office."
Prospective Patient: "Hello, I'm Mrs. Jones and new to the area. I would like to make an appointment with the doctor for myself and my family."
Medical Assistant: "I can schedule you for Thursday morning at 10:00 A.M."
Prospective Patient: "What does the doctor charge?"

OBJECTIVES:

You have just witnessed the making of a contract. After reading this chapter, you should be able to:

1. view the above conversation as a legal action.
2. understand the elements that make it a contract.
3. recognize the importance of the proper handling of telephone calls and scheduling of appointments by medical office personnel.
4. identify certain conversations between patients and medical office professionals that make for potential contract liability.
5. develop techniques for answering patients' questions that are consistent with what you have learned about contract law.
6. recognize the contractual nature of your employment.
7. identify situations of incapacity and how they affect the medical office.
8. understand the law of agency as it affects patients.

BUILDING YOUR LEGAL VOCABULARY

abandon	age of majority	contract
abandonment	agent	emancipated minor
accepted	conservator	express contract
adjudicated	consideration	guardian

implied contract	mature minor	principal
incompetents	memorialize	remedies
indigent	mental incompetence	specific performance
injunctive relief	minors	statute of frauds
insane	mutual assent	undue influence
legal disability	offer	warranty

The doctor-patient relationship is the keystone of medical practice. It is also contractual in nature. To demonstrate—an individual determines there is need to seek treatment for a medical problem. A telephone call, similar to the one in the quotation at the beginning of this chapter, is made to a physician's office, an HMO, or a clinic, and a contractual relationship is established between the patient and the doctor. The person answering the doctor's phone or making the appointment acts as the doctor's **agent** in forming the contract.

FORMATION OF A CONTRACT

A **contract** comes into being when an **offer** is made by one party, **accepted** by another party, and **consideration** passes between them. Parties enter into the contractual relationship by mutual assent. By entering into a relationship with a health care provider, the patient offers his or her person for treatment. By opening the doors or answering the phone and making an appointment, the health care facility accepts the patient. The patient promises to pay the fee, the physician promises to treat the patient, and with these agreements a contract is formed.

Contracts are fundamental in the business aspects of medical offices. If there is more than one physician in the practice, the entire practice is considered to have formed a contract with a patient. An HMO is held together through contract law: the same holds true for hospitals, nursing homes, and other facilities. Employees have a contract for employment stating that they are employed, at what rate, what the job consists of, and whatever other terms are necessary to define the framework of employment.

A breach of contract occurs when there is failure to perform the terms of the agreement by either party. Because contracts are legally enforceable by the courts, there are **remedies** for breach, including money, **specific performance,** and **injunctive relief.**

CLASSIFICATION OF CONTRACTS

A contract may be either implied or express. An **implied contract** gives rise to contractual obligations by some action or inaction without verbally expressed terms. For example, if an individual is taken to an emergency room unconscious, it is implied that the patient will accept treatment and that responsibility for payment of the treatment will be assumed by the patient. If a nurse prepares an injection, and a patient rolls up his or her shirt sleeve to receive the injection, it is implied that the patient is willing to undergo this treatment. The following is an example of an implied contract that imposed liability from a telephone call.

CASE STUDY   In this case, the plaintiff, Mrs. O'Neill, was the wife of the deceased. Her husband, on the day of his death, awoke at five in the morning with classic symptoms of a heart attack—severe chest pains, shortness of breath, perspiration, and an ashen complexion. The plaintiff walked three blocks with her husband to a nearby hospital and told the nurse that they were members of a prepaid medical group. The nurse replied that the hospital did not take care of patients from that group, then telephoned one of the doctors assigned to treat members of that hospital insurance plan who was in the hospital at the time the patient arrived. The doctor inquired over the telephone about the patient's symptoms, prior episodes, electrocardiograms, and other matters of importance in the patient's medical past. The physician told the patient to go home and call a physician from the medical group when the group's office opened in the morning. The hospital nurse and the physician refused any further attention to the patient who went home, attempted to disrobe, and dropped dead.

The appeals court held that a jury could have found that the physician accepted the deceased as a patient at the time he talked to him on the telephone. [Even though the doctor did not see the patient, he inquired about the patient's history and should have known the patient needed treatment.]

O'Neill v. Montefiore Hospital,
202 N.Y.S.2d 436 (1960)

An **express contract** is an actual agreement between the parties, the terms of which are openly stated in distinct and explicit language, either orally or in writing. In medicine, it is generally recognized that without an express contract, a physician or surgeon does not **warranty** the results of his or her work or contract to achieve a particular result. The facts in the following case demonstrate an express contract.

CASE STUDY   In the fall of 1963, the plaintiff was being treated by Dr. Klewicki for near-fatal bleeding due to a peptic ulcer. In January 1964, at the suggestion of Dr. Klewicki, the plaintiff went to see Dr. Campbell. The plaintiff states that the reason for the visit was that he "was curious about an operation, if I should have one or if I shouldn't have one." It was never indicated to the plaintiff that he must have an operation.

According to the plaintiff, at the first consultation with Dr. Campbell, the following conversation took place: "Once you have an operation, it takes care of all your troubles. . . . You can eat as you want to, you can drink as you want to, you can go as you please." The plaintiff also recalled that Dr. Campbell assured him that "there was nothing to [the operation]. That it was very simple [and] that he had performed the operation very often." The plaintiff was told he would be out of work "approximately three to four weeks at the most [and that] there was no danger at all in this operation." The plaintiff was assured that "after this operation you can throw your pillbox away. . . . Your Maalox you can throw away," and then the doctor stated, "In twenty years if you could figure out what you spent for Maalox pills and visits to doctors you could buy an awful lot. Weigh it against an operation."

Unfortunately, there were many problems. On March 4, 1964, the day following the operation, a "ruptured esophagus due to surgical trauma in doing the vagotomy, with bilateral effusion and mediastinal emphysema and mediastinitis" was diagnosed. The mortality rate from a ruptured esophagus is 50 percent to 75 percent. After the original operation, the plaintiff went through three subsequent operations, dropped from 170 to 88 pounds, was unable to sleep and required another admission for insertion of a drainage tube. At the time of trial, he was scarred badly from the operations, unable to hold down two jobs as he had prior to surgery, physically weak, and unable to be athletically or socially active.

The appeals court held that the trial court was correct in sending the case to the jury to determine the offer, acceptance, breach, and damages.

Guilmet v. Campbell,
385 Mich. 57, 188 N.W.2d 601 (1971)

The issue in this case was whether the doctor made a specific, clear, and express promise to cure or bring about a specific result that was relied upon by the plaintiff. The court determined that this was a possibility. By making a promise of a cure and not curing the patient, the doctor breached the agreement and, under contract law, could be found guilty of medical malpractice.

Consideration

In any contract, each party gives or does something in exchange for what is received. This is known as consideration. In the medical community, the accepted term for consideration is fee for service. Fee is the cost to the patient for the physician's services. Service is the cost to the physician for the patient's fee. A physician is free to withdraw from a case for nonpayment of fees but is liable for **abandonment** if proper termination procedures are not carried out or if the patient continues to need services. Once there is a contract between the physician and the patient, the issue of finances is totally irrelevant to the patients' care.

It is a general rule that the person who receives treatment is responsible for payment even if someone else requests the services. In certain circumstances—for example, in the care of **minors** and **incompetents**—others are responsible for the bill. In the situation of minor children, the parent is responsible; for those who are mentally incompetent, the parent or legal **guardian** is responsible. When an individual who is not legally obligated assumes responsibility for the doctor's fee, it is necessary that the agreement be in writing to satisfy the **statute of frauds.** This common law, according to *Black's Law Dictionary,* has been adopted by nearly all of the states in the United States in a more or less modified form. It comes from a very celebrated English statute passed in 1677. Its chief characteristic is the provision that no suit or action can be maintained unless there is a writing, signed by the party to be charged.

Mutual Assent

In order to have a contract, there must be clear understanding between the parties known as **mutual assent** or "meeting of the minds." Both the party who makes the offer and the one who accepts must be thinking and saying the same thing. The physician must be offering to treat the person as a patient, and the person talking with the doctor must view the situation as a patient seeking service. For example, when a hospital employee stopped the medical director of the hospital in the corridor and asked him a question about a personal medical condition, the court held that there was no mutual assent establishing a physician-patient relationship: "The physician never agreed to treat her or advise her as a physician. . . . [M]erely because the defendant was a physician and knew of the condition of the patient would not devolve upon him the duty of rendering to her medical care." (*Butterworth v. Swint,* 186 S.E. 770 (Ga. 1936)).

Mutual assent allows doctors to limit contracts with patients. For example, a physician may assent to treat patients only within a particular specialty:

CASE STUDY An internist, treating a patient unsuccessfully for bacterial colitis, referred the patient to a surgeon. The surgeon diagnosed appendicitis and performed an appendectomy. The patient, in turn, sued the internist for not having performed the surgery himself. The court held that the internist did not have to perform surgery because he had limited his practice to internal medicine.

Skodje v. Hardy,
288 P.2d 471 (Wash. 1955)

Physicians may limit their practice to a certain geographic area, for example, a town, city, or county:

CASE STUDY   A woman cut her leg in the middle of the night and telephoned her physician. The physician's partner was on call, sutured the wound, and directed her to return for another examination in two days. The next day, the patient went on vacation several miles away. While she was there her leg gave her difficulty and she demanded that the doctor who sutured the wound come to see her. He refused and referred her to a physician in the locality where she was vacationing. She sued him for refusing to attend to her needs. The court held that a physician is entirely justified in limiting his practice to his own community.

McNamara v. Emmons,
97 P.2d 503 (Cal. 1939)

Physicians may refuse to make house calls.

CASE STUDY   Several days following delivery of a baby, the patient called her obstetrician and asked him to make an immediate house call because she was having a problem. He informed her that he had an office full of patients and that she would have to come to the office. She became angry, went to a second obstetrician's office, and sued the doctor who had delivered her baby. The court held that the physician had the right to tell her that he would see her only at his office or at the hospital.

Rogers v. Lawson,
170 F.2d 157 (D.C. Cir. 1948)

Physicians have the right to limit the hours that they are available in their office and to take vacation time away from their practice. They also have the right to refuse to take a patient—to refuse to enter into a contractual relationship.

CASE STUDY   Hurley, at one time a patient of Dr. Eddingfield, became ill. He sent a messenger to the doctor with fee paid in advance and requested that the messenger bring the doctor back with him. The physician refused to return even though it was made clear to him that an emergency existed and no other doctor was available. The patient died.

The court held that the physician-patient contractual relationship is one depending on the assent of both parties and that a license to practice medicine does not compel a physician to contract against his will. The court pointed out that the physician probably could have saved the patient's life if he had responded to the request, that he was not busy at the time with another patient, but that he had the right to refuse to see the patient and was not, therefore, liable for the patient's death.

Hurley v. Eddingfield,
156 Ind. 416, 59 N.E. 1058 (1901)

Capacity of the Parties

Each party to a contract must be able to enter the agreement knowingly and without a legal disability. A person with a **legal disability** cannot form a contract because a contract cannot be made by or enforced against a person who does not have the legal capacity for mutual assent. Minors, incompetent persons, and individuals under the influence of a drug that alters their mental state are considered legally disabled. The capacity to contract is also affected when individuals are under duress or required to make an agreement while under undue influence. An exception is made when the contract is for necessities that are defined as things reasonably needed to continue life.

Minors

General Rule: Common Law

The general, common law rule in the treatment of minors is that a minor is incapable of giving effective consent for the administration of medical treatment. Therefore, without the consent of the parents or guardian, medical practitioners are liable for assault and battery. A minor is any person under the age of majority. Depending upon state law, the **age of majority** may be eighteen or twenty-one. Exceptions to the rule are made in medical emergencies and for mature and **emancipated minors.** Application of the rule may depend on the threshold issue of whether the medical treatment is for the benefit of the minor or for a third party. Almost every state allows minors to give consent for services that are for treatment of pregnancy, drug addiction, or sexually transmitted disease.

Exceptions

Medical Emergencies   Physicians are not liable for treating minors without consent when an emergency exists and it is dangerous to delay treatment in order to obtain consent. For example:

CASE STUDY   A physician was not found liable for performing a lumbar puncture on a five-year-old child without parental consent when the child was suspected of having meningitis. The child, born with achondroplasia, a condition causing dwarfism and hydrocephalus, had previously been admitted to the hospital for evaluation of his condition. The mother could not be located by phone. Consent of the grandmother had been given.

Plutshack v. University of Minnesota Hospitals,
316 N.W.2d 1 (Minn. 1982)

When a minor's condition is life threatening but immediate attention is not required, the courts have held that doctors are not entitled to provide treatment without parental consent.

Emancipated Minors   Under the laws of most states, a person can become emancipated from the legal restrictions of being a minor by:

1. marrying (in which case emancipation continues after separation, widowhood, or divorce),
2. becoming a parent for matters of parenting (even if not married),
3. joining the Armed Forces, or
4. living away from home and earning an independent living, managing one's own finances, and in general assuming an adult role. (*Nurses' Legal Handbook,* p. 131 (1985))

Statutory Adults   Recently legislatures in twenty-two states and the District of Columbia redefined minors as statutory adults at the age of fourteen for the purpose of receiving medical care. In these states, the statutory adult is regarded as similar to an adult for purposes of consent, privacy, confidentiality, access to medical records, and so on, while parents may still be financially responsible for the cost of care.

For children under seven years of age, the consent of parents is still required. For those between the ages of seven to fourteen years, the provider is allowed to use personal perceptions about the "minor's ability to comprehend the situation."

Under California statutes, minors fifteen years of age or older who live separate and apart from their parents or legal guardians and who manage their own affairs, regardless of source of income, can give consent to hospital care or any X-ray, anesthetics, medical or surgical diagnostic tests, or treatment. For example:

CASE STUDY   A seventeen-year-old minor lived away from home with a woman who gave her free room and board in exchange for household chores. The girl made her own financial decisions, and "managed her own affairs." Even though the minor's parents provided part of her income by paying for her

> private schooling and certain medical care, [she is] considered . . .
> [emancipated.]
>
> *Carter v. Cangello,*
> 164 Cal. Rptr. 361 (1980)

Generally, neither a minor nor parents may consent to sterilization, transplants, experimental medical care, or refusal or withholding of treatment without a court order. Yet, in the following action for damages from a vasectomy performed without the consent of parents, the court held that the minor could make his own decision:

CASE STUDY   A minor and his wife decided to limit their family, and at eighteen years of age a physician performed a vasectomy on the husband. The minor was married, completed high school, the head of his own family, earned his own living, and maintained his own home. Because he was afflicted with a progressive and incurable disease that could affect his future earning capacity and ability to support his family, the court held that the minor could make the decision without involving his parents.

Smith v. Sibley,
431 P.2d 719 (Wash. 1967)

Mature Minors   A **mature minor** is a nonemancipated minor in mid- to late-teens who has the intelligence and emotional maturity to be able to grasp the information necessary to make an informed decision. The complexity of the medical treatment may affect whether the minor is sufficiently mature to give informed consent. The standards determining a minor's maturity and an individual's capacity to give informed consent are closely related.

Constitutional Law Issues   Minors are persons and, as such, enjoy rights that belong to everyone from birth. One of these, the constitutional right of privacy, is fundamental in matters of abortion.

On June 25, 1990, the United States Supreme Court handed down two decisions affecting minors and the right to abortion. In *Hodgson v. Minnesota,* the Court upheld a state law that requires teenagers to notify both biological parents before obtaining an abortion or to seek a court order to waive parental notification. To obtain a court order, the minor must go before a judge with her request, at which time the judge makes a decision about the maturity of the minor to give informed consent to abortion. In addition, the Court upheld a mandatory forty-eight-hour waiting period between the time of the request and the time of the procedure.

In the second decision, *Ohio v. Akron Center for Reproductive Health,* the Court voted six to three to uphold a 1985 law requiring a physician to notify one of the parents of a pregnant minor before performing an abortion. If the minor is unable or unwilling to obtain parental permission, the minor must go before a judge and prove by "clear and convincing evidence" that she has sufficient maturity and information to make the abortion decision herself or that one of her parents has engaged in a pattern of physical, emotional, or sexual abuse against her.

Thirty-three states have laws requiring some form of parental consent or notification for teenagers prior to abortion.

Statute of Limitations   The statute of limitations defines the length of time a plaintiff has before he or she may no longer file a suit after injury. Included in the statute of limitations is usually a discovery rule that concludes that the statute of limitations does not begin to run until the child or the family knew, or should have known, that there was injury.

A minor does not have the capacity to sue in court and is dependent upon the parent to file complaints prior to the age of majority. For one reason or another, a parent or guardian may make the decision not to pursue a cause of action. To cover this possibility and safeguard the minor's best interest, many states have maintained a statute of limitations extending two years or more beyond the age of majority. If a state has this provision, health care providers must keep the records of pediatric patients longer than the time that is legally required for adults, or at least until the required number of years after the patient reaches majority.

Who Pays?

The relationship between physician and patient is one of fee for service. The physician provides the service, and the patient pays the fee. The reliability of this arrangement is essential to the fundamental principles of contract law and necessary to continuing commerce. Our economic system is built on the expectation that contracts between parties will be honored.

Children (minors) legally lack the capacity to contract without a parent or guardian's permission. The interest of the state in this matter is to protect children from the consequences of their unknowing acts.

If a minor contracts for basic necessities, such as food, shelter, and certain life-saving medical services, the policy of protection from unknowing acts is not urgent. When medical care is considered a necessity, the court will generally conclude that a fair trade was made and an implied contract will be upheld. The minor, or person responsible for the minor, must pay.

When a minor contracts for plastic surgery for cosmetic purposes, the issue of necessity may be questioned, and the need to protect the minor becomes more urgent. In this situation, the minor may or may not be obligated for the cost. It is reasonably certain that an emancipated or mature minor would be responsible for the fee.

A minor who arranges for medical care may, by statute, invoke the parent's responsibility because parents are responsible for children's necessities. Yet, under certain circumstances, even if a child is living with a parent or guardian, the liability for medical services may rest entirely on the minor if the services were rendered entirely on the credit of the minor. For example, when the expense of treatment was a material and substantial consideration in a judgment recovered by a minor as the result of litigation or settlement, the minor was liable for the medical bills.

Divorce, Minors, and the Single-Parent Family

Today's society offers particular challenges to the collection of bills for minors due to the number of divorces and "yours, mine, and ours" families. Divorce often means that the parent who brings the child to the physician is not the person who pays the bill. The party carrying the children's health insurance may be the noncustodial parent. In addition, there may be special arrangements for uninsured medical expenses.

In some cases, the divorced parties have maturely resolved their differences, and the payment of children's medical expenses is not the battleground for further argument. In other situations, this may be the one place where an unhappy, immature ex-spouse can still make a statement of anger by delaying or refusing payment. Sometimes medical insurance is deliberately allowed to expire. In any of these instances, the parents are responsible for the payment of the minor's medical necessities. The problem of the medical office is to collect the fee and remain impartial, unaffected, and independent of the continuing haggling between the parties. When a minor cannot get medical funds from the parents, the courts, under the doctrine of *in loco parentis,* usually assumes payment through child welfare departments.

Mental Incompetence

Mental incompetence exists when a party to a contract does not understand the nature and consequences of the contract at the time that it is formed. Some individuals are judged incompetent by the courts and have an appointed guardian. Many of the contract rules that apply to minors also apply to **insane** or **adjudicated** mental incompetents.

Incompetence alone does not absolve individuals of the consequences of their behavior. In the following case, the situation of an incompetent person is weighed against the good of the public.

CASE STUDY   Mr. Smalley had been hospitalized and undergone treatment for a manic depressive condition for many years. Dr. Giese, his psychiatrist, testified that while in the manic state, Smalley felt euphoric and invincible and his judgment and behavior were grossly affected. While in such a manic state, Smalley bought from Baker the privilege of selling a mechanical device to the government under a license that required extensive sales work from Mr. Smalley. Smalley testified that he thought he knew what he was doing when he made the transaction but also felt that he "could do anything," and was the "greatest salesman going." Mr. Barrett, Smalley's attorney, testified that neither he nor Mrs. Smalley intended to let Smalley go through with the deal, but thought it would be good therapy if he went through with the negotiations. Mr. Baker did not know about Smalley's condition.

The trial court found that Smalley did not have the required mental capacity to enter into agreements, and Mr. Baker appealed. The appeals court held that the desire to protect the mentally ill must be balanced with the need to keep business transactions stable and secure, and held in favor of Mr. Baker.

Smalley v. Baker,
262 Cal. App. 2d 824, 69 Cal. Rptr. 521 (1968)

Incompetence is not necessarily adjudicated for severe mental illness or retardation only. In some situations, an individual may be competent to care for himself or herself but unable to attend to personal finances. For such individuals, a **conservator** may be appointed to oversee property and/or finances. A conservator differs from a guardian in that a guardian is responsible for both the financial resources and the person.

Undue Influence

Undue influence occurs when one party in a contract improperly uses personal power over the other to cause actions not in the second party's best interests. In the doctor-patient relationship, physicians are in a position to influence their patients' decisions. When the physician uses the position to form an agreement that is more beneficial to the doctor than to the patient, the doctor is using undue influence. For example:

CASE STUDY   An elderly woman saw a psychoanalyst for many years before she died. During the period of treatment she gave him $116,050, and left him a large sum of money in her will. Part of the money was professional fees, part was a loan that he had never repaid, and $30,000 was a gift. After her death her heirs attempted to recover all the money except legitimate fees on the grounds of undue influence. The court ordered a hearing. The psychoanalyst had to prove that the transfers were "fair, open, voluntary, and well understood."

Estate of Reiner,
383 N.Y.S.2d 504 (1976)

BREACH OF CONTRACT

A breach of contract occurs when one of the parties does not keep a promise—by not performing, not paying for services, not keeping to schedule, or not doing the procedure as had been agreed. Breach of contract also occurs when one party prevents the other party from performing.

Examples of breach of contract occur in medicine when the patient does not pay the bill or when a physician makes a warranty that the patient will be cured. When the promised cure does not take place, the physician becomes liable for breach of contract regardless of whether there was negligence.

CASE STUDY   Scar tissue, which was the result of an electric wire burn nine years prior to the operation, was replaced with skin grafted from the plaintiff's chest. Prior to the operation, the plaintiff and his father went to the defendant's office and asked the doctor how long the plaintiff would be in the hospital. The defendant replied, "Three or four days, not over four. Then the boy can go home and it will be just a few days when he will go back to work with a good hand." Before the operation was agreed to, the defendant also said, "I will guarantee to make the hand a hundred percent perfect hand or a hundred percent good hand."

The defendant argued that even if these words were uttered by him, no reasonable person would understand that they were used with the intention of entering "into any contract whatever," and that they could reasonably be understood only as his expression in strong language that he believed and expected that as a result of the operation he would give the plaintiff a very good hand.

There were other factors that tended to support the contention of the plaintiff. There was evidence that the defendant repeatedly solicited the plaintiff's father for the opportunity to perform this operation. The theory was advanced by plaintiff's counsel during cross-examination of the defendant that the doctor sought an opportunity to "experiment on skin grafting," a field in which he had little previous experience. The defendant was held liable for breach of contract including a promise to cure.

Hawkins v. McGee,
146 A. 611 (N.H. 1929)

When the court determines there is a breach of contract, the objective of the court becomes making the injured party whole. The most common means for accomplishing this is to award the party monetary damages in an amount sufficient to offset the losses incurred. The major problem in achieving a just result is the difficulty in measuring damages.

AGENCY

When a person agrees to work for and under the direction or control of another, a principal-agent relationship is created. The **principal** is the employer, and the agent is the employee. In the medical office, the principal is the physician, and the agent is the medical assistant or other employee. Special rules, called the law of agency, govern this relationship. Business owners, physicians, hospitals, and other employers—who generally have greater financial resources than employees—are required to compensate persons who suffer injuries caused by their agents. An example of the power of an agent to bind the principal in contract follows.

> A middle-aged man was worried after a consultation with a surgeon. "Looks like I'll have to have a heart bypass," the patient remarked to the assistant at the front desk.
>
> "Don't worry," she assured him, "the doctor is very good at that procedure. You won't have any trouble. I can promise you that."
>
> The operation was prolonged by unexpected complications, and the patient died several weeks later. His family successfully sued the surgeon on the grounds that his assistant had made a promise that amounted to a warranty.
>
> Belli, Melvin M.
> *For Your Malpractice Defense* (1986)

Advance directives are effective because of the law of agency.

PATIENT SELF-DETERMINATION ACT (PSDA)

The Patient Self-Determination Act, sponsored by Senator John C. Danforth (R-Mo), requires health care facilities to provide written information to each adult admission concerning patient rights under state law to make decisions concerning the acceptance or refusal of medical or surgical treatment. Also called the Miranda Law for Patients, it requires documentation of the patient's receipt of this information in the medical record as well as whether a patient has executed an advance directive. Institutions cannot condition care on the provision that the patient execute an advance directive or agree to accept treatment. Examples of advance directives are the living will, the durable power of attorney, and the health care proxy.

Living Wills

The Danforth bill includes living wills in its list of acceptable advance directives. Forty-one states have living will statutes. These "natural death" statutes have differing requirements for the content of living wills.

Over the past ten years, living wills have been accepted by the courts, physicians, the President's Commission for the Study of Ethical Problems in

Medicine and Biomedical and Behavioral Research, and lawyers, but only approximately nine percent of the public have made living wills. According to the June 1989 issue of the *Journal of the American Medical Association,* there appears to be little use of them in clinical practice. Contact your local bar association or department of elder affairs for information appropriate to your jurisdiction.

Durable Power of Attorney

The American Medical Association (AMA) suggests a medical directive as a substitute for the living will and suggests further that these be made available in doctor's offices and hospitals and included as a part of the medical record. Assessing the relative merits of the living will and the durable power of attorney for health care, the AMA finds that the durable power of attorney can cover a broader range of illnesses than the living will, which is often linked to situations of terminal illness when death is imminent.

Nineteen states have durable power of attorney statutes. In a durable power of attorney, a principal, in writing, designates another as his or her attorney in fact. The document contains the words, "This power of attorney shall not be affected by subsequent disability or incapacity of the principal. . . . This power of attorney shall become effective upon the disability or incapacity of the principal," or similar words indicating the principal's intent that the authority conferred continue despite his or her disability or incapacity. This authority differs from that of a regular power of attorney, which terminates upon disability or death.

In most cases, the durable power of attorney is accepted for the clauses of instruction contained within the document. If there is no direction to the agent concerning right-to-die issues, the document is interpreted to mean that the agent has no authority on these issues. Occasionally, the agent may be looked to by a hospital or physician to assist in a decision, but as a general rule, without instruction for medical treatment, the document cannot be used for that purpose.

Health care durable powers of attorney direct the agent to serve as a surrogate in health care decisions under certain circumstances. Some legal practitioners suggest that everyone who has a living will should also execute a durable power of attorney. Again, each state is different in its requirements, and state bar associations have the pertinent information.

A health care proxy is a medical durable power of attorney. A durable power of attorney authorizes another to act as one's agent. It becomes effective in the event he or she should later become disabled.

TERMINATION OF CONTRACTS

A contract between a physician and a patient may be terminated in many different ways. The most satisfactory outcome is that the patient is treated, is cured, and pays the physician a fee for services, and both parties are satisfied.

Since the physician-patient relationship requires mutual assent by the parties, either party may terminate the relationship. Once a physician enters into a physician-patient relationship, the physician is obliged to attend the case as long as it requires attention unless the patient is given reasonable notice of the physician's intention to withdraw or the patient informs the physician that services are no longer desired.

If the physician desires to withdraw from the case, the reasonableness of notice becomes an issue that depends on the patient's condition, the availability of other competent physicians, the manner of notice, and, indirectly, the patient's educational and economic status. If a patient discharges a physician and the patient is in need of further medical attention, the responsibility lies with the doctor for protection from a charge of abandonment by confirming discharge by the patient. A letter to the patient confirming discharge using certified mail will protect the doctor. Some physicians follow this procedure when a patient does not keep an appointment or fails to follow their advice.

Abandonment

To **abandon** a patient means that the physician gives up completely—deserts the patient—and indicates that the physician intends to terminate the contractual relationship. Abandoning a patient is a breach of contract and a tort. There are various classifications of abandonment. A physician's comment that he or she will not take care of the patient is the easiest abandonment to prove, as in the following case.

CASE STUDY   Following removal of the patient's appendix, the physician saw the patient at regular intervals without any sign of the incision healing. When the patient remarked that there must have been something wrong with the operation, the doctor became furious and stated that if that was the way she felt about it she could get out of his office, and that he "would not do anything more for her." He then further threatened that if she did not leave the office he would call the sheriff to evict her.

The woman left the office and went to another surgeon. Another operation revealed that a gauze sponge had been left in her incision. The court found that the first surgeon was liable and determined that the surgeon owed her an obligation to continue to administer her needs until all the effects of the operation had subsided and that abandonment had occurred.

Gillette v. Tucker,
65 N.E. 865 (Ohio 1902)

Obligations imposed on the physician by the doctor-patient relationship continue until the relationship is ended by "mutual consent of the parties; by dismissal of the physician by the patient; patient's improved condition; or physician's proper withdrawal" (*Peterson v. Phelps,* 143 N.W. 793 (Minn. 1913)).

A patient may terminate the relationship with a physician at any time, but it is important that a physician acknowledge in writing any termination if the patient is still in need of medical care for a particular problem. When the doctor wishes to withdraw from a case before its completion, the patient must be afforded the opportunity to acquire the needed services from another physician.

Termination should be with a written notice sent by certified mail and should explain the patients medical problems. The terminating physician must allow time for the patient to receive medical care. The amount of time should be stated as well as the date of projected termination.

If a patient relationship is not properly terminated, the physician may be sued for a breach of contract, abandonment, or professional negligence.

Abandonment might also occur when a physician does not visit a patient in the hospital, as in the following:

CASE STUDY   The plaintiff was operated upon for varicose veins. The recovery was complicated by gangrene setting in. Following examination the surgeon informed the patient that amputation of his foot was necessry immediately. The patient consented. The patient thought that the operation would be performed at once but nothing happened. Four days later when the surgeon had neither returned nor communicated with the patient, the man insisted on being transferred to another hospital where another surgeon performed the amputation. The court held that the first physician had abandoned the patient.

McGulpin v. Bessmer,
43 N.W.2d 121 (Iowa 1950)

Once a physician has accepted a patient, the financial question is irrelevant to the patient's care. If the physician does not arrange substitute care for the patient, abandonment is held to have occurred. For example:

A patient who was **indigent** had a miscarriage and was treated by a physician the day of the miscarriage and for the following two days. Because she could not pay him, the doctor refused to see her again, even though he knew she had retained the placenta. The court held that the physician was guilty of abandonment.

Becker v. Janiski,
15 N.Y.S. 675 (1891)

SUMMARY

A contract is a promissory agreement between two or more parties that creates, modifies, or destroys a legal relationship. In order to have a contract, there must be an offer, acceptance, and consideration. An offer is a statement or other conduct by one party that invites acceptance by a second party. The offer may be accepted in an express or implied manner. Consideration is the money that is transacted for service or goods.

In order to have a legal contract, there must be mutual assent between parties with the capacity to contract. Minors, mental incompetents, and those under undue influence are able to engage in contracts only on a limited basis. In these situations, the court must weigh the rights of the individual with rules of contract law, balancing private and public interests.

Contracts not performed according to agreement are termed breached. A party who suffers from breach of contract is entitled to be made whole by the court. In the medical field, the most common remedy for a breach is monetary damages.

Employees are the agents of their employers and, under the law of agency, able to contract for the principal. Contracts made by an agent within the scope of employment are valid. The principal is usually held responsible for any damages.

Contracts are terminated upon completion of the agreement. In the contract between physician and patient, the patient may desire to change physicians before treatment has been completed. The discharged doctor should **memorialize** the patient's wishes by sending the patient a certified letter documenting the conditions of the discharge. If a physician terminates the relationship, further provisions must be made for the care of the patient or the physician will be guilty of abandonment.

SUGGESTED ACTIVITY

Look up the age of majority in your state. This may be found in the state's general laws, and should be located in the local library. While looking through the index, try to determine how many laws apply to minors in medical situations and for what conditions.

STUDY QUESTIONS

1. Go back to the first page of this chapter and reread the telephone conversation. Analyze each sentence, and list the questions that come to you based on the legal material you have just read. Rewrite the telephone conversation. Remember, *your words may form the contract.*

2. Give examples of implied and express consent to medical treatment in a hospital emergency room situation.
3. Write a skit detailing the conversation of a medical assistant making an appointment for a new patient.
4. A patient has just been informed by the doctor that she must have a hysterectomy and that there is a question of malignancy. As she leaves the office and you schedule her for hospital admission, she comments: "The doctor makes me feel so good about this. She says that I will be out of the hospital in four days and on my own within a week. Isn't she a wonderful person? She says that I will be completely cured following my surgery." How would you handle this situation?
5. A sixteen-year-old male comes to the office without an appointment and asks to see the doctor because he thinks that he has AIDS. He does not wish to give you his or his parents' names or address. You have seen him around town and know that he is a local resident. The doctor is not available but you expect her within an hour. As the agent of the doctor what is your responsibility in this situation?
6. A fifteen-year-old girl comes to the office with a diagnosis of first-trimester pregnancy. A year ago, she visited the doctor twice, and then miscarried. There is an outstanding fee to be collected from the patient. Her parents are also patients of the physician but do not know that their daughter is pregnant. It is your job to collect the fees from patients. What would you do as an agent of the physician in this situation?

CASES FOR DISCUSSION

1. A teenage boy suffered from a massive deformity of the face and neck. His appearance was so grotesque he was excused from attendance at school and therefore was illiterate. The condition could be corrected by surgery, but the mother objected to blood transfusions on religious grounds and would not consent to the surgery. (a) Did the minor have a right to surgery? (b) Did the mother have the right to refuse to enter into a contractual relationship with the physician?
2. A sixteen-year-old female was pregnant and wished to get married in order to give the child legitimacy. Her mother objected strenuously and took her daughter to a gynecologist to have an abortion. The gynecologist refused to enter into a contract to perform the abortion without a court order. Should the court allow the abortion?
3. The director of a drug treatment center called a physician friend and requested that he admit one of the center's patients to the hospital. The physician friend had been seriously ill and was at home recovering when he received the telephone call. He was in no condition to visit the patient in the hospital and conveyed that information to the director but did allow the patient to be admitted to the hospital under his name. The patient never saw the physician before she died of an undiagnosed

brain abcess within a few days after admission. Her father sued the physician, claiming that there was a physician-patient relationship between his daughter and the physician. Should the court agree with the doctor or the father?

4.   A woman was hit by a car and complained of injuries to her leg, knee, hip, and thigh. She was taken to the nearest hospital where, on the orders of a physician, she received X-rays of her arm and pelvis. No X-ray was taken of her leg, and she was released from the hospital on crutches. The pain in her leg increased and she went to another hospital some hours later where an X-ray was taken and revealed that her leg was fractured. She was admitted to the second hospital and remained an inpatient for a month. Ten days after admission to the second hospital, she received a letter from the first hospital telling her to return for a leg X-ray. She sued the first hospital and the radiologist. Does the radiologist, who never saw her, have a contractual relationship with the patient?

5.   A clinic patient was operated on by a hospital resident for removal of his gallbladder. It was later determined that a piece of gauze was left in the patient's abdomen. The defendant, in this case, was a consultant physician who saw the patient before and after the operation but who was not present at all times during surgery. He was not paid a fee for his services and did not expect payment. Was the consultant physician liable for the gauze in the patient's abdomen?

6.   A man had a vasectomy. He and his wife were the parents of two developmentally disabled children, and the vasectomy was desired to prevent the birth of another disabled child. After the vasectomy, another child was born who was developmentally and physically disabled. Should the surgeon who performed the vasectomy be liable for breach of contract?

7.   A woman went to a plastic surgeon for an operation to improve the appearance of her nose. Before the operation, the woman's nose had been straight but long and prominent. The surgeon undertook, with two operations, to reduce its prominence and shorten it, thus making it more pleasing in relation to the woman's features. Actually the patient was obliged to undergo three operations, and her appearance worsened. Her nose now had a concave line to about the midpoint, at which it became bulbous; viewed frontally, the nose from bridge to midpoint was flattened and broadened, and the two sides of the tip had lost symmetry. This configuration could not be improved by further surgery. Should the surgeon be liable for breach of contract?

8.   The plaintiffs engaged a physician to perform a sterilization operation on the wife. Some seventeen months later, the wife became pregnant, and nine months later, she was delivered of a child by caesarean section. At the time of this birth, one of her fallopian tubes was found to be intact. This is alleged to have resulted from the negligent manner in which the doctor performed the sterilization. The plaintiffs alleged a

breach of warranty. Should the court allow them to recover damages under a breach of warranty action?

9. An eighteen-year-old girl, one of ten children whose mother was a welfare recipient, was allegedly told by a county social worker that if she refused to be sterilized, her mother would lose her welfare payments. Although the state had an involuntary sterilization statute for mental incompetents residing in state institutions, there was no allegation that the plaintiff was developmentally disabled or incompetent. To the knowledge of the court, there had not been any intelligence tests administered. There was no court order. After her mother's death and upon reaching legal age, the plaintiff filed suit against the social worker who had required sterilization, the county welfare department, the physician who performed the sterilization, and the hospital in which the operation was performed. Was the plaintiff unduly influenced, causing her to consent to a sterilization procedure?

10. A patient was hospitalized for mental illness and as part of the treatment received electroshock therapy. When the psychiatrist realized that the patient could not pay his hospital bill, the doctor sent the patient home immediately following electroshock treatment. The patient was prescribed a heavy sedative. The patient, confused from the combination of the drug and the effects of the treatment, fell asleep and ignited himself with a cigarette. He suffered nearly fatal third-degree burns over a wide area of his body. Did the physician have the right to discharge the patient from the hospital because he could not pay his bill?

11. The plaintiff, a blind person, accompanied by her four-year-old son and her guide dog, arrived at the defendant's "medical office" on a Saturday to keep an appointment "for treatment of a vaginal infection." She was told that the doctor would not treat her unless the dog was removed from the waiting room. She insisted that the dog remain because she "was not informed of any steps which would be taken to assure the safety of the guide dog, its care, or availability to her after treatment." The doctor "evicted" the patient, her son, and her dog, refused to treat her condition, and failed to assist her in finding other medical attention. Because of this conduct on the part of the physician, the patient was "humiliated" in the presence of other patients and her young son, and "for another two days while she sought medical assistance from other sources," her infection became "aggravated" and she endured "great pain and suffering." The plaintiff demanded damages resulting from "breach of the physician's duty to treat." Should she be awarded damages?

Chapter 5

Anatomy of a Medical Malpractice Case

"I didn't mean to do it."

OBJECTIVES:

The above statement is the essence of negligence. Even though the person making the comment meant no harm, our legal system is based on the premise that everyone is responsible for the consequences of his or her actions. After reading this chapter, you should be able to:

1. distinguish between a cause of action for negligence and one for malpractice.
2. list the elements of a civil malpractice cause of action.
3. identify when there has been a breach of duty to a patient based on an inappropriate standard of care.
4. analyze the legal cause of a patient's injury and assess accountability of the employee.
5. give examples of the defenses available to the defendant.
6. appreciate the legal, moral, and ethical aspects of informed consent.
7. recognize the need for malpractice insurance.
8. be able to analyze emergency situations and determine whether or not a situation is covered by a good samaritan statute.
9. distinguish between invitees, licensees, or trespassers and the duty of care owed to them for maintenance of equipment and premises.
10. define strict liability in tort.
11. identify a product liability cause of action.

BUILDING YOUR LEGAL VOCABULARY

adversary	ethical	pharmacopoeia
affirmative duty	expert witness	product liability
assumption of risk	grossly negligent	proximate cause
burnout	idealistic	psychosomatic
comparative negligence	insurance	reasonable care
consumer	invitee	res ipsa loquitur
contributory negligence	latent defect	sample
defensive medicine	licensee	sanction
delegated	malfunction	sociological
depression	nonverbal	statute of limitations
emergency	communication	suit-prone
empathy	patent defect	trespasser
entrepreneur	peer review	

NEGLIGENCE OR MALPRACTICE?

When an act performed on an individual results in injury in a situation where there is no intent to injure, it is called negligence. *Negligence* is defined as not doing something that a reasonable person would do or doing something that a reasonable person would not do. In a trial for negligence, the jury decides the facts of the case, including whether a reasonable person would commit the act. Malpractice differs from negligence in that it is a professional's negligence.

When deciding whether an act resulting in injury should be labeled negligence or malpractice, the training and experience of the individual committing the act is taken into consideration. *Malpractice* is a term associated with any professional misconduct and implies a greater duty of care to the injured person than the reasonable person standard. The term implies that a doctor, nurse, or other health care professional has special knowledge, which raises the expectations of society. For example, a surgeon performing an appendectomy is held to a higher standard of care than a general practitioner performing the same operation. The surgeon has special knowledge, education, training, and experience, which indicates to society that he or she is better qualified to perform an appendectomy. An **expert witness** is required to testify in court to set a standard for the surgeon.

The expert witness informs the jury whether the manner in which the surgeon operated was acceptable to a majority or respectable minority of other surgeons practicing under similar circumstances. Expert witnesses come from the ranks of a profession. In order to be labeled professional, an expert witness must belong to a certifying or qualifying organization with professional standards against which a defendant's adequacy may be compared. This might present a problem in assessing the conduct of medical assistants.

The American Association of Medical Assistants maintains a national certifying program; therefore, there is a certifying organization. Difficulties arise, however, because the medical assistant works under the supervision of a physician or other health care professional and performs **delegated** tasks. The variety of procedures performed, the varying educational levels of medical assistants, and the differences in state statutory requirements make it difficult to establish a national professional standard for the medical assistant. In addition, medical assistants are emerging health care professionals working to carve out professional recognition in the health care delivery system. They are hybrid professionals performing tasks of nurses, secretaries, and technicians. When performing the work of a secretary or receptionist, the medical assistant may be regarded as a reasonable person and charged with negligence; however, when performing clinical procedures, such as giving an injection or doing blood tests, the medical assistant may be regarded as a professional and charged with malpractice. These same guidelines may be used in establishing the standard of care for all cross-trained professionals.

The courts—recognizing that for the plaintiff hiring expert witnesses is expensive and, in certain cases, evidence of what occurred is not available to the injured person—developed the doctrine of **res ipsa loquitur.** Translated as "the thing speaks for itself," res ipsa loquitur requires the following three conditions:

1. In the normal course of events, the accident would not have occurred if reasonable care had been used.
2. The defendant had exclusive control over the cause of the injury.
3. The plaintiff did not contribute to the occurrence of the accident.

Following is a classic example of res ipsa loquitur:

CASE STUDY On July 23, 1945, a 45-year-old soldier had undergone an operation for gallbladder trouble at Fort Belvoir, Virginia. In January, 1946, he was discharged from the Army. On March 8, 1946, he went to Johns Hopkins Hospital in Baltimore, Maryland, complaining of nausea and vomiting that he had for two weeks and which was getting worse. On March 13, 1946, he was operated on at Johns Hopkins. The surgeon found a well-healed medical scar. When he operated through the scar the surgeon came upon a towel which had eroded into the intestine. The towel was removed, measured and photographed. It read "Medical Department, U.S. Army." It was two and one-half feet long by one and one-half feet wide. The court held that this evidence indicated negligence on the part of "agents or employees of the government."

Jefferson v. United States,
77 F. Supp 706 (Md. 1948)

ELEMENTS OF A CIVIL MALPRACTICE SUIT

In order to have a civil medical malpractice lawsuit, the patient must show that:

1. there was a relationship between the physician and the patient;
2. this relationship established duty by the physician to the patient;
3. the duty had been upheld at a professional standard of care;
4. the physician breached the duty to the patient;
5. the patient had a resulting injury; and
6. the physician's breach was the **proximate cause** of the patient's injury.

Relationship

The relationship between the physician and the patient is established by contract law, which was covered in the preceding chapter. If there is no professional relationship between the doctor and the patient—for example, if the doctor is at a cocktail party and, during a social conversation with the patient, discusses an illness or some symptoms that the patient reveals—there is no malpractice, even if the patient suffers injury from something that was said during the conversation.

The relationship establishes duty by the physician to the patient when it can be shown that the patient consulted the physician for medical advice and the elements of a contract were met: offer, acceptance, consideration, and mutual assent. The duty required by the physician is established by the profession and/or the expectations of society and is termed the standard of care. Once a contract is made between a doctor and a patient for medical care, the physician has a duty to the patient that must meet a professional standard of care.

Breach of the duty by the physician, by action or inaction, is measured against the standard of care. For example:

CASE STUDY   A patient visited his doctor because of chest pains. While in the office an electrocardiogram was taken. The physician did not tell the patient about the results nor did he prescribe rest or other treatment. A week later the chest pains recurred, were more severe, and the patient called the doctor. The physician told him to go to the hospital. The doctor did not tell him to go in an ambulance. The patient walked down several flights of stairs and rode to the hospital in his own car. Examination revealed that he had a heart attack several days before and open heart surgery was necessary to repair the heart damage. The patient sued and recovered damages from the physician. The court held that a duly careful, reasonably prudent physician would have told his patient about the electrocardiogram results and would have hospitalized the patient immediately.

Armstrong v. Svoboda,
49 Cal. Rptr. 701 (1966)

Duty

The first breach of the physician's duty occurred when he did not inform the patient of the irregularities in the electrocardiogram and of the possibility that he had or was at risk of having a heart attack. The second breach of duty occurred when the doctor did not advise the patient to go to the hospital in an ambulance. A majority of physicians would have called an ambulance and sent the patient to the hospital. Therefore, the doctor performed below an acceptable standard of care. In addition, it is the expectation of society that a patient will be informed of a life-threatening situation, especially when simple modification of the behavior of the patient could save his or her life.

Standard of Care

Standard of care is undergoing many changes. In the past, physicians were held to a local standard because of inequities in education and funding for the latest technology between urban and rural localities. Subsequently, the trend in the court was a shift toward a national standard due in part to advances in communications technology allowing for physicians any place in the United States to access training experiences. More recently, standards of care appear to be reverting back to a local standard of care with the utilization of the practice guidelines of HMOs and other managed care organizations as the basis. Theoretically, doctors should be protected from malpractice actions by following these recognized practice guidelines because the law sets the standard of care according to minimally accepted medical practices. The guidelines usually set ideal levels of competency, and the law recognizes different medical practices as long as they are generally accepted. There have not been enough cases tried in the courts to accurately assess this trend, but as the managed care networks grow larger and encompass broader areas of the country, the standard of care may again focus on national acceptance.

Injury

The patient must have an injury in order to sue for malpractice even if the physician has made an error. Without an injury, there is no case, as is seen in the following:

CASE STUDY   A child had Perthes disease in one leg. The physician, by mistake, placed a cast on the other leg. No harm was proven to have occurred as a result of the error; therefore, no damages were awarded.

Redder v. Hanson,
338 F.2d 244 (1964)

Causation

The physician's breach must be the cause of the injury. There are two definitions of the legal cause of injury. The first is "but-for" causation. This means that, but for the action of the physician, the injury would not have occurred. In addition to "but-for" causation, proximate cause must be established. Proximate cause differs in that it takes into consideration any incidents that may have occurred between the original negligent act and the outcome that is the basis for the lawsuit. For example:

CASE STUDY   The plaintiff was involved in an automobile accident and fractured a cervical vertebra. The fracture was not discovered for two months and it was determined that a bone graft was necessary. The patient sued the doctor for failure to discover the fracture immediately. A witness for the defense, at the trial, testified that the treatment would have been the same whether or not the fracture had been discovered immediately and that it would have been necessary to perform a bone graft. The court held that no proximate cause existed because a graft would have been necessary even if the fracture had been discovered immediately. The period of time between the accident and treatment did not cause further injury.

Rudick v. Prineville Memorial Hospital,
319 F.2d 764 (1963)

The elements of a medical malpractice case are the same whether the defendant is the physician, as in the above cases, or a nurse, therapist, technician, medical assistant, or other defendant. In order for the plaintiff-patient to win, each element must be met by a preponderance of the evidence. This means that the jury or the judge must find that the plaintiff has enough evidence to continue the trial. Enough evidence is admitted if the trier of fact, the judge, or the jury questions the defendant's innocence. If the plaintiff does not have enough evidence for each element, the case is dismissed. Today this rarely happens because most medical malpractice actions are brought before a hearing officer or a tribunal to determine whether the plaintiff has met the burden of proof and has brought forward adequate evidence before being scheduled for trial.

Knowing the elements of a malpractice action is not enough. It is necessary to understand how these elements are incorporated into a case.

INFORMED CONSENT

Informed consent is an important part of medical practice today. Physicians are often sued for malpractice because of failure to adequately inform patients of drug reactions, possible adverse surgical results, or alternative forms of treatment. Many times, the office staff is actively involved in the consent process. In the next case, the physician was charged with medical malpractice because he did not adequately inform the patient.

Breach of Duty

CASE STUDY   A patient consented to a laminectomy, excision of a portion of the spinal column. The court found as a fact that the patient did not understand what laminectomy meant. If the patient did not understand the meaning of laminectomy, the court reasoned that the patient could not have understood what was involved in the procedure. The patient was paralyzed after the operation. Paralysis is a complication of a laminectomy. There was no evidence that the surgeon indicated to the patient that paralysis could be a result of surgery. The court found that there was no informed consent and that the surgeon was liable.

Gray v. Grunnagle,
23 A.2d 663 (Pa. 1966)

Analysis of the elements of this case results in the following:

1. Relationship: The relationship between the doctor and patient is established. The doctor offered services, the patient accepted, consideration was implied, and the fact that surgery took place indicates there was mutual assent.
2. Duty: The surgeon-patient relationship establishes a duty of the physician to inform the patient about the procedure to be performed, the associated risks, and the prognosis.
3. Breach of duty: The surgeon did not communicate to the patient the nature of the operation. It can be inferred that the surgeon did not inform the patient of the risks he was taking, and therefore, the patient could not decide whether to have the operation and assume the risk.
4. Injury: The patient suffered paralysis, establishing injury.
5. The breach was the cause of the injury: There is no claim that the physician was negligent in the operation. The cause of action is that the physician was negligent for not telling the patient what was going to happen to him during surgery or the risks involved. There was no informed consent. The patient had no opportunity to decide whether he was willing to take the risk of surgery; therefore, because the patient might have decided not to undergo surgery, the breach was the cause of the injury.

Informed consent is a legal tightrope on which physicians must walk. On one side is the doctor's medical judgment about what information the patient needs to have to make a decision, and on the other side is the patient's right to know every possible outcome. The issue of consent is based on the common law enforcement of the concept of personal autonomy and self-determination. In earlier days, the courts determined that an operation performed without the patient's consent was a battery. Today, when there is a breach by the physician in obtaining consent, the case is usually tried as negligence. Traditionally, the physician made the decision about how much information was given to the patient. Today, the patient and society exercise the patient's right to know, often requiring the doctor to reveal more information than was thought necessary in the past.

Informed consent enters medical practice in many instances. Patients carrying the "breast cancer" gene have the opportunity to have their own vulnerability to the disease exposed. In a study by the New England Medical Center, fifty percent of patients who had a history of breast cancer in their family refused the test. Of the remaining fifty percent, forty-seven percent made the decision to receive the results of the testing. The others did not wish to be informed. Their decision is informed consent to be uninformed. But what about those with diseases like Huntington's cholera where symptoms of the disease, which is hereditary in nature, become evident between thirty and thirty-five years—for many, after childbearing years have ended. The pain of informed consent under these conditions is documented in the book *Mapping Fate* by Alice Wexler. In addition, under certain circumstances, physicians may make the judgment that for "therapeutic" reasons a patient should not be informed about his or her condition.

Another aspect of informed consent occurs when a doctor has an "impairment" and has to decide whether to inform the patient. For example, the doctor may have an infectious disease or a number of malpractice actions may have been brought against the physician for whatever reason. In the case of former actions, there may have been a conviction or a plea to dispose of the case. In Massachusetts, the Massachusetts Medical Society initiated legislation to publish the malpractice history of all physicians registered in the Commonwealth. This was a controversial decision, but the bill was passed and took effect in September 1996.

The following is an example of an issue of informed consent:

CASE STUDY   The plaintiff, Mr. Cobbs, was admitted to the hospital in August, 1964, for treatment of a duodenal ulcer. The surgeon, Dr. Grant, made the decision to operate and informed Cobbs of the nature of the operation but not the risks of surgery. After a two-hour operation, the ulcer disappeared. Cobbs' recovery appeared to be uneventful and he went home eight days later. He had to be readmitted for emergency surgery, however, when it was discovered he was suffering from internal bleeding due to a severed artery in his spleen. Injuries to the spleen compelling a second operation are found in approximately five percent of surgery such as Cobbs had undergone but the surgeon had not informed the patient of this possibility. The spleen was removed by Dr. Grant.

Four months after discharge from the hospital, Cobbs developed a gastric ulcer and half of his stomach was removed. The evolution of a second ulcer is another risk inherent in surgery performed to relieve a duodenal ulcer. Cobbs had to be hospitalized again when he began to bleed from the premature absorption of a suture, another inherent risk of surgery.

The court held that . . . when consent is given and an undisclosed potential complication results, the trend is to find the physician liable for negligence, not battery. . . . [T]he doctor may have failed to meet his due care duty to disclose pertinent information in obtaining the consent.

Cobbs v. Grant,
8 Cal. Rptr. 505, 502 P.2d 1 (1972)

There are ethical and moral implications in informed consent, especially when a drug or procedure is in the research phase and physicians are experimenting on patients. Physicians' comments and studies reveal that some patients do not want to hear bad news from the doctor. In addition, when the risks of a procedure or medication are communicated to a patient, the patient often does not remember what is said. In some situations, a patient may selectively remember comments by the physician and selectively forget other important statements. The sicker the patient, the less accurate the memory for details of pending treatment. The less educated the patient, the less accurate the recall of information. In some situations, a physician may determine that it will be harmful to the future care of the patient if he or she is informed of possible side effects. Lawyers develop forms for patients to sign indicating that they have been informed of possible adverse reactions, but studies have shown that in order to be understood, many of these forms require an education at the level of a doctorate in a scientific area.

The Medical Assistant and Informed Consent

Medical assistants cannot be delegated the responsibility of receiving informed consent from a patient. However, the medical office staff is in a position to protect, or at least warn, the physician of potential malpractice actions when there is doubt whether the doctor adequately informed the patient. Keeping accurate records, providing adequate documentation, and relaying patient misunderstanding to the physician can help prevent such actions. These efforts also support the patient's right to self-determination.

Physicians are legally responsible for obtaining informed consent from a patient. The primary responsibility of the medical office staff is to be certain that copies of informed consent forms are available to the physician, that they are properly dated and signed, and that they are accurately and promptly filed in the medical records. Following discussion with the patient, the doctor should document the fact that the patient has been informed and the patient's reactions. Following the visit, a check of the record by the staff offers the physician a second chance to legitimately update the record.

In addition, many times a member of the office staff knows the patient well enough to function as a sounding board for the physician. Patients often express confusion and ask questions of the staff that they will not ask of the doctor. **Nonverbal communication** can cue the staff that something is amiss. Medical assistants should communicate with the doctor and document personal observations on a sheet attached to the medical record but not part of the record. This information is for the physician only and gives the doctor an opportunity to follow up the first discussion and correct a patient's inaccurate perceptions and misunderstandings.

A patient may decide to withdraw consent. This is the patient's right even after the authorized treatment has begun. The presence of a third person offers assurance to the patient that his or her preferences will be honored.

IMPACT OF MEDICAL MALPRACTICE SUITS

It is a devastating experience for doctors to be sued by patients for whom they have done their best. Physicians may feel that everyone is pointing a finger; they may feel disgraced in the community. They may be afraid that one claim of poor treatment will negate all the good performed in a lifetime.

In a recent study of 154 physicians who had been defendants, a majority suffered from **depression** or other **psychosomatic** illnesses, and 8 percent actually came down with physical ailments. Nearly 20 percent reported a "loss of nerve" in some clinical situations after the suit had been resolved. Fifteen percent said they'd lost confidence in themselves as physicians.

Belli, Melvin M.,
For Your Malpractice Defense, p. 19 (1986)

Families are affected by a medical malpractice suit. Emotional tension increases in the home as a result of stresses such as children defending a parent to other children. The fact that the doctor can be **ethical,** honest, and competent and still be sued is seldom remembered as the defendant and others ask the question, "What has gone wrong?"

Nurses, pharmacists, therapists, and other professionals voice the same disbelief when informed that their actions and professional behavior are in dispute. For the most part, these are **idealistic** individuals who have tried to improve society by choosing a medical vocation to help relieve suffering of others.

Emotions of a defendant may fester and potentially poison relations with patients. Embittered physicians can also have an impact on their colleagues.

Doctors and patients can begin viewing each other as **adversaries** rather than as partners working together to defeat a common enemy, ill health. The ultimate result is that medical care becomes a business—an impersonal, cold, monetary transaction—rather than a trusting relationship between the healer and the sick.

Once a malpractice case has been initiated, a defendant loses even if he or she wins the case. The substantial amount of time used to prepare for litigation, the stained reputation, the diversion of society's resources, and the emotional harm to the community can never be recovered or undone.

When malpractice litigation rose sharply in the 1970s, the threatened medical profession instinctively struck back. Physicians accused the public of greed and insensitivity and lawyers of unscrupulous behavior. They lashed out at laws they perceived as protections for the public but not for physicians and blamed insurance companies for seeking excessive profits. Retaliation came in the form of **defensive medicine.**

Defensive Medicine

Doctors, afraid that they might be accused of unscrupulous practice, ordered every known test in search of a definitive diagnosis when presented with specific symptoms. Following the old adage—the best defense is a good offense—they requested more and more laboratory tests, X-rays, assorted diagnostic procedures, hospitalizations, consultations, and referrals. Many hospitals and most experienced physicians, when confronted with an accident victim, cynically "X-rayed 'em wherever they hurt."

The practice of defensive medicine led to increased specialization because general practitioners were no longer willing to deliver babies, and fewer general surgeons were willing to repair broken bones. The increased use of specialists served to increase the psychological distance between doctor and patient. The gap between the patient and the physician began to widen. Each viewed the other as a potential enemy. By continually guarding against litigation, patient hostility—of which doctors constantly complain—became a self-fulfilling prophecy. The trusting relationship the patient wanted was met with a screen of suspicion and wariness. The warm, intimate family doctor relationship changed as the doctor looked at every patient as a potential malpractice suit. **Entrepreneurs** published lists of patients who were known to have been involved in malpractice actions against physicians. Medical magazines published articles describing **suit-prone** patient behavior in an attempt to alert physicians that particular kinds of patients should be avoided.

Although it is not known whether the practice of defensive medicine aids in preventing professional liability suits, physicians are now caught between protecting themselves by ordering tests and being **sanctioned** for ordering unnecessary procedures by professional **peer review** in a society that is extremely interested in containing medical costs.

Economics

Practicing defensive medicine, in short, transformed the malpractice crisis into a vicious circle. Not only did it cause an inevitable deterioration in the doctor-patient relationship, but it contributed to the spiraling cost of medical care.

If each accident victim has twenty dollars' worth of medically unnecessary but legally advisable x-rays, it does not take calculus to elicit a staggering bill of waste. At from fifty to hundreds of dollars a day, excessive hospitalization swiftly mounts to NASA levels.

Brooke, James W.,
Willamette Law Review 6:225, 232 (1970)

When you go to the hospital, you lose decision-making power. You get naked and that's it. . . . [T]he doctor decides what tests to order . . . what course of treatment to pursue . . . and few patients are qualified to argue.

Stevens, William K., "High Medical Costs,"
New York Times, pp. 1, 50 (March 28, 1982)

Physicians have a stake in selling a lot of health care because they get paid on a piecework basis. An example is the yearly physical.

Some doctors may resist curtailing the annual checkup for economic, as well as medical, reasons. Many of them perform several of the exams, such as electrocardiograms and X-rays, in their offices, and the charges for these tests are often an important source of income.

Bishop, Jerry E., "Physical Isn't Needed Yearly,"
The Wall Street Journal, p. 1 (December 16, 1981)

An example of the cost of defensiveness was shown in an article in the *New York Times:*

An elderly patient was admitted to the hospital late one night suffering from bronchitis and running a fever. In the judgment of the reporting doctor . . . her illness could have been safely and effectively treated at home. . . . Initial x-rays and electrocardiogram would have been justified in view of the woman's age . . . instead she was kept in the hospital for nine days. She was given $575 worth of intravenous infusions, $657 worth of electrocardiograms, $1,454 worth of x-rays, and $944 worth of laboratory services. The total hospital bill came to $9,065.10.

Stevens, William K., "High Medical Costs,"
New York Times, pp. 1, 50 (March 28, 1982)

The reporting doctor stated that in his opinion, "no fraud was involved, rather the doctors were simply doing what they were trained to do."

The excessive number of tests ordered by physicians to ensure accurate diagnosis is passed on to the patient in the form of dollar cost and lost time, and to the American public as a major contributory cause of inflation.

The nation's medical care bill has grown tenfold over the last two decades, from $27 billion in 1960, to $274 billion last year [1981]. The cost of the average stay in the hospital has soared to $2,119 from $670 since 1971, far outstripping the rate of inflation elsewhere in the economy. . . . Almost one dollar in every ten generated by the American economy goes for medical care today, as against one dollar in twenty two decades ago. . . . Taxes increase, health insurance premiums increase, and the physician's fee increases.

Bishop, Jerry E., "Physical Isn't Needed Yearly,"
The Wall Street Journal, p. 1 (December 16, 1981)

Doctors, employers, patients, and insurance companies become paper shufflers, adding to the fixed costs of the medical industry. As inflation spirals upward, the American public succumbs to stress-produced illnesses, anxiety states affecting mental health, and despair that hurts the economy by reducing the nation's productivity.

For the physician, one of the immediate effects of the increase in malpractice litigation is seen in higher malpractice insurance premiums and the decline in the number of carriers willing to assume the risk. As the size of awards and number of suits increase, insurance companies suffer losses. Small companies have dropped out of the medical malpractice insurance coverage arena altogether or are selective about who they insure. Everyone knows that insurance companies are in business to make money and realizes that physicians are also. Since physicians cannot absorb the burden of additional insurance premiums, the public again picks up the tab.

Negative Defensive Medicine

When the penalty for unsuccessfully performing a procedure becomes too high, the thinking person avoids the act. Some physicians today are shying away from the treatment of difficult cases with a potentially poor result. Many physicians have refused to take emergency room duty, which has given birth to another specialty in medicine. Fear of malpractice action may prevent a physician from attempting new procedures or employing new drugs. Doctors have protested the hike of medical malpractice insurance premiums by refusing to treat certain classes of patients, primarily obstetric and orthopedic cases.

Seeking to avoid the high cost of malpractice insurance premiums, some physicians are choosing early retirement, increasing the shortage of trained personnel in some parts of the country. Provisions have not yet been made for older physicians to continue on a part-time basis and obtain less costly coverage for limited practice. This is expensive to the American public.

Another example of physicians taking the path of avoidance is the so-called conspiracy of silence. In some situations, it is difficult, if not impossible, to find a practitioner who is willing to testify against another doctor. The reasons for failing to testify are many. Physicians have lost hospital privileges and had their malpractice insurance canceled as the result of testifying for a plaintiff. Others think of their own vulnerability when asked to testify against another doctor and react with, "There but for the grace of God go I." On the other hand, there are physicians who make it a habit to testify and are labeled "professional witnesses" by their angry colleagues. In some cases, a physician will testify against another doctor as a matter of conscience because the substandard treatment the patient received is an insult to the profession.

Increased Specialization

It is rare today that a person suffering from a major illness will be treated by one family doctor. When several physicians are called in, the doctors usually see the patient on a very limited basis, and the trust that is necessary for a good physician-patient relationship never has a chance to develop. As a result, when some unexpected complication occurs, the patient is more likely to believe that the physician did something wrong. Even the process of a routine physical examination, which in the past required direct doctor-patient contact and active cooperation, has been delegated to nurses and technicians, with a growing number of diagnostic procedures being performed in laboratories away from the physician.

ANALYSIS OF THE PROBLEM

A malpractice cause of action usually arises from two factors: the objective, which is the injury suffered by the patient; and the subjective, which is the alienation, anxiety, frustration, and potential anger in the patient. While malpractice as a legal concept requires both injury and negligence, the injury alone does not usually bring about the intense hostility that a lawsuit expresses. A majority of malpractice suits are brought because of:

> . . . patient, or patient-family, anger over something totally peripheral to the event leading to the claim damages. . . . [T]his may be hostility, inattentiveness, abruptness, or any one of the many other human characteristics which would cause any of us to turn hostile.
>
> Brittain, Robert S., "Physician Defines Role of Medical Profession in Claims Prevention," *Lawyer's Medical Journal* 7:203–205 (1978)

Statistics support this statement when the number of actual suits is compared to the number of potential suits. A study by James L. Peterson conducted in 1972 found that over forty percent of the **sample** had experienced some form of negative medical care. Of those, over eighty-five percent believed that some kind of medical failure had been involved, but only eight percent considered seeking legal advice. Of those who had suffered major permanent injury, approximately thirty-five percent considered consulting a lawyer. In 1974, a Louis Harris poll reported that fifteen percent of those interviewed felt that they or someone close to them had been the victim of malpractice, but only six percent attempted to bring suit. Over a twenty-year period, a hospital association's risk management program conducted by Buddy Steves produced about 700,000 reports of unusual incidents such as equipment failures, anesthesia deaths, and slips and falls. During that same period, only 15,000 malpractice claims were filed, and eighty-five percent of those involved unreported incidents. Although these studies are not exhaustive, there is enough evidence to indicate that injury alone does not cause a lawsuit.

The Suit-Prone Physician

It has been suggested that the working habits and personality of any particular physician can make the difference between a dangerous, unhappy patient and a friendly, satisfied one. The Richardson Commission warned that there is a suit-prone physician. They portrayed the doctor as follows:

> One who cannot admit his own limitations. . . . When such a doctor is confronted by a dissatisfied patient, he dismisses the complaint as being trivial instead of making the patient feel less angry, afraid or depressed by showing understanding and explaining matters.
>
> Wilson, Paul T., "Anesthesiology and Malpractice Lawsuits," *Medical Trial Technique Quarterly* 76:73

An attorney who specializes in defending doctors in malpractice suits describes the typical physician who gets sued for malpractice as:

> . . . the surgeon who will read the *Wall Street Journal* while the jury is out. He's got the businessman's personality and it shows in the way he runs his practice. He's usually the one who has eight patients in six rooms, with half a dozen more in the waiting room, and with a flock of nurses checking Blue Shield cards. He is also arrogant, egotistical, condescending, and aloof.
>
> . . . The doctor who wants to get in trouble after an incident of actual malpractice can do so easily. All he has to do is avoid the patient, blame the patient for the bad result, refuse to talk to the family, refuse to apologize, refuse to listen in humility to patient castigation, and then to send his bill as usual.
>
> Landers, Louise, "Why Some People Seek Revenge Against Doctors,"
> *Psychology Today,* p. 94 (July 1978)

The Patient Litigator

Can a doctor spot the patient who will sue? An unnamed general practitioner commented in a poll taken by *Medical Economics,* "I have a list above the phone of suit-prone patients who are not to be given appointments." In trying to recognize the patient who is a potential troublemaker, a well-known anesthesiologist has found that patients in the lower middle class tend to be more demanding about medical activities before and after surgery. Likewise, when a patient's family situation may be emotionally disturbing, there is a greater tendency or predisposition to initiate a lawsuit. Other studies of the patient litigator describe the individual as:

> . . . an emotionally immature neurotic who has subconscious fears of illness, doctors, and death. He wants to have complete faith in the physician, who is a father figure to him, and he sues as a hurt child when the treatment fails to restore him to health quickly.
>
> Brant, Jonathan, "Medical Malpractice Insurance,"
> *Valparaiso University Law Review* 6:152, n. 41, 157, n. 31

Being sick is uncomfortable, often painful, often embarrassing, frequently terrorizing, and involves one's self-image. If there is a malignancy involved, the emotions of the patient, as well as those of the family, are highly charged.

> Immediately after diagnosis, both the patient and relatives go through a time of intense anxiety. This anxiety may be manifested by hostility and anger toward health professionals. Paradoxical though it may seem, a supportive physician or surgeon may find the patient ventilating hostility and resentment directly toward him. . . . As a natural reaction, the physician would like to increase the psychological

distance between himself and the patient at just the time when the patient's need for a trusting relationship is the greatest.

Mittleman, Michael, "What Are the Chances When
Malignancy Leads to a Malpractice Suit?"
Legal Aspects of Medical Practice, p. 42 (February 1980)

Breakdown of Doctor-Patient Relationship

In the good old days, the family physician conjured up an image of a kindly, sympathetic, respected friend. Although today's physicians are better equipped to deal with the problems of illness, the very technology to which they have access increases the distance between the patient and the physician. Today's patient senses that the relationship with the doctor is not a relationship of one person to another, but of a person (the doctor) to a thing (the disease).

A serious aspect of malpractice is the loss of trust and faith in the physician. The family physician practiced medicine as an art, and missing today are many intangibles and unknowns that worked to the patient's advantage in the past. The one-to-one relationship between physician and patient is being replaced by third parties, such as employers, hospitals, insurance companies, and paramedical personnel. Doctor-patient communication is a social interaction, and, as in any interpersonal relationship, it is painful to unmask the underlying dynamics preventing harmony.

Insults in the Medical Office

It has been said that a malpractice suit is a sort of reverse class action suit—one individual suing the entire medical profession to revenge all the psychic insults of long delays in crowded waiting rooms and doctors with too little time to give each patient. John A. Appleman, attorney for the plaintiff in *Darling v. Charleston Community Hospital,* has summarized several factors he feels contribute to the problem. First on his list—the physician guilty of overbooking the number of patients that can be seen in a day. Many schedule all patients for a given hour. Patients who are depressed may have to wait two hours or more while being exposed to other patients who are coughing or sneezing. Following up on this subject, an insurance carrier's newsletter to doctors warns them against subjecting patients to long waits:

A wait of more than fifteen minutes means to patients not that the doctor is a little behind or a little disorganized, but that he does not care. . . . This sets the stage for anger and revenge and the patient is left feeling "His time is too precious to risk wasting five minutes, but he doesn't care a hoot about mine." These same doctors try to maximize their revenue by processing a large number of patients per hour. They master the art of dismissing the patient by looking at the wall above the patient's head, cooling the voice response, and getting out of their chair to signify the end of the interview, skills that swell the [pocketbook] but leave the patient dissatisfied.

Appleman, John Alan, "Malpractice Insurance Rates—What's the Answer?"
Journal of Legal Medicine, p. 37 (November/December 1975)

The following demonstrates a layperson's experience with a preferred provider organization (PPO). The woman reporting this experience is thirty-five years of age.

My frustration with the health care system began when I became a member of what has come to be known as a "PPO." I'm not even quite sure what all the initials stand for, all I know is that it has something to do with a primary care organization. Supposedly my plan works with a minimum co-payment of $10 per visit. I theoretically can go to my primary health care physician, get the care I need, and when they are unable to provide it they refer me to a specialist where I again pay another $10 fee. It all sounds fine, the only catch is getting in to see your primary care physician.

Once I signed on with my "PPO" I needed to choose a physician. The criteria I looked for in a primary care physician was convenience to my home and office, and gender. I wanted a female doctor. I checked with a local "PPO" and the doctor that I chose was accepting new patients, so I became her patient in January of 1996. In early May of 1996 I began experiencing some chest pain and dizziness and felt it best that I see my new doctor right away. I called the "PPO," when, after waiting on voice mail hold for some ten minutes, a young sounding female answered the phone. I realized as soon as I called that she was one of several "receptionists" that the "PPO" had on a switch board. I explained my problem and that I wanted to see the doctor as soon as possible.

After a short delay and some clicking on a computer, the receptionist said the doctor would be available to see me on May 30th. I said, "That is nearly a month away, don't you think the doctor should see me sooner?" The receptionist clicked on her computer a little longer and said, "No, that's the first appointment available with the doctor. Would you like to see the nurse practitioner?" I replied, "Maybe I should. When can I see her?" Again more clicking and then the receptionist responded, "She can see you next Tuesday."

I was very surprised by the lack of concern over my potentially serious medical condition, but realizing that there didn't seem to be any way to get in to see the doctor any sooner, I arranged for my appointment for the following week with the nurse practitioner. I then asked, "While I have you on the phone, I would like to arrange to have that appointment on May 30th with the doctor." The receptionist responded, "O.K., that will be for a diagnostic." "Can she give me a full check up while I am there?" I asked. "Oh, no," she responded, "a diagnostic is only a half hour appointment. If you want a physical we will need to schedule an hour appointment." "O.K." I said, "When is the first appointment for that?" Some more clicking and then, "June 23," she responded. "June 23rd," I said, "That is almost two months away. Can't she see me any sooner than that?" More clicking, and then she said, "No, that is the first available hour long appointment." "O.K.," I said, "I better book it." "O.K." the receptionist said, "You're all set with the nurse practitioner for next

Tuesday and with the doctor for May 30 for a one half hour diagnostic and on June 23rd for a one hour physical." The receptionist then recapped everything with me. I thanked her, although I wasn't sure why, and hung up.

When I arrived at the "PPO" the following Tuesday, I was first relieved that I made it through the week and lived, and then I was convinced they were going to rush me off to the hospital and scold me for not coming in sooner. Before I could see the nurse, I had to fill out forms, give them a copy of my license and wait for nearly forty-five minutes, although I wasn't sure why because my appointment was at 7:00 P.M. and no other patients appeared to be present.

Finally, when the office worker appeared to be done with me, I was ready to pay my $10 co-payment. I attempted to hand her a twenty dollar bill since that was all I had with me, but apparently this created a massive dilemma since nobody there knew where change was kept and no one had that kind of money with them. After about fifteen minutes of rushing around, the worker pleaded with me to let her send a bill. I agreed, reluctantly. Needless to say, nearly three months later I have yet to get a bill. I'm sure I'll see it in about a year.

Anyway, after all the formalities were completed, I went in to see the nurse practitioner. She was very gracious and professional and after I explained my symptoms she explained that she felt it best to rule out any chance of heart disease and said she could do this by going over the risk factors. I agreed, so the questioning began: "Do you have heart disease in your family?" "Yes," I responded. "Does your mother have heart disease?" "Yes," I said. "Did she develop it before the age of 60?" "Yes," I said. "Does your father have heart disease?" "Yes," I said. "Did he develop heart disease before the age of 60?" "Yes," I responded. At this point I noticed that the nurse had developed a very concerned look on her face and although there apparently were several more questions on the check list, she stopped short and asked if she could take a chest x-ray. Evidently no reason to fool around with this much heart disease in one family.

Fortunately my chest x-ray was normal. The nurse seemed to think my discomfort was probably related to indigestion and stress more than anything else. The nurse practitioner spent at least an hour with me and after I left I did feel that I received adequate medical care.

Debbie Segal
(Permission to quote, Debbie Segal, 1997.)

The saga for an appointment with the doctor continued. For some reason the patient's name was removed from the computer. There were problems with times and dates of future attempts to see the doctor and processing the appointments through the receptionists. The patient and her primary care physician finally met for a physical examination on July 9, 1996, six months after the doctor responsible for the patient's care was engaged as the primary care physician.

Lack of Empathy

Empathy is a form of communication that is one level deeper than understanding. Empathy requires vicariously experiencing the feelings or thoughts of another person. Health care professionals cannot identify with each patient but can communicate, through nonverbal cues and listening skills, their recognition of the patient's situation.

> According to the results of several recent surveys, patients have little complaint with the competence and expertise of their physicians, but they are dissatisfied with the human element. They want a chance to talk, to be listened to and to be told as much as possible, but this frequently doesn't happen.
>
> Krupat, Edward, "A Delicate Imbalance,"
> *Psychology Today,* p. 22 (November 1986)

Often the physician's casual attitude indicates a lack of empathy for his patients. Because members of the office staff pick up their cues from the physician for acceptable behavior toward patients, too much casualness may lead to a situation that implies contempt for the patient and the patient's complaints. On the other hand, too formal an atmosphere may inhibit the staff's freedom to share their observations about the patient with the physician, as well as give the office a snobbish, uncaring, cold environment.

Empathy is often crucial in treating illness that does not have an organic basis. The family physician knows his patients well and is aware of the stress that can produce psychosomatic complaints. Often the only treatment available is listening, rest, and reassurance.

Today's practice involves a group of physicians with a primary care doctor assuming the role of the family physician. The rules of managed care schedule a certain number of minutes for each patient visit with little flexibility to allow for lengthy conversation in any area. Some patients can express their concerns about their health in this time frame, but others require a few minutes to establish or reestablish a trusting relationship in which to reveal troubling problems. It is difficult to exhibit empathy for a patient's situation when the subject causing distress is never broached.

The public's reaction to a physician lacking in empathy is documented well in the following Ann Landers column:

Dear Ann Landers:

I would like to use your soapbox to appeal to all those doctors out there who deal with this sort of thing every day. I work for two fine physicians and know how busy doctors are. I have tremendous respect for them. But why does it have to take an eternity to relay test and procedure results to the parents?

During my daughter's three-week hospital confinement she had seven major procedures, each of which was supposed to give us "the answers we were looking for." Every procedure was done before 10:00 A.M. [for fasting reasons] and all results were evident at the time of the procedure. We never saw our doctor before 8:00 P.M.

Victim in Youngstown

Ann Landers' response:

Your letter struck a raw nerve. For a long time I have been angered by the very thing you are complaining about. . . . There is no good reason people should be kept waiting for days to learn the results of tests and biopsies. Why then does it happen? Because too many doctors are insensitive to the needs of their patients and their families. You can be sure when THEIR loved ones have lab tests that determine whether there is a serious illness, they don't wait around. The results are in their hands at the earliest possible moment.

Landers, Ann, "The Inhumanity of Some Doctors,"
The Boston Globe, p. 33 (March 19, 1982)

The Effect of a Prescription

Today's physician has at hand a **pharmacopoeia** that dazzles the imagination. One need only spend a weekend with an elderly grandparent to see an array of pills that will match a flower garden in full bloom for color, and a precious gem display for variety in size and shape. It is estimated that in the mid-seventies, three-quarters of all visits to general practitioners, internists, and family practitioners were concluded with the doctor prescribing at least one drug.

Patient and physician typically collude in the substitution of the drug for the relationship. . . . For a physician, writing a prescription is easy, but to come to an understanding with people is difficult. With the prescription, the doctor is an "activist-technologist" who acts upon the patient's body rather than teaching the patient how to give the body's healing powers a chance to act. When a patient visits a doctor there is the expectation of something tangible to make him feel better. He or she feels cheated when a physician advises rest, inhalation of steam, and letting the virus run its course.

Landers, Louise, *Defective Medicine,* p. 3 (1978)

The American public is impatient, sees serious illnesses "cured" in thirty minutes on television soaps, and anticipates being back in the swing of things the next day if the proper pill is prescribed. If the prescribed drug does not work against a particular illness, the patient becomes angry at the doctor. Even worse, if the prescribed drug causes an allergic reaction, it is the doctor's fault for prescribing the medication. In certain segments of the population, the doctor is viewed as a dispensing technician and trust is placed in the drug, not the doctor.

One of the most serious outcomes of our prescription-conditioned society is that patients do not properly take prescribed medication. Again, the physician is battling the time problem. Doctors do not take, or do not have, the time to explain to patients the importance of properly taking medication and continuing to do so once they feel better. If the physician cannot take the time or does not feel comfortable explaining details to the patient, someone else should be delegated to provide patient instruction.

For many elderly, the taking of pills is a ritual performed whenever indicated by the clock. It is sometimes viewed as the continuing care of the doctor, extending the doctor-patient relationship into their daily lives, yet:

> More than three out of four times the physicians failed to give explicit instructions about how regularly or how often drugs should be taken. And even when instructions were given, they were often ambiguous. Does "Take one capsule every six hours" mean that a total of four should be taken each day, with the patient waking up to take one in the middle of the night? Or does it mean that the capsules should only be taken during waking hours, totaling three a day?
>
> Krupat, Edward, "A Delicate Imbalance,"
> *Psychology Today,* p. 24 (November 1986)

Problems arise when more than one physician is involved in the prescribing and incompatible drugs are ingested or complications result from a double dosage of the same drug. Many elderly have blind loyalty to the doctor, little understanding of the purpose of a particular medication, and fear of asking questions that might brand them as "stupid." When trouble comes, angry relatives enter the picture and view the physician as negligent.

The changes that have taken place in the delivery of health care have affected pharmacies and the dispensing of medications. Where there used to be a small pharmacy on Main Street in every town, there are businesses, such as CVS (Consumer Value Stores), Walgreens, and so on, dispensing pharmaceuticals from mega stores strategically situated to draw customers from a defined geographical area. A national drug chain has its advantages when the customer is away from home and forgets a prescription, but it also has impacted the personal relationship that pharmacist and customer enjoyed in the past. Large pharmaceutical stores coach their personnel to be friendly and helpful and to interact with customers as part of the health care team, but often this is a bit much and becomes offensive rather than helpful. Following is an example of the history of a small pharmacy and its demise:

> Joe W. was in a Boston hospital recovering from a heart attack when his neighborhood pharmacist called every night with a heavy dose of good cheer. Janet H. was recuperating from surgery at home when the same pharmacist and his wife, George and Marjorie Miller, hooked up a basket trolley that carried hot coffee to her third-floor apartment window, and shut-ins across South Quincy could count on the Millers to deliver prescriptions to their doors. But customers who called Miller's Pharmacy this week are getting no answer. After 70 years in business, Miller's has given way to the inevitable and been sold to CVS across the street.
>
> Like other small pharmacies in the state, the Millers were hurt by changes in the health care industry. More than 500 pharmacies in Massachusetts have closed in the past decade, many because they lost business to chains with exclusive contracts with HMOs. A big blow for Miller's came four years ago when the city

made Pilgrim Health Care its sole insurer for employees. The health plan allows prescriptions to be filled only at certain pharmacies, which drew 50 to 100 regular customers away. The mayor said that the change in medical insurers has saved the city about $15 million since 1992, but city officials didn't realize when they made the switch how it would affect smaller pharmacies.

"We are now in a situation where everything is cost-driven," he said. "As a society when something like Miller's closes or a corner store closes, something in that community dies. It never will be the same" . . . "It's like a part of your life is gone," said Barbara B., a former nursing supervisor at Quincy Hospital and long-time customer of the pharmacy. "It leaves an empty space."

Davis, Maia, "An Empty Feeling,"
The Patriot Ledger, p. 15 (August 1, 1996)

Fee

It is generally agreed that money can become a catalyst of intense patient anger, but high fees alone are not necessarily the problem. An Ohio woman is quoted as saying:

I don't begrudge our doctor a penny of his fees . . . as long as he practices good medicine and puts financial considerations last instead of first. He charges a bit more than other doctors, but doesn't make a big thing about money.

Landers, Louise, "Why Some People Seek Revenge Against Doctors,"
Psychology Today, p. 96 (July 1978)

Patients are often reluctant to discuss fees with physicians. It has been suggested that patients fear that if they initiate the subject, the doctor may disapprove of them. Another stated reason is that the public is culturally conditioned to hold the physician apart from everyday concerns of others, including money. A surgeon observes that he is sometimes viewed like a man of the cloth, and just as people never know quite how to discuss a fee with a minister at a marriage or funeral service, they do not know how to discuss money with a doctor.

Impact of Public Communications Media

The American public has spent many hours enmeshed in the romantic life of Dr. Marcus Welby and watching soap operas like *General Hospital.* What has become known as the "Marcus Welby syndrome" places the average physician at a disadvantage:

First of all, he is not as photogenic, does not have a staff of writers to plug in the appropriate lines, is not able to travel from hospital to house call in ten seconds and cannot garnish himself with an adoring flock of attractive nurses, studious technicians, and admiring house staff. Secondly, he cannot effect every cure within the thirty-minute program time slot. On television . . . the hospital illness situation is romanticized . . . and real life incidents, for the most part, are hidden from the camera's eye. The female physician does not stand a chance with the afternoon soap opera crowd.

Roth, Neal, "The Medical Malpractice Insurance Crisis,"
Insurance Counsel Journal 41:469–73 (1977)

Influencing the American public are commercials for drugs that bombard the television, videos glamorizing the drug scene, and newspaper articles about physicians accused of rape, fraud, and other criminal acts. The media focuses on the dramatic and traumatic moments of life, both of which are routine in the daily experience of health care professionals.

PRACTICING PREVENTIVE MEDICINE IN THE MEDICAL OFFICE

As can be seen, anger is the thread running through the entire medical malpractice saga. The patient is angry, the doctor is angry, relatives of both are angry, and the American public is angry about the spiraling medical costs, illness, and the inevitability of old age and dependence.

Within the past twenty years much has been done to prevent injuries, but attention is just beginning to be drawn to the skills necessary to prevent patients from becoming angry and hostile in their relationships with health care professionals. Legally, the first element of the malpractice case that must be proven is that the doctor-patient relationship exists. The case, at this point, turns on the physician's assertion that the relationship exists or does not exist. Psychologically and **sociologically,** the first element of the malpractice case again involves the physician-patient relationship. Here, the question is not whether a relationship exists but what kind of relationship exists. Again the onus is on the physician.

As can be seen from the preceding analysis of the medical malpractice problem, no amount of defensive medicine will aid in reducing the irritants that interfere with a friendly relationship between physician and patient. As can also be readily acknowledged, without a harmonious interpersonal relationship, the patient's inclination to sue skyrockets, and the resulting malpractice situation becomes increasingly destructive to doctor and patient alike. In an effort to dissipate the patient's anger and prevent hostility from ruling, physicians practice assertive preventive medicine.

According to a 1980 Aetna Insurance Company study, seventy-five percent of oncology malpractice cases originate in the physician's office. Fortunately, physicians are becoming aware of the need for a friendly office environment. This is reflected in the "Help Wanted" section of local newspapers in advertisements for medical assistants and secretaries, where adjectives such as "warm," "mature," and "friendly" are used among other qualifications for the position. This is a beginning, but it is not enough.

A professional office staff can complement the physician in all areas. The physician's staff stands in the physician's corner. Most are working in the health care field for ethical reasons, as are most physicians, and from this common ground they can work together on a common problem. Just as patients prefer to stay with one doctor, stability in the office staff adds to the sense of security and continuity. A medical assistant or office nurse who knows the patients can alleviate some of the anxiety associated with a visit to the doctor and fill gaps caused by the doctor's schedule. Training in the art of making immediate contact with patients and basic skills in good human relations will help the assistant meet the patient's needs, avoid confrontations, and contribute to a cheerful office environment.

Burnout is both a result and cause of many problems between people working with the public and the public they are serving. A burnt-out health worker only adds fuel to the fire if a patient is incubating a malpractice action. Burnout can be addressed in an office by staff meetings and training sessions to help the employees support each other. They can work together rather than drain personal resources coping with interoffice interpersonal insensitivity. Without dwelling further on the intricacies of informed consent, a well-trained office staff can minimize the difficulties in educating patients.

Physicians don't always deliberately leave patients in the dark; sometimes they think they've told the patient more than they actually have. Howard Waitzkin, a professor of medicine and social science at the University of California at Irvine, and John Stoeckle, an internist at Massachusetts General Hospital, recorded the interactions of more than 300 patients and their physicians both in their offices and in hospitals. They found that during a visit averaging about twenty minutes, little more than one minute was actually spent giving information. But when asked to estimate the time they spent giving information, the physicians said nearly one-quarter to one-half the visit. Later, when asked to estimate their patients' desire for information, 65 percent of them underestimated how much information the patients wanted.

Krupat, Edward, "A Delicate Imbalance,"
Psychology Today, p. 24 (November 1986)

A well-educated office staff can either assist the physician in informing a patient or refer the patient to an educational center for instruction. They can tactfully question the patient after the physician's explanation to assess the patient's comprehension and state of acceptance. Many times a patient feels more comfortable asking a nurse or other assistant questions because he or she is not intimidated. Hospitals are educating personnel to prevent malpractice claims. Medical societies are educating physicians in the "art" of practicing medicine. It appears logical to extend this educational process to those office personnel who are at every patient's entrance into the maze of modern medical care. "An ounce of prevention is worth a pound of cure."

Melvin Belli, an internationally known attorney who has practiced extensively in medical malpractice, wrote a chapter in his book for physicians, *For Your Malpractice Defense,* on the medical office staff and titled it "Is your staff leading you into legal hot water?" Following is the beginning of that chapter:

A woman once came to me with a complaint that she'd been incorrectly treated by a "dumb doctor."

"How do you know he's dumb?" I asked her.

"Because everybody who works for him is dumb."

It's common for patients to relate a doctor to his or her staff. Therefore, quite often, patient dissatisfaction with an office assistant will put the doctor on a malpractice spot.

Belli, Melvin M.,
For Your Malpractice Defense, p. 47 (1986)

DEFENSES TO A MEDICAL MALPRACTICE CAUSE OF ACTION

The five defenses available to a defendant in a medical malpractice cause of action are tolling of the **statute of limitations, contributory negligence, comparative negligence, assumption of risk,** and **emergency.**

Statute of Limitations

If a physician is sued, an attorney will first determine whether the statute of limitations has run out by determining how much time has passed since the injury or at what point the patient should have known there was injury. The statute of limitations determines a particular number of years within which one person can sue another. In medical malpractice actions, the statute of limitations is specified in each state's medical malpractice law. Statutes of limitations are necessary because as the years go by, evidence vanishes, witnesses' memories dim, and witnesses die. By setting a time frame within which a lawsuit may be initiated, there is assurance that relevant evidence is available for a judge or jury to decide a case.

The statutes of limitations of medical malpractice law usually give the patient two years to sue for damages. This does not necessarily mean that the medical practitioner is free from concern about malpractice two years after an incident occurs. In most states, the statute begins to run when the injured patient becomes aware of the injury. In the case of minors, the statute may not begin to run until the minor reaches the age of majority; therefore, if a child is injured at the age of one year and eighteen years is the age of majority, it may be nineteen or twenty years before the statute of limitations has run out.

In some states, the statute of limitations for negligence is longer than that for malpractice. This may be an issue for medical assistants, depending on whether the medical assistant is viewed as a layperson or as a professional. If the medical assistant is held to be a layperson, the negligence statute of limitations determines the length of time between the injury and the filing of a cause of action. If the medical assistant is held to be a professional, the malpractice time frame will rule. Following is a case that demonstrates how the statute of limitations defense works:

CASE STUDY   A patient has pain in her leg which began immediately following surgery on her kidney. For several years following surgery she knew that she had phlebitis. She went to another surgeon, who informed her that a vein in her leg had been severed at the time of her first operation. She filed a malpractice action against the first surgeon. The court determined that the pain in her leg and other symptoms put her on notice that something was wrong, and that she should have filed an action immediately. Her failure to do so within the statutory period eliminated her right to sue.

Crawford v. McDonald,
187 S.E.2d 542 (Ga. 1972)

Contributory Negligence

Contributory negligence is a term used to describe any unreasonable behavior on the part of the patient that contributed to the cause of injury. In other words, if a patient does anything that contributes to his or her suffering and constitutes behavior that is non–self-preserving, the patient is contributorily negligent. For example:

CASE STUDY   Two men, following arrest, were taken to the emergency room following their declaration that they were heroin addicts. The doctor on duty observed one of the men writhing, twitching, and moaning, and behaving in a manner that gave the appearance of a person suffering withdrawal symptoms. The physician administered methadone to both men. An hour later one patient stated that he was still having difficulty and the physician gave him an additional dose. The police returned both men to jail. The next morning one of the men was found dead in his cell of an overdose of methadone.

Investigation revealed that one of the men was a drug addict but that the one who died was intoxicated from the combination of Librium, beer, and methadone. The dead man's family brought an action against the emergency room physician. The court held that a patient has a duty to be truthful to a physician, and that failure to do so, in this case, was the sole cause of the death. The dead man had stated he was an addict when he was not an addict. The patient's negligence, or more accurately, his intentional misconduct, barred a malpractice action.

Rochester v. Katalan,
320 A.2d 704 (Del. 1974)

The above case gives an example of a patient contributing to his own suffering by giving a physician false information. What follows is an example of a patient unwilling to follow the doctor's directions and, as a result, contributing to the injury:

CASE STUDY   The physician advised his patient that an X-ray was necessary to determine whether or not his tibia had been fractured. Because of the cost of the procedure, the patient refused. The patient then sued the physician, stating that he had been negligent in not ordering an X-ray. The court held that "the patient . . . cannot attribute to the physician the damages which resulted from his own failure to have something done when this was caused by his own conduct."

Carey v. Mercer,
132 N.E. 353 (Mass. 1921)

Comparative Negligence

In states that allow the defense of contributory negligence, the plaintiff is unable to recover any damages for injury if he or she has contributed in any manner to the injury. Under comparative negligence, the plaintiff is allowed to recover damages proportionate to the defendant's fault, at least in a situation where the plaintiff's negligence is less than that of the defendant.

Assumption of Risk

Assumption of risk is defined as voluntarily accepting a known danger. The consent to assume risk may be expressed or implied. This is a defense similar to the doctrine of informed consent in that the only way a patient may assume the risk of a procedure is if the patient is informed of it by the physician. Assumption of risk is a complete defense. The following is an example of assumption of risk in an employment situation:

CASE STUDY   A private-duty nurse was engaged by the wife of a patient. After the patient had gone to the bathroom alone he was heard calling, weakly, for assistance. The private-duty nurse responded and was assisting him back to bed when her leg twisted; the patient fell on her and she suffered a fracture of the leg. The nurse sued the hospital for damages, claiming it had been negligent. The court found for the hospital, holding that the private-duty nurse assumed the risk.

Pearch v. Canady,
52 Tenn. 343, 373 S.W.2d 617 (1963)

Emergency

Both common law and the good samaritan acts protect health care professionals when they respond to an emergency situation. Under common law, the elements of a medical malpractice action are applied to the emergency situation. For example, if a medical assistant witnesses an automobile accident and no one else is available, is the medical assistant liable for what happens to the victim?

1. Relationship: No contractual relationship exists between the medical assistant and the victim as long as the medical assistant does not stop to give help. As soon as help is offered—merely stopping a car may prevent someone else from coming to the aid of the victim—a relationship is established with the victim.
2. Duty: As long as the medical assistant passes the accident, he or she has no legal duty to assist the victim. Once a medical assistant stops, the victim cannot be abandoned unless care is being provided by someone with comparable or better training, or until the police arrive on the scene and assume responsibility for the victim. This reasonable person duty applies whether the good samaritan is a health care professional or a layperson.
3. Standard of care: In an emergency situation, in order to encourage trained people to stop and assist, states have enacted good samaritan statutes to protect the rescuer from liability. The level of training of the good samaritan and the standard of care is important to the person being rescued, but the rescuer will only be held liable for reckless behavior.
4. Breach of duty: If a person passes an accident, no breach of duty exists because no relationship with the victim from which a duty arises has been established. If a helper stops and assists, he or she will be held to a standard of care appropriate to the individual's training and experience. If the procedures are performed below standard, the usual question of the court is whether the actions increased the injury of the victim.

5. Injury: The victim is already injured. The good samaritan has a responsibility to help the victim, but in order for the helper to be held liable for the injury, the helper's acts must cause a considerable amount of additional harm.

6. The breach was the cause of the injury: Under negligence law, the victim must prove that there is a greater than fifty percent chance that the help offered incorrectly caused injury. Since the victim is already injured, the helper's behavior would have to be **grossly negligent** to increase the victim's injuries.

As can be seen from the preceding analyses, there is only a slim chance of being charged with malpractice under common law for aiding an accident victim. The reason courts are reluctant to find those who help accident victims guilty is that the public has an interest in encouraging people to stop and aid someone who is injured. Pursuing this reasoning one step further, the states have enacted good samaritan laws to encourage trained professionals to provide services at accident scenes.

Good samaritan statutes provide immunity to volunteers at the scene of an accident as long as they do not intentionally or recklessly cause the patient further injury. It is important to remember that the basis of negligence law is that everyone is responsible for the consequences of his or her own acts. The immunity of the good samaritan statutes offers protection for all but those who are grossly negligent.

Office emergencies usually do not fall under the protection of good samaritan laws. For example, someone walks into a medical office off the street, obviously ill, and requests medical help. Add to this scene the facts that the potential patient is dirty and has no money, and the doctor has asked the medical assistant to get rid of the bum. It will probably not go well for the physician in court if the patient sues for not receiving emergency medical care. It is the public's expectation that emergency care will be provided; therefore, the patient should be treated prior to arranging for transportation to the closest emergency room.

MALPRACTICE INSURANCE

Malpractice **insurance** is a subject that has been making headlines because of rising rates. In a society where many are willing to litigate situations that they feel violate their rights and where there is the opportunity to do so, it is understandable that the premiums for coverage increase. The subject is complex. Litigation is very expensive, and the damages that are awarded to successful plaintiffs are rising.

Malpractice insurance is required for a professional practicing medicine. Hospitals, health care facilities, doctors, nurses, and other health care employees carry malpractice insurance. Because a medical assistant works under the direct supervision of the physician and is not licensed to practice, the physician's insurance usually covers the assistant. The reasoning behind this is that a medical assistant extends the effectiveness of the physician.

Problems arise when an assistant is named a codefendant in a lawsuit and the physician's insurance will not represent the assistant, or the positions of the assistant and the physician conflict. The cost of hiring an attorney is high, especially in a lengthy defense. Malpractice insurance for medical assistants is available and especially important for a medical assistant where the physician employer or health care facility employer does not carry insurance for the assistant.

PRODUCTS LIABILITY

A medical malpractice case involves negligence on the part of a professional and, because it is negligence, does not include intent as an element of the case. A products liability case is negligence against a manufacturer, a distributor, or some other supplier of goods. Products liability becomes of concern in the medical office when equipment malfunctions, proper instructions are not given for medication, or supplies utilized in a procedure are defective. The basic theories of recovery are negligence and breach of warranty. In some states, an action filed under strict liability is allowed. Examples of product liability include the following:

A pediatric nurse checks on a patient, then leaves the room. She returns later to discover that the child has been crushed to death by the automatic lowering device on his electric bed. Several children at other hospitals have been killed by activating such bed-lowering buttons.

A nurse in the post-anesthesia care unit breaks a left-atrial catheter while trying to remove it from a patient's chest after open heart surgery. A piece of it remains permanently embedded.

An ICU patient dies when nurses fail to hear a ventilator disconnect alarm through the plate glass doors. Respiratory therapists rig a remote alarm system. Four more patients die before it's debugged.

A nurse's aid manages to keep a patient from falling when the caster drops off a shower chair, but sustains disabling injury herself.

Tammelleo, A. David, "Who's to Blame for
Faulty Equipment?" *RN,* p. 67 (October 1990)

Products liability cases have surfaced in court when patients have been injured by tampons, pacemakers, wrinkle cream, implant prosthetics, and so on. Even peanut butter manufacturers have been sued because of the "dangerousness" of the product to a young child. Within the past few years, common products have become the object of these suits: blood transfusions, Tylenol, silicone breast implants, and tobacco. Those who have standing to sue include persons injured by the product, their relatives in certain circumstances, employees, and, in the national class-action lawsuit against leading tobacco companies for causing smoking-related problems, flight attendants in the so-called "second-hand-smoke case."

Products liability actions that will be faced by workers in medical offices most often include those classified as "failure to warn" suits. Medical office personnel are often responsible for educating patients about the medications that the physician has prescribed. In information researched by *The Wall Street Journal,* it was stated that:

A new study found that 11% of the statements that drug industry sales representatives made in pitches to doctors falsely described the benefits of their products. The report, based on 13 lunchtime sales presentations sponsored by drug companies at the University of San Diego School of Medicine, said the inaccurate statements contradicted information in federally approved labeling for the drugs in the companies' own brochures.

In one case, a sales representative said an anti-inflammatory drug had a low incidence of "gastro-intestinal upset," when the product's own package insert said that minor problems "are common" and that fatal bleeding is possible. [Another] was an assertion that monitoring a patient for potentially dangerous blood-count changes should be at a doctor's discretion, when the insert actually advised taking daily blood counts and included a boxed warning to draw attention to the side effect.

The findings offer a new glimpse of the pharmaceutical industry's controversial and enormously effective marketing practices, particularly the thousands of sales people known as drug detailers who visit doctors' offices, hospitals and medical meetings to tout the industry's products.

Winslow, Ron, "Drug-Industry Sales Pitches to Doctors Are Inaccurate 11% of the Time, Study Says." *The Wall Street Journal,* p. B6 (April 26, 1995).

The plaintiff in a products liability suit may include a passenger in an automobile accident if a physician fails to warn the driver about mixing the drugs Prolixin and Thorazine with drinking and driving.

The driver, a hospital patient, was given the drugs by two psychiatrists, the day he was discharged from the hospital. He then had an alcoholic drink and drove his car into a tree, permanently injuring his passenger.

The court held that the drug manufacturers, doctors and the hospital had a duty to warn the patient of the drugs' adverse effects. What happened was 'within the realm of reasonable foreseeability absent a pertinent warning.' The burden of preventing injuries to the general public is not undue in light of the great risks to the public, it continued, declaring that 'the fast pace at which new drugs are presently being introduced and utilized demands that the public be protected from their varying adverse effects.'

Kirk v. Michael Reese Hospital,
No. 81-2408 (Ill. App. Ct. August 28, 1985)

The duty to warn is so important in the dispersement of medications, the question arises, should the warnings be bilingual? A California court felt that this is a question that should be tried in the courts, and if the decision is to be made to grant immunity, "such a sweeping grant of immunity should come from the legislatures."

The suit was brought on behalf of a child who contracted Reyes Syndrome after he was given aspirin for a respiratory ailment. The child became blind, quadriplegic and severely mentally retarded as a result of the illness. The aspirin package contained a warning in English about the danger of Reyes Syndrome, but the child's mother, who could only speak Spanish, was unable to understand it.

Some persuasive factors in *Ramirez v. Plough, Inc.,* were that the aspirin manufacturer knew that Hispanics were an important part of its market and advertised heavily in Hispanic media.

American Bar Association Journal,
p. 83 (January 1993)

Duty to Provide Adequate Warnings and Directions for Use

A manufacturer is obligated to provide adequate directions for use of a product. The extensive written material that accompanies a prescription drug is an example of the manufacturer's duty to give directions for use and to warn of any untoward results. Directions are primarily to secure the efficient use of a product. Where a departure from the directions may create a serious problem, a separate duty to warn arises. The following is a case in point:

CASE STUDY Heat blocks are used to help revive injured persons. Instructions to wrap the blocks in insulating material before using were given, but there was no statement that if used without insulation, the blocks would cause serious burns. The plaintiff was seriously burned by the blocks. The court, in dictum as to the need for warning, observed that "instructions, not particularly stressed, do not amount to a warning of the risk at all . . ." and found against the defendant.

McLaughlin v. Mine Safety Appliances Co.,
11 N.Y.2d 62, 226 N.Y.S.2d 407, 181 N.E.2d 430 (1962)

Responsibility of Business to the Public for Equipment

There have been many cases brought by plaintiffs against hospitals and physicians when equipment used in diagnosis or treatment has caused patient injury. Whether the defendant is liable is based on whether the **malfunction** or defect in the equipment could be detected or should have been known by the operator prior to the incident. For example:

CASE STUDY   A patient was in the dentist's office. During the examination the dentist pulled an x-ray machine, held to the wall by a bolt, over the patient's face to take an x-ray of her teeth. The machine came off the wall and fell onto the patient's face causing serious injury. It was determined that the bolt that held the machine to the wall was broken. The court found for the plaintiff.

Bence v. Denbo,
183 N.E. 326 (Ind. Ct. App. 1932)

In the above incident, the attachment of the machine to the wall was entirely within the control of the dentist. The defect would be called a **patent defect** because the malfunctioning bolt could be seen by the physician on cursory examination of the unit prior to use. The following is an example of a **latent defect,** or one that the physician could not detect with reasonable investigation.

CASE STUDY   A patient was injured when an x-ray table collapsed under him. . . . [T]he cause of the accident was found to be a broken pin in the sealed gear box. The court held that while a physician would have a duty to make reasonable checks of equipment for obvious defects, there was no requirement to investigate the components of the gear box. Because the physician was not put on notice that there was a problem in the gear box prior to the accident, the patient could not recover damages against the doctor.

Johnston v. Black Co.,
91 P.2d 921 (Cal. 1939)

Strict Liability

Strict liability is used in product liability cases in which the seller is liable for any and all defective or hazardous products that unduly threaten a **consumer's** personal safety. Strict liability may arise when the product is defective and unreasonably dangerous. To prevent the product from being unreasonably dangerous, the seller may be required to give directions or warning, on the container, as to its use. For the most part, actions in strict liability are not applied to physicians and hospitals because of the requirement that there be a sale of goods. Health delivery is primarily a sale of services. However, there have been exceptions. For example:

CASE STUDY   In Texas a patient was injured when his hospital gown caught fire after the patient dropped a lighted match on it. The court held that where a hospital supplies a product unrelated to the essential professional relationship with the patient, it cannot be said that, as a matter of law, the hospital did not introduce the harmful product into the stream of commerce for purposes of a strict liability cause of action.

Thomas v. St. Joseph Hospital,
618 S.W.2d 791 (Tex. Civ. App. 1981)

Problems of strict liability arise in medicine with use of drugs. For the most part, physicians and health care facilities are not liable under strict liability, but drug manufacturing companies are. The courts have to balance the risk of taking the drug versus the risk without it, and whether the physician and/or patient was warned. If the drug has known side effects and the physician warns the patient of these, the patient *assumes the risk* of the treatment.

Legal actions against drug manufacturers is a threat that helps keep inferior products off the market. On the other hand, it may also keep needed products off the market. For example:

CASE STUDY   Thanks to a long-standing program of immunization, few American children today contract whooping cough, a serious and sometimes life-threatening illness. But now there are shortages of the whooping cough vaccine and Lederle Labs, the only manufacturer, says it may stop production because of 150 legal cases charging that the vaccine caused brain damage. Any such connection has yet to be proved, but juries have awarded large damages in two cases.

Even if rare side effects were found, the protections offered over many years have far outweighed the risks. Obviously there is something wrong with a legal system in which a type of lawsuit ostensibly designed for public protection in fact endangers a broad public. . . . Whooping cough vaccine, when available, has tripled in price in a year.

"Tort Law's Victims,"
The Wall Street Journal (April 2, 1985)

Premises Liability

Corporations, partnerships, and individual practitioners are responsible to the public for their offices, laboratories, buildings, and equipment, as shown in the following:

A Connecticut woman has sued Norwalk Hospital, claiming that she bumped her head when she fell out of the back of a moving ambulance whose doors flew open as it turned a corner.

An Indiana woman has filed suit against Morgan County Memorial Hospital and its board of trustees, claiming that she stumbled and fell on a wheelchair ramp at the front entrance to the hospital. The woman contends that the wheelchair ramp was unmarked and had a deep and sloping depression.

A New Jersey woman has filed a lawsuit against Community Memorial Hospital claiming that she was injured when the ceiling of her room, which was located in the hospital's new 115,000 sq. ft. wing, collapsed.

Biomedical Safety and Standards
(Quest Publishing Company, Brea, CA)

Property owners must observe certain standards of care for the protection of others, whether they come onto the property legally or not. Persons coming on property are classified as either **invitees, licensees,** or **trespassers.**

Trespassers

Someone who enters property illegally is a trespasser. Despite the fact that such a person is not invited and probably not wanted, the owner and the occupier have obligations for the safety of this person. There is a duty to warn of dangers and a duty to reduce and eliminate dangers existing on the property. This duty should be carried out with **reasonable care.** The care necessary to fulfill the duty required, in most cases, is merely giving warning of the activity or condition. There is a stricter responsibility to trespassing children because they are often unable to recognize danger. The law limits the extent to which property may be protected against trespassers as shown in the following:

CASE STUDY   The house was inherited from the defendants' grandparents and had been unoccupied for some time. There had been a series of intrusions and the defendants had boarded up the windows and the doors in an attempt to protect the property. They had posted "no trespass" signs on the land, the nearest one being thirty-five feet from the house. On June 11, 1967, the defendants set a "shotgun trap" in the north bedroom. After Mr. Briney cleaned and oiled his 20-gauge shotgun, defendants took it to the old house, where they secured it to an iron bed with the barrel pointed at the bedroom door. It was rigged with wire from the doorknob to the gun's trigger so it would fire when the door was opened. Briney first pointed the gun so an intruder would be hit in the stomach, but at Mrs. Briney's suggestion it was lowered to hit the legs. He admitted he did so "because I was mad and tired of being tormented" but he did not intend to injure anyone. He gave no explanation of why he used a loaded shell and set it to hit a person already in the house.

The plaintiff entered the old house by removing a board from a porch window which was without glass. . . . As he started to open the north bedroom door, the shotgun went off striking him in the right leg above the ankle bone. Much of his leg, including part of the tibia, was blown away. Only by . . . assistance was the plaintiff able to get out of the house and then to a hospital. He remained in the hospital 40 days.

The trial court held that an owner may not protect personal property in an unoccupied boarded up farmhouse against trespass by use of deadly force. This decision was affirmed by the appeals court.

Katko v. Briney,
183 N.W.2d 657 (Iowa 1971)

Licensee

A licensee differs from a trespasser in that a licensee enters property with implied permission. Examples of licensees include public servants, such as the police and firefighters, those who may cross property to take a shortcut, social guests, those who come into the office to get out of the rain, traveling salespersons, and charitable solicitors. There is a duty to warn these people about any dangerous conditions that they would not anticipate or easily see.

Invitees

Invitees are persons who enter property for business as a result of express or implied invitation. Store customers; patrons of restaurants, banks, and places of amusement; delivery persons and plumbers; and electricians and carpenters doing work at an owner's request are all invitees. The duty owed to invitees is higher than that owed to trespassers or licensees. Generally, it is to make the premises safe by exercising reasonable care to warn the invitee of known defects in the property, or of those which could be discovered with reasonable care. This includes an **affirmative duty** to protect the invitee. Reasonable care may include inspection of the premises to discover possible defects, an example of which is seen in the following:

CASE STUDY   A mother took her five-year-old son to the pediatrician's office. After the visit she left by the back door, stepped into a hole and hurt her ankle. The hole was hidden by some very high grass and neither she nor the pediatrician had noticed it on prior trips through the door. The court found that she was an invitee, even though she was not herself a patient, but held that there was no evidence that the physician had known of the hole.

Goldman v. Kossove,
117 S.E.2d 35 (N.C. 1960)

With snow and ice on the sidewalk, liability for falls is a concern for landlords. In the following case, the court ruled in favor of the physician:

CASE STUDY

A patient left the physician's office after dark following a late afternoon appointment. When she got to the parking lot she fell. While she had been in the office during her time of her appointment, a mixture of snow and rain had fallen. She slipped as a result of the slush on the ground. The court pointed out that snow is so obvious a danger that invitees are presumed to protect themselves from falling while walking in it.

Jeswald v. Hutt,
239 N.E.2d 37 (Ohio 1968)

Premises owners are increasingly being held liable for injuries intentionally inflicted by third parties unrelated to the victim or the premises owner. For example:

CASE STUDY

The father of Shannon Lowney, one of two women killed in attacks on two Brookline reproductive clinics, filed a wrongful death lawsuit this week against the landlord of the building where she worked. Lowney, 25, was a receptionist at the Planned Parenthood clinic in a building at 1031 Beacon Street. The lawsuit alleges negligence and says [the owner] should have provided more security.

The lawsuit, which seeks unspecified damages, is the second filed by families of the victims of the December 30, 1994, attacks in which John C. Salvi walked into two clinics and opened fire with a .22 caliber rifle. In March 1995, the family of Lee Ann Nichols, 38, a receptionist at Preterm Health Services, sued that building's landlord for unspecified damages.

Leung, Shirley, "Father of Shooting Victim Sues
Owner of Clinic Site," *The Boston Globe*, p. B8 (August 10, 1996)

SUMMARY

When one person hurts another without intent, the legal cause of action is negligence. Professional negligence is known as malpractice. The difference between negligence and malpractice is the standard of care required of the injuring party. If the act is negligent, the defendant is a layperson who is held to the reasonable person standard. If the act is malpractice, the inflicting party is a professional who is held to the standard of a profession with prescribed education, training, and experience. An expert witness sets the standard for the profession with testimony in court.

Medical assistants are hybrid health care professionals. Receptionist and secretarial duties are categorized under a layperson standard, and clinical tasks may be labeled professional. In either case, the responsibilities extend the effectiveness of a physician and are delegated by the employer. The American Association of Medical Assistants is the national certifying body, and membership would be recognized in the qualifications of an expert witness. The expense involved in hiring expert witnesses for trial has motivated the courts to develop the doctrine of res ipsa loquitur.

The elements of a civil medical malpractice cause of action include the following:

1. injury;
2. a relationship between the physician and the patient;
3. a duty by the physician to the patient;
4. the duty must be held to professional standard of care;
5. breach of duty by the physician and the breach is the cause of the injury to the patient; and
6. injury to the patient.

Informed consent requires that a physician communicate information to a patient concerning the treatment he or she is about to receive. The patient has a right to refuse treatment; therefore, the physician must provide enough information to allow the patient to make an informed decision. Only a physician can accept consent from a patient. The medical assistant performs the duties of preparing and filing the consent forms, as well as listening and observing to determine whether the patient understood and accepted the proposed treatment plan.

Five defenses are available to a defendant in a medical malpractice cause of action: tolling of the statute of limitations, contributory negligence, comparative negligence, assumption of risk, and emergency. Medical malpractice insurance is available for defense as well as awards against the defendant. Medical assistants may or may not be covered under a physician's insurance. Insurance is available for the protection of a medical assistant.

Corporations, partnerships, and individual practitioners are responsible to the public for their offices, laboratories, buildings, and equipment.

Different standards of responsibility are required for trespassers, licensees, and invitees. The standard of maintenance of the property for a trespasser is reasonable care. The standard of maintenance increases for licensees. The highest standard of maintenance is due invitees and requires affirmative behavior on the part of the landlord or occupier to warn the invitee about dangerous conditions or activities that are known or could be discovered with reasonable effort.

SUGGESTED ACTIVITY

Play the childhood game of rumors. Begin by giving directions for taking medication. As the rumor travels around the circle, document the changes. After fifteen minutes, attempt to remember the directions first given. This will give each player an opportunity to learn about some of the confusion a patient experiences in the informed consent process.

STUDY QUESTIONS

1. Describe a situation that might place a medical assistant in the position of being negligent.
2. Describe a situation that might cause a medical assistant to be charged with medical malpractice.
3. List the qualifications for an expert witness in a legal action involving a medical assistant who works in a pediatrician's office.
4. Define and give an example of res ipsa loquitur.
5. Distinguish between defensive medicine and an exhaustive search for a diagnosis.
6. What is meant by, "Even if a doctor wins, he or she loses in a medical malpractice lawsuit"?
7. List four conditions that have contributed to the breakdown of the doctor-patient relationship.
8. Role play. Show empathy to a patient who has just learned that he has cancer of the larynx.
9. The doctor has not been able to cure a patient. A large hospital bill is outstanding. The bill is not covered by insurance, and the patient is having difficulty paying. The patient also owes the physician money for services provided. The patient is in the office in an agitated state, unhappy about the results of treatment. How will you handle collection of the doctor's bill?
10. What relationship is necessary between a physician and patient to establish duty of care for the doctor?
11. List the elements of a medical malpractice cause of action.
12. A newly diagnosed cancer patient comes to your desk after being informed of two alternatives for treatment, one involving surgery, the

second involving chemotherapy. He asks your advice. How do you handle the situation?

13. List, define, and give examples of the five defenses available to a defendant in a medical malpractice suit.

14. An automobile accident occurs in front of your office. You hear the crash and go to the door to see what has happened. One of the passengers in the car is walking around the street in a daze with blood dripping from a facial laceration. What do you do?

15. Prepare a question for your employer to determine whether his or her malpractice insurance covers a medical assistant working in the office.

16. An individual comes onto the office property, is drunk, has been told to leave, but remains in the building. There is a floor board in the front hallway that everyone knew needed to be fixed, but nothing has been done about it. The individual falls when the board gives way and breaks his leg. What is the responsibility of the medical corporation?

17. Every day a postal employee delivers mail to the office. The mail carrier always comes inside and chats with the staff. Is this person a trespasser, licensee, or invitee?

18. The weather report has predicted snow. A patient comes to the office in the early afternoon and leaves later in the day. As she is leaving the office, she falls on the front steps and breaks her arm. The snow has covered ice that is left from the last storm the day before. Who is responsible for the injury?

19. While sitting in the waiting room of a medical office, a patient falls when the chair gives way under him. The man is a very heavy person and chose to sit on a regular chair. There was a large chair available for him. The patient ends up in the hospital for observation and later for pneumonia related to his inactivity. Who is responsible for the pneumonia?

20. The physician orders an electrocardiogram for a patient. The medical assistant performs the test. He notices that there is something wrong with the machine but continues with the tracing. The tracing is read by a cardiologist, who notices there are problems. The doctor requests a second test for a patient. Who has to pay for the second electrocardiogram?

21. The manufacturer is responsible for injury to a patient under products liability under what conditions?

22. Tylenol was removed from the market because someone was injured when the cap of the product was removed and a poison substituted for the original material. Why was the manufacturer responsible?

CASES FOR DISCUSSION

1. A negligence action was brought by a mother on behalf of her minor daughter against a hospital. It alleged that when the mother was thirteen years of age, the hospital negligently transfused her with

Rh-positive blood. The mother's Rh-negative blood was incompatible with and sensitized by the Rh-positive blood. The mother discovered her condition eight years later during a routine blood screening ordered by her physician in the course of prenatal care. The resulting sensitization of the mother's blood allegedly caused damage to the fetus, resulting in physical defects and premature birth. Did a patient relationship with the transfusing hospital exist?

2. The patient was admitted to the hospital for a "D and C." The defendant was an anesthesiologist who injected sodium pentothal into the patient. The patient developed a laryngospasm, which prevented oxygen from entering the lungs and bloodstream. Attempts were made to break and relax the spasm but were unsuccessful. The plaintiff suffered severe and disabling brain damage. Conflicting evidence was submitted with regard to whether the defendant left the operating room to attend another patient before or after an equally qualified physician arrived to provide patient care. Was the physician at liberty to withdraw from the patient?

3. A woman was in labor. The nurse on duty refused to call the obstetrician. Instead, the nurse sat and read a magazine, ignoring repeated requests from the patient and her husband to call a doctor. The husband informed the nurse when his wife was about the deliver, and the nurse told him to sit down. The woman delivered before the obstetrician arrived and she was injured. Was the hospital liable for the nurse's negligence?

4. The plaintiff first consulted the defendant for myopia in 1959. At that time, the plaintiff was fitted for contact lenses. The plaintiff consulted the defendant again in 1963, 1967, and 1968, complaining of irritation caused by the contact lenses. Until the end of 1968, the defendant considered the plaintiff's problems to be connected with the contact lenses. On the visit in 1968, the defendant tested the plaintiff for glaucoma for the first time. The patient had glaucoma, which is relatively symptomless until the damage is done to the eyes. At trial, the expert witness stated that it was usual practice not to test patients for glaucoma until they were forty years of age. The plaintiff was thirty-two. Testimony also revealed that the test should be given if the patient's symptoms so indicate prior to forty years of age. Should the defendant be guilty because he did not give the plaintiff the glaucoma test?

5. A sixteen-year-old boy was hit by an automobile while riding his bicycle. He was taken to the emergency room by a parent; the physician on call looked him over and sent him home. The boy died a few hours later. Autopsy revealed that he had a massive skull fracture. Was the physician's lack of a thorough examination the cause of the patient's death?

6. A male patient was admitted to the hospital with pneumonitis. He was ill with a high fever and in his confusion walked out on the balcony outside his room and told construction workers below that he was

going to jump. They notified the nurse on the patient's floor, who called his physician. The physician told her to watch and restrain the patient. The nurse called the patient's wife and told her what was happening. The wife explained that she had to get a babysitter before she could get to the hospital but that the patient's mother could be there in five minutes. The wife asked the nurse to stay with the patient until a family member could get there, but the nurse stated that they were too busy. The man jumped or fell from the balcony. Was the nurse guilty of malpractice?

7. The plaintiff was a twenty-one-year-old student who severely injured his right index finger while working in a bakery. He is left-handed. The defendant, a board-certified orthopedist who specializes in hand surgery, testified that the value of the hand had been reduced by some forty percent. At the plaintiff's request, the defendant took over the case. There were two operations. The first went well, but after the second, circulation could not be restored to the finger and it had to be amputated at the base. With the amputated finger, the plaintiff had eighty percent use of the hand, which was more than prior to surgery. The plaintiff sued, alleging that the defendant did not inform him of the risks of the operations and that he might lose his finger. Should the court find the defendant guilty of malpractice?

8. The plaintiff, Bonner, was a fifteen-year-old Washington resident who had a severely burned cousin. The cousin was brought to the defendant, a plastic surgeon, for treatment. The doctor advised a skin graft. After many unsuccessful attempts to find a donor, Bonner's aunt asked him to go to the hospital for a test to see if his blood would match with that of his cousin. He went to the hospital, had the test, and his blood matched. The defendant performed the first operation on Bonner's side. Bonner's mother, with whom he lived, was ill and knew nothing of the operation. Bonner later returned to the hospital for a second operation. He told his mother that he was going to have his side "fixed up." Instead, Bonner remained in the hospital, where an unsuccessful graft was attempted. In the course of the operation, Bonner lost a lot of blood and skin and had to remain hospitalized for two months. There was sufficient evidence for the jury to believe that Bonner's mother never knew the exact nature of the operations or consented to them. Once his mother did learn of the operations, she made no attempt to prevent them but instead allowed Bonner to return to complete them. Bonner was a minor. Must the parents of a minor give consent before an operation for the benefit of another may be performed?

9. Kennedy, the plaintiff, consulted the defendant, a surgeon. The surgeon diagnosed appendicitis and recommended an operation to which the plaintiff agreed. During the operation the defendant discovered some enlarged cysts on the plaintiff's left ovary, which he punctured. After the operation, the plaintiff developed phlebitis in her leg, which caused her considerable pain and suffering. The plaintiff alleged that the puncturing

of the cysts on her ovary was unauthorized, and she brought an action for damages. Can a surgeon extend an operation without consent?

10. The plaintiff, Anderson, was undergoing a back operation. During surgery, the tip of a forceps-like instrument broke off in Anderson's spinal canal. The surgeon was unable to retrieve the metal, and the patient suffered significant and permanent physical injury caused by the fragment, which lodged in his spine. The plaintiff-patient sued the defendant-surgeon for medical malpractice, the hospital for furnishing a defective instrument, the medical supply distributor for furnishing the defective instrument to the hospital on a warranty theory, and the manufacturer on a strict liability theory for making a defective product. The trial court held that there was no cause to the surgeon and the other defendants. Did the appeals court support the trial court's decision?

11. The plaintiff's minor daughter was given a dose of Sabin oral polio vaccine at a county health clinic. It was produced by Wyeth Laboratories. The wife of the plaintiff was present when the vaccine was administered but testified that she had received no warning about the vaccine and she either did not read or understand a release form she had signed. Two weeks after the vaccine was administered, the plaintiff's daughter developed polio. The plaintiff brought the suit against Wyeth Laboratories for products liability, alleging that his daughter had developed polio from the live virus in the vaccine and that the drug manufacturer's failure to warn him or his wife of the risk associated with receiving the live virus caused Wyeth to be liable for his daughter's injuries. Was Wyeth liable for the child's injuries?

Chapter 6

Health Care Is Big Business

The total U.S. health-care expenditures in 1990, according to the Health Care Finance Administration (HCFA), was $666.2 billion dollars, 12.2 percent of the gross national product. A study published in the New England Journal *of Medicine put the administrative cost of U.S. medicine at 22 percent of total health expenditures. . . .*

American Hospital Association, 1992

OBJECTIVES:

After reading this chapter, you should be able to:

1. recognize the importance of the business aspect of the health care industry.
2. identify three alternative health care delivery systems.
3. recognize the complexity of the government influence on the practice of medicine.
4. recognize the influence of managed care organizations on medical malpractice litigation.
5. describe the importance of understanding basic discrimination law when hiring, promoting, and terminating employees.
6. identify five social security entitlements.
7. recognize the importance of OSHA regulations.
8. describe the relationship between union and management.
9. define job descriptions, procedures, manuals, and handbooks.
10. define ERISA.
11. understand basic collection law.
12. recognize situations affected by the American Disabilities Act.
13. identify provisions of the Family Medical Leave Act.

BUILDING YOUR LEGAL VOCABULARY

assets	dividends	partnership
bargaining unit	facially neutral	per capita payment
bylaws	fee-for-service	probable cause
capital	good faith	profits
capitation	impact	prospective
collective bargaining	inference	quality assurance
comparable	interstate	retirement benefits
comprehensive	investment	risk management
conglomerate	joint ventures	shares
corporation	levy	sole proprietorship
creditors	management	stockholders
debts	mitigating	subscribers
diagnostic related groups (DRGs)	negligent per se	tendered
	negotiated fee schedules	tracked
directors	notice	utilization review
discrimination	officers	venue
disparate		

During the past decade, there has been dramatic change in the delivery of health care. The causes for the change are many and are rooted in technological advances with resulting escalating costs. Technology has provided medicine with diagnostic capabilities and procedures to assist in the treatment of many illnesses. These advances, coupled with the competition in business and the medical needs of an aging population, have set the climate for today's health care delivery system. On one side, there is the demand for medical care, while on the other, there is the need to curb costs. The delivery of health care has changed in an effort to achieve a reasonable balance between needs and costs.

The health care industry in its attempts to operate as a business, does not exist in a vacuum. While doctors, nurses, hospital employees, and others attempt to achieve personal financial gains, the insurance industry, employers paying for the insurance, the government, and the consumer all try to get their "money's worth."

Two basic ways of controlling health care costs are competition and regulation. Competition is "the American way" and represents an attempt by both provider and insurer to control costs by individually increasing their share of the consumer market. This competitive approach has given rise to the "alphabet soup" of the eighties (HMO, PPO, and so on). The regulation approach attempts to control costs by using resources efficiently and effectively and is imposed upon the provider by the payer. During the eighties, the payers were primarily the insurance companies, both private and government, and they attempted to control costs by controlling the amount they would pay; hence, the appearance of **DRGs (diagnostic related groups),**

prospective payment, and so on. The large number of patients (consumers) on Medicare and Medicaid encouraged the federal government to take the lead in regulating health care expenses.

As regulatory factors become increasingly influential in the type and amount of care a patient receives, physicians are being put under increasing economic and professional pressure. Their role is changing. Traditionally doctors have been placed on a pedestal, but currently because of the elevation of other health care professionals and the entrance of a more sophisticated consumer taking a more active part in personal health care decisions, physicians are experiencing the pain of transition.

BUSINESS STRUCTURES OF MEDICAL PRACTICE

A business is a commercial or industrial establishment. Legally, it is either a **sole proprietorship, partnership,** or **corporation.** In the medical profession, the business structure may be a simple solo practitioner operating from an office, or it may be a large group of corporations, known as a **conglomerate,** controlling hospitals or other health care facilities. As business entities, each is subject to specific laws.

Sole Proprietorship

A sole proprietor is a single physician, therapist, or other licensed health care professional operating a business alone. This is known as private practice. The individual who chooses this business structure does so for two main reasons. First, individual ownership is the simplest and most basic business structure and appeals to a person who is independent and likes to "run the whole show." Second, any financial rewards from the practice are for the owner and do not have to be shared with anyone else.

On the other hand, any losses are also the owner's. Legally, sole proprietors are responsible for the obligations or debts incurred in the course of the business. Their liability is not limited solely to the amount of **capital** invested in the business but includes personal savings, automobiles, and all other **assets.** This is known as unlimited liability and is the main reason that most individuals do not choose the sole proprietorship business structure.

Partnership

A partnership is two or more people who combine their work, money, and talents to do what one could not do alone. It is a more complicated form of business organization than individual ownership. A partnership is formed when an agreement is executed and a document—identified as a "certificate of doing business as partners"—is filed in the county clerk's office. The agreement forms a legal bond between the partners, and the certificate serves as **notice** to the public that they are doing business together. Unless the terms of the partnership provide otherwise, each partner has a right to participate in managing the business and making decisions.

A high degree of mutual trust and confidence must exist between partners. For example, if one partner's personal **debts** become so large they cannot be satisfied by his or her private assets, **creditors** may go after that partner's share of the business property, thereby threatening the partnership.

In conducting the affairs of a partnership, all partners are bound by the acts of one. This affects them as individuals. If, for example, one partner places an order for equipment beyond the financial means of the partnership, the other partners are required to share payment of the bill, possibly by using their personal funds. Partnership law is changing and may offer additional advantages in the future.

Corporations

A corporation is primarily a means by which a group of people can band together and create an artificial being, or entity, that can do something that the members of the group could not do individually. An individual may also incorporate in order to make use of corporate tax and legal advantages.

A corporation is formed by filing a certificate of incorporation in the state in which the organization has its main place of business. Another name for the certificate is a corporate charter. The charter describes the corporation's purpose, the method of finance (number and value of **shares,** for example), the name, the number of directors, and the names and addresses of the original directors and the corporation.

Much thought is often given to the corporate name. The corporation may use any name, provided it has not been taken by some other firm in the state or does not too closely resemble the name of an existing firm. Health care providers usually try to choose a name that will instantly indicate to the public the services they provide.

The life of a corporation does not end upon the death of its **officers, directors,** or **stockholders.** Even if all died in a common disaster, the corporation would continue until it was dissolved by legal process. This is true even in a one-person corporation in which all of the stock is held by one individual.

One of the most desirable features of a corporation is the protection that is given to investors; for example, if the corporation loses money and the debts become greater than the assets, the creditors may not collect from the individual owners, known as stockholders. Only the capital of the corporation is available for the payment of debts. The most an individual investor may lose is the amount of the original **investment.** This differs from individual or partnership organization, where the investor is personally responsible for the debts of the business.

Management responsibility is in the hands of the board of directors in a corporation. The number of directors is usually set in the **bylaws** of the corporation, which are drawn up and adopted at the first stockholders' meeting. Directors answer to the stockholders, who elect and terminate them. A member of the board of directors is expected to be loyal to the corporation. It is improper for a director to have an interest in any business that competes with the corporation. Officers of a corporation include the president, vice president, treasurer, secretary, and any other officers the board of directors appoints. They are employees of the company and need not be stockholders. **Profits** of a corporation are distributed as **dividends.**

Alternative Delivery Systems

The two basic forms of alternative delivery systems are the health maintenance organization (HMO) and the preferred provider organization (PPO). In the HMO, the member physician assumes financial risk for services delivered or provided. In the PPO, the member physician does not.

Health Maintenance Organization (HMO)

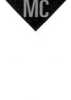

There are two types of HMOs, the prepaid group practice (PGP) and the individual practice association (IPA). Prepaid group practices (PGPs) are groups of physicians who agree to provide comprehensive health care services for a fixed prospective **per capita payment** to a definite population. The staff model and the group model are two forms of PGPs. Under the staff model, the physicians are employees of the HMO, are salaried, and may at the end of the fiscal year receive a portion of any profit. In the group model, the physicians are organized as a partnership or corporation in a group practice. The group contracts with the HMO to provide care for HMO **subscribers.** The group receives **capitation** payment and a share of the HMO's net income as a group and pays participating physicians on a **fee-for-service** or salary basis.

Individual practice associations (IPAs) are groups of physicians who join together and enter into agreement with other organizations to provide medical services to a defined population. In this structure, the physicians practice in their own office on a fee-for-service or capitation basis. Comprehensive health benefits are provided to the designated population for a fixed periodic payment.

Health Maintenance Organizations (HMOs) are regulated under the HMO Act of 1973 (42 United States Code section 300c-300e-17 (1976 and Supp III 1979)). Under this act, member physicians must agree to give at least one-third of their time to HMO subscribers. Employers with more than twenty-five employees must offer an HMO as an alternative choice to conventional medical care coverage if such a choice is available in the area.

Preferred Provider Organization (PPO)

Preferred provider organizations (PPOs) are associations of physicians and hospitals (providers) that contract with employers, insurance companies, or third-party administrators to provide **comprehensive** medical services on a fee-for-service basis to subscribers. A PPO may be sponsored by a hospital, physician, employer, and insurer, or it may be a **joint venture** between a hospital and a medical staff. The mechanisms used to control health care costs include **negotiated fee schedules** and **utilization reviews.**

Prominent economic theorists predicted that none of these "alphabet soup" organizations would be around after the mid-1990s. Because of the high cost of health care, the estimated 37 million Americans who are uninsured, and the perceived American value that a single human life is important, it was expected that Congress would enact some form of national health care. This, however, has not happened. Regulations offering health care are increasing at the state and federal level, with the most significant being Congress passing legislation to prevent insurance companies from denying insurance to applicants with a "preexisting condition" and mandating the continuity of health insurance when transferring from one job to another.

MANAGED CARE

Managed care is a term used to describe a system of integration of the financing and delivery of health care to provide comprehensive services to an identified segment of the population. In the past, the typical managed care organization (MCO) was a nonprofit, prepaid HMO made up of consumers from unions, business groups, or other organizations who contracted with the MCO for health care. An example of this type of MCO is Kaiser Permanente. Lately MCOs have included preferred provider organizations (PPOs) and independent practice associations (IPAs) who contract with insurers to provide services at a volume discount and assume varying degrees of financial risk.

With the perceived need to control the cost of health care, primary care physicians are utilized as gatekeepers by MCOs in an effort to control the cost effectiveness of services offered to the membership. Gatekeepers control access to health care by denying approval for certain procedures and allowing payment for others. They make decisions that reduce the number of hospital admissions, shorten the time until discharge, control the number of expensive diagnostic procedures, and, in the mental health field, to substitute medication for therapeutic counseling treatment. When gatekeepers are given an incentive to deny referrals to specialists, limit diagnostic treatments, and shorten hospital stays, the integrity of the physician-patient relationship is called into question. When insurance companies make the decision to allow or deny diagnostic testing and hospital admissions, the doctor-patient relationship is further eroded, and the well-being of the patient becomes an issue.

In managed care, the actual care a patient receives is influenced by the policies and procedures of the managed care plan. It therefore follows that the MCO should become vicariously liable for the acts of its physicians and other employees.

Although case law on MCO "corporate liability" is scanty, corporate liability claims could be made against MCO's on several potential grounds:
- negligent credentialing of contracted providers,
- negligent or excessive utilization review,

- failure to implement specified quality assurance programs or redress identified deficits,
- use of aggressive cost-control incentive designed to reduce utilization, or
- denial of benefits or "bad faith" by the plan.

> Gillespie, Karen, "Perspectives: Malpractice Law
> Evolves under Managed Care" (The Robert Wood
> Johnson Foundation, Princeton, NJ, January 1997)

Managed care brings another dimension into the economics of health care:

> The future may consist of just a few mega-managed-care plans serving millions of people in multi-state territories. HMO's are trying to get bigger to become more cost efficient: Well Point Health Network with 700,000 members is trying to buy Health Systems International, with 1.6 million members, in what would be a $1.78 billion transaction. Consumers could benefit because big health plans are likely to offer members a wider choice of doctors and hospitals. But rapid consolidation may leave only a few jumbo health plans dominating each local market, free to raise premiums and less likely to compete in price and quality.
>
> Winslow, George and Ron, "The HMO Trend: Big,
> Bigger, Biggest" *The Wall Street Journal*, pp. B1, B4 (March 30, 1995)

Managed care will affect the development of medical malpractice law in the future. Currently, most cases will be tried in state courts with MCOs operating in more than one state. These may be decided in the future without the benefit of precedent-setting case law. "With the rapid restructuring of the health care delivery system, medical malpractice litigation and other consumer protection mechanisms are in a state of flux." (Winslow, *Id.*)

TELEMEDICINE

Telemedicine is a way of practicing medicine when the patient is in one location and the treating physician is in another, possibly thousands of miles away. It is not new. Telemedicine techniques were used at the Logan International Airport in Boston in the 1950s after the victims of an airplane accident there could not be transported to the city's hospital and medical professionals because of traffic tie-ups in the Callahan Tunnel that connects the airport and the city.

In medicine's present cost-cutting environment, telemedicine has become prominent. It offers a way to provide quality care to patients in rural areas or in need of specialized diagnostic evaluation. A physician in one state "telepractices" treatment to a patient in another state. As with any new process, legal questions arise. For example, in which state is medicine being practiced—where the patient is ill or where the physician is located? Does the physician need a license to practice medicine in each state where he or she consults with a patient? Some issues affect the physician engaged in practicing. Others affect the medical profession as a whole:

> Much of the resistance to the proliferation of telemedicine is generated by local physicians who fear that the technology may be used to establish networks to shut them out. The fear is not necessarily far fetched. For example, in Melbourne, Fla., the Harris Corp., a worldwide electronics firm, requires its employees to use a teleradiology network for nonemergency outpatient imaging. Medical Technology Transfer Corp. established a teleradiology facility in Florida that is hooked up to UCLA. Images are first read in the Florida facility, and then are sent to UCLA for an over-read. Harris entered this agreement because it concluded that it would be more economical and would offer a higher quality of care as compared with using local radiologists.
>
> Cepelewicz, Barry B., "Telemedicine: A Virtual Reality, but Many Issues Need Resolving," *Medical Malpractice Law and Strategy,* p. 4 (July 1996)

In addition to legal and economic issues, telemedicine tests current concepts of confidentiality and standard of care. These are arguments on each side of these issues. Telemedicine will likely become more visible in the future, as is evidenced by the Telecommunications Act of 1996. It fits into the goals of managed care as a cost-effective approach to the "prevention and early detection" of health problems.

GOVERNMENT REGULATION OF THE MEDICAL PRACTITIONER

Medical Practice Acts

The business of practicing medicine is controlled professionally by medical practice acts passed by state legislatures to establish a state medical board with the authority to control licensing. In all states, individuals who are not MDs are prevented from practicing medicine, yet not every state defines medical practice. When there is no definition of medical practice and a disagreement erupts, the matter is taken to the courts on a case-by-case basis. Medical practice acts may include nursing practice acts, or the two may exist independently. The position of other health professionals and licensure depends upon individual state policy.

Licensure statutes were originally required to exclude incompetents from the practice of medicine. In *Hawker v. New York,* 170 U.S. 189 (1898), the United States Supreme Court extended physician licensure decisions to include standards of behavior and ethics holding that in a doctor, "character is as important a qualification as knowledge."

Licensing boards not only grant licenses but also renew and revoke licenses. They may fine, reprimand, and censure. In so doing, the board must follow due process. Due process requires that a practitioner be put on notice that there is a pending suspension or revocation, be given an opportunity for a prompt hearing, and be given the rights to confront the accuser, prepare an effective defense, retain counsel, and cross-examine any witnesses.

One of the grounds for the revocation or suspension of a medical license is permitting unlicensed personnel to perform medical procedures normally restricted to physicians. Physicians should consider the consequence of loss of license when assigning procedures to allied health personnel in medical offices.

State Board of Registration

Licensing statutes regulate the State Board of Registration. Complaints about physicians are brought to the board's attention by anonymous communications, newspaper articles, patients, hospitals, other physicians, insurance companies, and employees. The board has the power to perform investigations and adjudications but may not prosecute a case. The board may have access to records concerning the health care provider's practice—prescriptions, hospital records, reimbursement claims—as long as the patient's identity is withheld.

Some states require physicians to carry medical malpractice insurance. In Idaho, this requirement has been held as reasonable by the courts because liability insurance ensures that the patient will be cared for if the physician makes a mistake.

Mandatory Reports

Physicians are required to submit reports on a regular basis to various governmental agencies. To whom and when the reports are submitted are factors that vary from state to state. Certain reports are required by all practicing physicians, and these include births, deaths, and communicable diseases. Generally, physicians are required to report injuries and suspicious or "unnatural" deaths to the coroner or medical examiner. In many states, misdemeanor charges may be filed for failure to report the following:

---

1. all manner of violent deaths, including thermal, chemical, electrical, or radiational injuries;
2. death due to criminal abortion, whether apparently self-induced or not;
3. deaths occurring when a physician was not in attendance;
4. deaths of persons after unexplained comas;
5. medically unexpected deaths during the course of a therapeutic procedure;
6. deaths of prisoners at penal institutions;
7. deaths of those whose bodies are to be cremated, buried at sea, transported out of state, or otherwise made unavailable for pathological study.

American College of Legal Medicine, *Legal Medicine: Legal Dynamics of Medical Encounter*, p. 27 (1988)

Controlled Substances Acts

Controlled substances acts restrict the distribution, classification, sale, and use of certain drugs, often defined as "drugs of abuse." The controlled substances acts cover everyone from criminals, who are not involved in health care delivery, to physicians, who have the license to write prescriptions. Not every drug that is controlled is considered to have the potential to be abused. Because different states have varying prescription and over-the-counter drug regulations, the Uniform Controlled Substance Act was implemented and has been adopted by most states.

Statistically, malpractice suits involving drugs usually involve prescriptions. This is important for medical office personnel because nurses, medical assistants, and other medical office personnel (with the exception of nurse practitioners in some states) are not allowed to write prescriptions. Renewing existing prescriptions, and even advising a patient to take aspirin, is treating patients and is considered practicing medicine.

Abuse

Physicians, nurses, and other health care personnel are mandated in most states to report abuse of children, elderly, and patients. In 1973, Congress passed the Child Abuse Prevention and Treatment Act. This act requires states to meet certain uniform standards in order to be eligible for federal assistance in setting up programs to identify, prevent, and treat problems caused by child abuse and neglect. It also protects the reporter against liability and includes a penalty clause that will prosecute the professional who has knowledge of but does not report abuse.

Elder abuse is handled at the state, not the national, level, and as of 1985, nine states had no law that mandated reports of elder abuse. In seventeen states, reporting laws protected abused elders, and twenty-one states included the protection of the elderly with that of the disabled. Although there are similarities in the laws, there are also differences. For example:

In Alabama, a nurse who, on a home visit, sees signs that an elder has been abused and does not report it can be found guilty of a misdemeanor and fined up to $500, or jailed. In California, the same nurse, although still guilty of a misdemeanor, could be fined up to $1,000. In Maine, the nurse would be subject to licensing penalties. In many other states there is no provision for any penalty.

Anderson, M.T., "Reporting Elder Abuse: It's the Law,"
AJN, p. 371 (April 1985)

In 1992, in Massachusetts, there were more than 4,000 reported cases of suspected elder abuse, about a third involving physical abuse. More than a quarter involved neglect, another quarter emotional abuse, and the rest financial exploitation.

In nursing homes, studies by sociologist Karl Pillemer of Cornell University indicate that forty percent of staff admit to psychologically abusing patients, and ten percent admit to committing physical abuse.

EMPLOYMENT LAW

Laws to protect employees often have both positive and negative effects. Years ago, hospitals were thought of as "charity" employers. They would hire individuals who were otherwise unemployable—the aged, the handicapped, and homeless off the street. Often there was housing within the hospital structure that completed the employment picture, offering the employee a bed to lie in, food for the stomach, and a place in society. By offering this employment package, hospitals not only acted like today's social service agencies, but they also kept the price of hospitalization down by paying employees less than prevailing wages.

This hiring pattern set the stage for present health care employment. Tradition dies slowly. The paternalistic attitude of hospital employers, particularly large-city teaching hospitals, combined with low wages provide fertile fields for the development of employee unions. Recently there has been an increase in the organization of health care workers at all levels, from the unskilled to the professional.

Hiring Process

Interviewing

Discrimination law has initiated many changes in the employment interview situation. Employers are not allowed to ask questions concerning race, religion, age, or even to inquire whether a woman is pregnant. Because of the importance of the employment interview in getting the job, there is considerable dissention among employment specialists as to the handling of these matters. For example, *The Wall Street Journal,* on February 13, 1990, ran the following on the front page:

> Title VII of the Civil Rights Act of 1964 bars companies from asking applicants about family plans. But Felice Schwartz, president of Catalyst, suggests women confront the issue in job interviews: Open discussion of child-rearing plans, she contends, moves an interview "from insistence on the rights women had achieved . . . to a partnership with an employer. . . ."
>
> She's right, some say. But many protest. . . . Marnee Walsh, employment manager at Boston Edison Co., believes volunteering information could be "career suicide. It's an outrageous question for an interview that has nothing to do with a woman's capabilities on the job." Madelyn Jennings, senior vice president of personnel at Gannett Co., ventures "employers might as well start asking men if they have a family history of heart attacks." Besides, says Betty Bessler, vice president at Mary Kay Cosmetics, Inc., "Personal plans change."

Preemployment Testing

Employers are allowed to test potential employees as part of the hiring process, but such tests must be carefully constructed, usually by experts, to ensure that they only measure the skills and abilities necessary to do the job. In *Griggs v. Duke Power Company,* a landmark case in discrimination law, the United States Supreme Court established a strict standard, called the business necessity test, for business practices that have an adverse impact on minorities. Testing was determined to be a subtle means of discrimination:

CASE STUDY   Duke Power Company, a large power-generating corporation in the Carolinas, for years limited blacks to the labor department, the lowest-paying area of the company, and refused to approve requests for transfers to other departments. When Title VII was passed the company instituted a policy which stated that employees who wanted transfers from the labor department had to present a high school diploma or pass a high school aptitude test. Black employees sued, contending that the company was trying to lock them into their jobs as laborers by imposing unnecessary transfer requirements that they would be unable to meet because of unequal educational opportunities.

The U.S. Supreme Court found that the transfer policies were unlawful because "neither the high school completion requirement nor the general intelligence test was shown to bear a demonstrable relationship to successful performance of the jobs for which it was used." Under Title VII, the Court declared, "practices, procedures, or tests, neutral on their face, and even neutral in terms of intent, cannot be maintained if they have a discriminatory impact on minorities and are unrelated to measuring job capability." Selection practices that are fair in form but discriminatory in operation can be used only if they are justified by a "business necessity."

Griggs v. Duke Power, 401 U.S. 424 (1971)

Drug Testing

Another area of preemployment testing in which the Supreme Court has made decisions relates to drug testing. Because many hospital employees have responsibilities that directly affect patient care, an argument could be made that drug testing is needed to ensure the public's safety. On the issue of safety, *National Treasure Employees Union v. Von Raab* could be analogized to the situation of health care workers. The Court determined in this decision that mandatory drug tests for applicants and employees seeking promotions to sensitive positions in the United States Customs Service were constitutional. The Supreme Court had previously ruled that drug testing of employees is a "search and seizure" within the realm of the Fourth Amendment; each case must be resolved on a case-by-case basis using a balancing test between individual rights and public safety. The *Von Raab* decision considered public policy with public safety outweighing concerns about employees' rights to privacy.

> . . . where safety is not a concern (e.g., with clerical workers, mail carriers, or teachers) the courts refuse to allow random testing and sometimes allow testing on suspicion. Where safety is a concern (e.g., with police, firefighters, transportation workers, or prison guards) the courts usually allow testing on suspicion and sometimes allow random testing.
>
> Holthaus, David, "Employer's Power to Fight Drug Use,"
> *Trustee,* p. 20 (October 1989)

The law specifically requires tests that provide "qualitative data" on the presence of drugs and alcohol. The intent of the law is to determine whether the employee is fit for duty. New performance tests are being developed and private experiments being run to measure the employee's hand-to-eye coordination, spatial perception, reasoning ability, and judgment. These are expensive software programs purchased for computer use, but they overcome the objection to "urinating in a jar." They also offer immediate feedback as to the employee's ability to function safely. (McGinley, Laurie, "Fitness Exams Help to Measure Worker Acuity," *The Wall Street Journal,* B1, B9 (April 21, 1992).)

It is of interest that the Estelle Doheny Eye Hospital in Los Angeles was court-ordered to cease drug testing of workers but was allowed to continue the testing of job applicants.

Equal Opportunity Employment

In the United States, there is a myth that everyone has an equal opportunity to be hired for a job and, once hired, to be president of the company. Realistically, everyone cannot reach the highest rung on the corporate ladder, but, according to the Civil Rights Act of 1964, the opportunity to do so cannot be denied employees on the basis of race, color, religion, sex, or natural origin.

Title VII of the act prohibits employment discrimination and applies to all employers of fifteen or more employees whose business involves **interstate** commerce, to labor unions of fifteen or more members, to employment agencies, as well as to state, local, and federal employees. The Equal Employment Opportunity Commission administers and enforces Title VII. Illegal discrimination may be shown by either **disparate** treatment or disparate **impact.**

Disparate Treatment

The most obvious form of discrimination occurs when an employer treats similarly situated employees differently because of their race, sex, religion, or national origin. Because of the difficulty in proving a disparate treatment situation, courts allow plaintiffs to prove disparate treatment indirectly. **Inferences** may be drawn from the acts of the employers. In other words, if an act looks discriminatory, it may well be discriminatory. If an employer has been shown to discriminate in the past, the inference will be stronger that the present act involves conscious discrimination.

Disparate treatment cases are proven by the plaintiff establishing a prima facie case, the elements being (1) the plaintiff must be a member of one of the groups protected by Title VII, (2) the plaintiff must be capable of doing the job, and (3) he or she must have been discriminated against.

Disparate Impact

Some employment policies are **facially neutral,** in that they appear to treat all employees equally, but have a "disparate" or "adverse" impact on a particular protected group. For example, a minimum height requirement may discriminate against women, or a minimum education requirement may discriminate against minorities.

An employer, faced with the charge of disparate impact, may counter that the policy is justified by business necessity and is related to job performance. In the following case, an employer's business necessity defense was upheld by the court:

CASE STUDY   Gregory Backus, R.N., requested placement as a full-time registered nurse in the labor and delivery section. The hospital refused the request on the basis that it did not employ male R.N.s on the obstetrics and gynecology units and gave as a reason concern for female patients' privacy and personal dignity. Backus filed a sex discrimination complaint with the Equal Employment Opportunity Commission (EEOC), alleging that the hospital's refusal to transfer him to the labor and delivery section was discriminatory based on sex.

Testimony in the hospital's defense relied on its policy of recognizing and respecting the privacy right of its patients. Hospital policy required that catheterizations be performed by individuals of the same sex as the patient. The hospital's policy of restricting nursing positions in labor and delivery came from the fact that obstetrical patients continually have genitals exposed and that there are few duties that a nurse performs which are not sensitive or intimate in nature.

The court decided against Backus and found merit in the hospital's argument that the majority of women patients would object to intimate contact with a member of the opposite sex in the labor and delivery room. The court commented that "in addition to offending patients, a male nurse would necessitate the presence of a female nurse to protect the hospital from charges of molestation. . . . The court refused to consider a male nurse analogous to a male doctor because the doctor, and not the nurse, had been chosen by the patient."

It follows that it is reasonably necessary to the normal operation of the hospital's business that delivery room nurses be female.

Backus v. Baptist Medical Center,
510 F. Supp. 1191 (1980)

Sexual Harassment

Sexual harassment is unwanted sexual attention from anyone the victim may interact with on the job where the victim's response may be restrained by fear of reprisals. This can include peers, subordinates, supervisors, customers, and clients. The range of behavior includes verbal comments, subtle pressure for sexual activity, leering, pinching, patting, and other forms of unwanted touching as well as rape and attempted rape. Some harassers identify their own behavior as flirting, but there is a distinction between flirting and sexual harassment. Flirting is often described as instinctual and natural between genders, whereas sexual harassment has elements of premeditation and persistence. Flirting offers pleasure to both parties, whereas in most cases, a male harasses a female against her wishes. The looks between the parties engaged in flirting attract and complement, while the look or stare of a harasser makes the victim feel invaded, shamed, naked. Flirting is a mutual interaction between the parties, whereas sexual harassment involves obscene suggestions and hints, often followed with pinches, pats, and grabs.

Sexual harassment has always been a problem for women at work. In the past, it was kept quiet because women who were in the workplace desperately needed their jobs and there was no support for their position as the victim. *Redbook* magazine, in a 1976 national survey of nine thousand employed women, found that nine out of ten respondents had experienced sexual harassment at work. Of those who experienced harassment, seventy percent found it embarrassing and demeaning. Sexual harassment was painfully brought to the nation's attention in the Clarence Thomas/Anita Hill confrontation. Anita Hill accused her former boss, Supreme Court nominee Clarence Thomas, of sexually harassing her. All of the elements of a sexual harassment case were brought before the public on national television in the Senate confirmation hearings. Anita Hill was a credible witness, and Clarence Thomas, the epitome of a respected conservative nominee. Someone had to be lying. The ninety-eight percent male Senate confirmed Clarence Thomas for the position of Supreme Court Justice. The majority of working women believed in their hearts that Anita Hill was telling the truth. Sexual harassment is not a problem confined to the United States alone:

A nursing home employee in Quebec alleged that she missed five weeks of work because of depression and stress caused by "sexist remarks, insistent and vicious looks, and unwanted touching" by a security guard at work.

Quebec's Worker Compensation Board originally ruled against her claims but decided after a review that there appeared to be no other cause for her depression aside from her encounters with the guard.

The Board ruled that she had a period of extreme stress provoked by the climate of work. It also ruled that Quebec's law defines an accident to include any event which occurs at work and causes injury, illness or death. It said the woman was entitled to benefits for a work-related accident.

The Wall Street Journal, p. 1 (July, 1982)

RN Magazine addressed the issue with the following:

A well-known surgeon at a Chicago hospital tells off-color jokes to nurses and anyone else within earshot. He's been doing it for years. Some nurses avoid him entirely and others pretend not to hear, but no one ever tries to stop him.

Then one night, following surgery, when he and an OR nurse are alone, joking progresses to groping and grabbing. As she struggles to break free, her uniform rips.

Screaming she runs to her supervisor's office and reports the incident. When confronted with the allegation, the surgeon admits to the transgression and the hospital slaps him with a six-month suspension.

Horsley, Jack E., "Legally Speaking: Don't Tolerate Sexual Harassment at Work," *RN*, p. 69 (January 1990)

Filing with the Equal Employment Opportunity Commission (EEOC)

Most EEOC actions begin with the filing of a complaint by an individual who believes he or she has been discriminated against. A complaint may not be successfully filed after a 180-day period following the incident. Once a complaint is filed, the EEOC will contact the employer, and within ten days, an investigation will be initiated.

If the EEOC finds **probable cause** and that Title VII may have been violated, attempts are made to conciliate the matter. If the parties are not able to reach agreement, a "right to sue" letter is issued to the complaining party who is free to pursue federal court action. Under certain conditions, the EEOC may initiate a federal lawsuit.

FAMILY AND MEDICAL LEAVE ACT (FMLA)

The Family and Medical Leave Act of 1993 (FMLA) requires employers of fifty or more people to provide up to twelve weeks of unpaid leave each year for the "serious health condition" of an employee or member of the employee's immediate family or for the birth or adoption of a child. The FMLA covers:

- all public employers;
- private employers who have fifty or more employees on the payroll during each of twenty or more calendar workweeks in either the current or preceding calendar year; and
- employees who have been employed for at least twelve months and who have worked at least 1250 hours in the twelve months preceding commencement of the FMLA leave.

Verbal notice is all that is required to make an employer aware that the employee needs family medical leave (FML). After taking the leave, the employee must be returned to his or her former position or to an equivalent one with the same pay, benefits, and working conditions. When the FMLA was enacted, there was considerable concern by business management about abuses by personnel, but a recent government survey has shown that few are making use of it.

Only 2% to 4% of workers eligible to take time off under the FMLA have done so, says a study by the Labor Department. Of 2254 workers surveyed, 59% of the leave takers said they did so to attend to their own health, not to care for elderly parents, sick spouses, or children.

"Family Leave: A Government Survey,"
The Wall Street Journal, p. 1 (March 26, 1996)

AMERICANS WITH DISABILITIES ACT (ADA)

The ADA covers physical as well as mental disabilities in employment, public services, public accommodations, and telecommunications. A disability is defined as a physical or mental impairment that substantially limits one or more of the major life activities of an individual, or a record of such an impairment, or being regarded as having such an impairment. The ADA covers conditions ranging from infection with the AIDS virus to cancer to mental retardation, but excludes homosexuality and active illegal drug use.

Title I of the act prohibits employment discrimination and places the burden on an employer to prove that the requirements of a specific job could not be changed to accommodate a disabled applicant.

Titles II and III of the act guarantee the disabled access to the workplace. Professional offices of health care providers are identified as public-sector and, as such, require an employer to make "reasonable modifications" for the disabled to gain access.

Title IV requires all telecommunications carriers to provide a relay system that will allow the hearing impaired to communicate with a hearing individual by wire or radio.

The ADA was scheduled to be phased in for businesses of twenty-five or more employees on July 26, 1992, with the telecommunications requirements to be in place within three years.

The EEOC has issued detailed guidelines defining *disability* under the ADA. The employee may have a past impairment or simply be "regarded as" having an impairment. The guidelines provide examples of conditions that are not impairments, for example, pregnancy, physical characteristics like hair or eye color, common personality traits, and normal deviations in height or weight. Perhaps the most significant example of these conditions is found in the *Cook* case:

CASE STUDY   Bonnie Cook, 5'2" tall and weighing over 200 pounds, was turned down for a job as an institutional attendant for the mentally retarded at the Ladd Center, a residential facility for retarded persons. Ms. Cook had passed the Ladd Center's physical examination and the Center acknowledged that she was capable of performing the job adequately despite her "morbid obesity." However, the center worried that Ms. Cook's morbid obesity would hinder her ability to evacuate residents in an emergency and put her at greater risk of developing future serious ailments which would result in her being absent from work and possibly filing workers' compensation claims. At trial, Ms. Cook claimed that, regardless of whether "morbid obesity" is a "handicap," the Ladd Center "regarded" her morbid obesity as a handicap. The jury agreed and awarded her $100,000.

Cook v. Rhode Island,
10 F.3d 17 (1st Cir. 1993)

Under the ADA, an employer has a duty to provide reasonable accommodation to the known mental or physical limitations of a qualified individual with a disability. In *August,* the court upheld an employer's right to fire an employee whose handicap—major depression—kept the employee out of work for months with no clear indication of when he could return.

CASE STUDY   Mr. August requested, as accommodations, permission to work parttime, to miss some morning meetings, and to report late for work. His employer refused. The court suggested that, in some cases at least, an employer might be obliged to provide such "reasonable accommodations," but that in Mr. August's case it was not clear that he would have been able to perform capably even with these accommodations.

August v. Offices Unlimited, Inc.,
981 F.2d 576 (1st Cir. 1992)

In *Griece Mills v. Derwinski,* 967 F.2d 794 (2d Cir. 1992), a hospital was not required to accommodate the request of a head nurse suffering from depression to report to work at 10:00 A.M., as such accommodation would have imposed "undue hardship" on the hospital. In defining *undue hardship,* the ADA requires consideration of the following factors:

- the nature and cost of the accommodation needed
- the overall finances of the facility
- the overall resources of the covered entity
- the type of operation or operations of the covered entity

An employer is obligated to accommodate only "known" physical or mental limitations of a disabled worker. Discriminating against someone who is HIV positive is illegal.

> The administration of a hospital learned that Doe [a pharmacist] was infected with HIV and sought to bar him from preparing IV or hyperalimentation solutions, citing the risk of transmission. Condemning the job restriction as unnecessary and detrimental to his career, Doe filed suit. In finding that Doe did not present a significant risk to others in the workplace, [the court ruled in Doe's favor].
>
> [A nurse was found to be a significant risk to others in the workplace.] The court found that IV's, catheterizations, and dressing changes . . . are invasive procedures and because AIDS is fatal, even a minute risk is unacceptable.
>
> Kelasa, Eileen V., "HIV vs. a Nurse's Right to Work," *RN,* p. 63 (January 1993)

In another AIDS case, a dentist who refused to treat two patients who were HIV positive paid $120,000 under the ADA in a settlement with the Justice Department. The dentist argued that the AIDS patients posed a "significant risk" and required specialized dental care beyond his expertise. But a United States Court found that he had engaged in "blatant discrimination." There is no such thing as a "specialist for the purposes of cleaning teeth," the court said. The dentist "would not have refused these persons but for their disability." (*United States v. Morvant,* 843 F. Supp. 1092 (E.D. La. 1994).)

TELECOMMUNICATIONS

The ADA required the availability of Telecommunications Devices for the Deaf (TDD) by 1995. Among the services provided by public safety agencies is the 911 telephone response service. The law required that "telephone emergency response services, including 911 services, provide direct access to people who use TDDs and computer modems. Maintenance of this equipment is also mandated by the ADA.

Using these devices requires special knowledge involving communication with TDD system. Following is an example of abbreviations commonly used by TDD callers:

GA = Go ahead (it's your turn)

SK = Stop keying (ready to hang up)

GASK = Go ahead/hang up

SKSK = Stop keying/hang up now

XXX = Erasing the error—typing XXX indicates to disregard the previously typed word. Then the word is retyped.

Q = Question mark

Example of a call:

911:	"Okay what address for an ambulance q ga"
Caller:	"112 EVERG GA"
911:	"Spell everg ga"
Caller:	"EVERGREEN GA"
911:	"Where are u now q ga"
Caller:	"MY HOUSE 105 EVERG PLS. HURRY GA"

Rubin, Paula N., and Dunne, Toni, "The ADA: Emergency Response Systems and TDD's." *National Institute of Justice: Research in Action*, pp. 1–7 (February 1995)

FEDERAL AGE DISCRIMINATION ACT (FADA)

The Federal Age Discrimination in Employment Act of 1967 (290 *United States Code* sections 621–634) covers age discrimination and protects the rights of older workers. It provides that workers over the age of forty cannot be arbitrarily discriminated against because of age in any employment decisions. This includes hiring, discharge, layoff, promotion, wages and other terms and conditions of employment, referrals by employment agencies, and membership in and activities of unions.

The FADA applies to employers with more than twenty employees, and to public and private employers, including state and local governments and their agencies. States individually may have separate law further protecting workers. The act is administered by the EEOC.

EQUAL PAY ACT

Violations of the Equal Pay Act are a form of sex discrimination actionable under Title VII. The act was passed in 1963 to end the practice of paying women less than men for the same job. Equal work is defined as work requiring substantially similar "skill, effort, and responsibility." It does not mean equal pay for **comparable** work. The comparable worth theory is based on the premise that particular jobs have been traditionally underpaid because they have been held primarily by women.

FAIR LABOR STANDARDS ACT (FLSA)

State and federal laws regulate employee's wages, hours, and working conditions. The FLSA establishes a federal minimum wage, mandates extra pay for overtime work, regulates the employment of children, and is administered by the Department of Labor.

Under the FLSA, Congress periodically adjusts the minimum wage rate. The minimum wage applies to all employers who are involved in interstate commerce but exempts executives, administrators, professional employees, outside salespersons, state employees, and agricultural workers. Overtime is considered as any hours worked in excess of forty hours per week and must be compensated at one and one-half times the employee's regular rate of pay.

The medical office is often confronted with issues involving overtime pay. Overtime must be paid for work permitted but not necessarily required. For example, an employee may voluntarily work overtime without being required by the employer to put in extra hours, or it may be necessary for an employee to work through lunch and/or after hours to complete the job. In either case, the employee is entitled to overtime pay. Supervisory and professional employees are exempt from the law.

Registered nurses (RNs) qualify as professional employees and as such are exempt from overtime payment requirements, as are supervisory employees such as office managers.

WORKERS' COMPENSATION

Workers' compensation law reimburses employees for losses sustained because of work-related injury or disease, regardless of fault. Losses include the cost of medical care, lost income, and rehabilitation expenses. It also provides continuing payments to the spouses and/or children of workers who die of occupational disease or injury. The law applies to all industrial, service, private, state, and local government employees and is paid for by the employer.

SOCIAL SECURITY

Social security is several different but related programs: retirement, disability, and dependent's/survivor's benefits. Each part has its own set of rules concerning who is qualified to receive benefits and has its own schedule of payment of benefits. Benefits are paid to the retired or disabled worker and/or the worker's dependent or surviving family. The amount paid is based on the worker's average wages while working in employment covered by social security during his or her working life.

In order to receive social security benefits, an individual must accumulate a predetermined number of work credits in qualified employment. Work credits are measued in quarters of a year (three months) during which time the individual was employed earning the required minimum wage or more.

Retirement Benefits

Retirement benefits require a total of forty quarters or ten years of work credit from covered employment. An individual becomes eligible for retirement benefits at age sixty-two. If the person chooses to retire at sixty-two years of age, the monthly benefit payment will be considerably less than if retirement takes place at sixty-five years of age. Under new regulations, retirement benefits will not be available until sixty-seven years of age.

Disability Benefits

Disability benefits are paid to individuals who are disabled. Any medical condition that prevents an individual from being gainfully employed may be considered a disability, particularly if it is included on the list of disabling conditions found on the Social Security Administration's list. There are special provisions for people who are blind.

Dependent's Benefits

Certain dependents of a retired or disabled worker are eligible for monthly dependent's benefits if the worker is eligible for retirement or disability benefits.

Survivor's Benefits

Surviving family members of a deceased worker may be entitled to survivor's benefits. In order to distribute survivor's benefits fairly and equitably, survivors who are eligible are listed by the Social Security Administration.

Medicare

Medicare is a federal insurance program for people who are entitled to Medicare from their social security contributions and payment of premiums. It is for almost everyone sixty-five years of age or older, rich or poor, for certain people on social security disability, and for some individuals with permanent kidney failure.

Medicare Hospital Insurance provides basic coverage for inpatient hospitalization and posthospital nursing and home health care. There is a yearly deductible.

Medicare Medical Insurance, known as Part B, pays eighty percent of "reasonable" charges for doctors' fees, outpatient hospital and laboratory work, medical equipment and supplies, home health care, therapy, and so on. A monthly premium is charged for Part B.

Medicaid

Medicaid is a federal-state cooperative program with rules that vary from state to state. Medicaid is provided for low-income and needy individuals and is obtainable through local social services or welfare departments. Medicaid reimburses for Medicare deductibles and for the portion of "reasonable charges" not paid by Medicare (twenty percent). In many states, Medicaid will cover a number of services and costs that Medicare does not cover, including prescription drug costs, dental care, diagnostic and preventive care, eyeglasses, and the Medicare premium. Some states now require Medicaid clients to become enrolled in managed care organizations.

EMPLOYEE RETIREMENT INCOME SECURITY ACT (ERISA)

The Employee Retirement Income Security Act (ERISA) protects and regulates pensions. A pension is an agreement between an employee and an employer under which each contributes a certain amount of money while the employee works for the employer. These contributions create a fund from which the employee is paid a certain amount of money upon retirement, usually at the age of sixty-five.

In the past, many employers and employees contributed to pension plans, but employees often did not collect or benefit at retirement for the following reasons: people changed jobs and had to leave their pension rights behind; workers were "let go" just before they reached retirement age; and pension plans, or whole companies, went out of business.

Since the passage of ERISA in 1974, some of the abuses of pensions have been controlled. The act sets minimum standards for pension plans guaranteeing that a worker's pension rights cannot be unfairly denied.

The Health Insurance Portability and Accountability Act of 1996 amends ERISA by guaranteeing renewal and transferability of health insurance coverage to those already with coverage and to their dependents. As in any legislative act, there are clauses that require further interpretation on administrative appeal or litigation in court, and the wording regarding insurance eligibility promises these types of issues. For example:

The Act prohibits medical underwriting: it bars health insurers from using, as rules of eligibility, an individual's health status, medical or mental conditions, claims experience, medical treatment history, genetic information, disability or evidence of insurability. Health insurers may, however, select in a non-discriminatory basis, the coverage and benefits they wish to offer. For example, a health insurer may exclude benefits for AIDS or cancer in its policies, but cannot deny

coverage to an individual with AIDS or cancer when its policies otherwise offer
AIDS or cancer coverage.

Roverner, Jack, "Analysis of the Provisions of
the Health Insurance Portability and Accountability
Act of 1996," *The Health Lawyer* 9(3):1 (1996)

OCCUPATIONAL SAFETY AND HEALTH ACT (OSHA)

Congress enacted the Occupational Safety and Health Act (OSHA) in
1970. This act now is in effect in hospitals and other health care delivery
facilities. The OSHA rules and regulations are intended to prevent injuries
and promote job safety, and OSHA is authorized to enforce its standards
through complaint, inspection, and investigation.

The Occupational Safety and Health Act places employers under the
general duty to provide a workplace free from "recognized hazards," for
example, undue exposure to toxic substances, inoperable safety equipment,
poor air quality, and excessive noise levels. In addition, OSHA requires
detailed records of job-related injuries and may conduct unannounced workplace inspections to assess an employer's compliance.

Penalties of up to $1,000 for each violation and as high as $10,000 for
repeated or willful violations may be assessed by OSHA. Although OSHA
protects employee's rights, it also imposes responsibilities on employees.
Employees may not be discharged or discriminated against for filing a complaint or testifying against an employer due to violation of OSHA regulations.

Right-to-Know Laws

Right-to-know regulations, originated by OSHA for the protection of
industrial workers, now extend to cover health care workers. The right-to-
know legislation grew directly out of concerns about hazardous substances
and their health effects. The underlying purpose of the law is to make certain
that all employees have an opportunity to know what chemicals they are handling, the potential health effects of those chemicals, and ways to prevent or
reduce health risks.

These regulations give each employee the right to (1) a complete list of
all hazardous chemicals used in the workplace, (2) the contents of every
product and the hazards involved in its use, (3) education about hazardous
chemicals with which an employee may come in contact, and (4) protective
equipment to use when handling dangerous chemicals.

The law addresses toxic and poisonous chemicals, corrosive irritants,
flammable materials, and carcinogens. It requires that each product be
labeled. There are three types of labels: written labels with extensive information about the chemical; an encoded label with fire, reactivity, and health
hazards categories coded 1–4 for severity; and symbolic labels.

Material Safety Data Sheets (MSDSs) on every product must be made available to each employee. These sheets list every ingredient in the product. The MSDSs must be kept for future reference by the employee and the employee's family (for thirty years in Massachusetts).

Special regulations concerning chemical spills prevent workers from cleaning up a spill until the MSDS has been checked to determine whether there are any hazards or necessary precautions. Each spill requires an incident report listing the name of the chemical and the details of the spill— where it took place, the time, date, who was involved, and what was done to clean it up.

Regulations for Blood-Borne Pathogens

The AIDS epidemic has focused the health care industries safety concerns on blood-borne infections, including HIV and hepatitis B. Approximately 5.6 million employees who "reasonably could be expected" to come into contact with human blood or other potentially infectious material are affected by these regulations. The regulations cover both administrative and clinical aspects of practice.

The regulations order employers to offer hepatitis B vaccines free of charge to every employee who can be reasonably anticipated to have skin, eye, mucous membrane, or parenteral contact with blood or other potentially infectious materials.

Potentially infectious materials, in addition to products made from human blood, include semen, vaginal secretions, cerebrospinal fluid, synovial fluid, pleural fluid, pericardial fluid, saliva in dental procedures, any body fluid that is visibly contaminated with blood, and all body fluids in situations where it is difficult or impossible to differentiate between body fluids.

Regulations require universal precautions: a written exposure control plan; a list of all job classifications in which employees have occupational exposure; engineering and work practice controls; procedures for disposal of waste and sharps; availability of protective equipment, including gloves; a written schedule and method for housecleaning and decontamination, including laundry; postexposure evaluation processes; and employee training. Orange-red or fluorescent orange warning labels with the Bio-Hazard legend must be affixed to containers of regulated waste, to refrigerators and freezers containing infectious materials, and to containers used to transport them.

MEDICAL WASTE

The Medical Waste Tracking Act, passed by Congress in November 1988, tracked for a two-year period the movement of medical waste in the District of Columbia and five states: Connecticut, Louisiana, New Jersey, New York, and Rhode Island. Other states, such as Massachusetts, have passed strict medical waste regulations through their departments of public health.

Medical waste includes human organs, dressings, bandages, diapers, needles, scalpel blades, laboratory cultures, and specimens. Pictures of syringes, test tubes, and other medical waste that had washed up on public beaches, coupled with the public's fear of AIDS, brought demands for regulation of the disposal of medical waste. According to the Environmental Protection Agency, ten to fifteen percent of the 800 million pounds of medical waste produced by hospitals each year is infectious. Most of this trash is burned either at hositals in their own incinerators or at the incinerator of a trash-disposal company. Hospitals also generate about two-third of the low-level radioactive waste in the country, the other third being generated by industry and nuclear power plants.

According to the new law, waste must be separated from the other trash and garbage, placed in specially designated lead or puncture resistant containers, and tracked from the hospital to the landfill or incinerator through a system of logs, tracking forms, and identification labels.

UNIONS AND HEALTH CARE WORKERS

The history of the organization of health care workers goes back to 1919 when the first known attempt to organize hospital employees took place in San Francisco. The issues were shorter hours and improved working conditions. In 1936, the American Federation of Labor organized engine-room, laundry, and dietary employees; nurses' aides; and orderlies in three San Francisco hospitals. Since 1946, the American Nurses' Association (ANA) has supported **collective bargaining,** and most registered nurses have chosen their state nurses' association as their collective bargaining representative. In August of 1974, Public Law 93-360 amended the National Labor Relations Act (NLRA) to include nonprofit hospitals and health care institutions. By bringing hospitals, convalescent homes, health maintenance organizations, health clinics, nursing homes, and extended care facilities under the NLRA, Congress set the stage for the collective bargaining relationship between management and employees in these institutions.

People join unions for many reasons, primarily because of the dissatisfaction with wages, benefits, or working conditions. The job one holds determines the **bargaining unit** one may join. Once a union is organized, the employer is obligated to bargain in **good faith** with the employees. The employees, through their representatives, must bargain in good faith with management. When there is no collective bargaining relationship between management and employees, management has the absolute right to set wages, hours, and working conditions and to promote and discipline at will, subject to state law. Once there is an obligation to bargain, there are limits to how management may exercise these rights.

Many professionals feel that they cannot be professional and join a union. Critics of unions for health professionals feel that unionization tarnishes their image by shifting attention from meeting the patients' needs to concern about economic status. They have concerns about the destructive effect a strike could have on sick patients and fear that the presence of a union might become a barrier to communication between management and other professionals.

Among nurses, collective bargaining is relatively well established but still is a controversial and emotion subject. Unions are just beginning to attract hospital clerical personnel. Health maintenance organizations and other alternative health-delivery systems offer a fertile field for union organizers. Whether to join a union is a personal decision that depends on an individual's philosophy. It requires considerable self-examination and a weighing of the positive and negative aspects of union membership.

WORKING CONDITIONS

The working conditions in a medical office should be defined in individual job descriptions, an office handbook, and procedures manuals.

Job Description

Every position in an office should have a job description. Some job descriptions are divided into two parts: the responsibilities required of each employee, and the listing of tasks to be performed by each employee. Examples include:

The front desk personnel will:

1.   answer the telephone.
2.   make appointments for new patients.
3.   make appointments for returning patients.
4.   weigh all patients before they see the doctor.
5.   assist in preparing patients for examination.
6.   complete other tasks as assigned.

The clinical personnel will:

1.   answer the telephone if the medical assistant and the secretary are not available.
2.   prepare all injections for the physician.
3.   educate patients as to self-injection of insulin.
4.   complete other tasks as assigned.

The administrative personnel will:

1.   interview clients and obtain their insurance plan and identification numbers.
2.   complete all third-party billing forms.
3.   transcribe letters dictated by the physician.
4.   maintain, control access to, and file patients' medical records.
5.   complete other tasks as assigned.

Remember, the above is just an example. Job descriptions are an essential part of written standard office procedures and establish authority and responsibility for carrying out procedures.

Procedures Manual

In addition to the job description, each office should have a procedures manual. A procedures manual describes in detail the manner in which a task in the job description should be carried out. It is important as an educational tool for new employees as well as a resource for substitutes when a regular office employee is ill or on vacation. Written standard office procedures help maintain high standards of patient care, protect against the omission of important steps, ensure compliance with government and third-party regulations, and decrease the possibility of malpractice action. They aid in achieving the **risk management** goals for the office as well as maintaining **quality assurance.**

If a patient is injured during a procedure and the guidelines for performing the procedure as written in the procedures manual were not followed, the health care employee could be **negligent per se** without **mitigating** circumstances. If an employee is injured during the performance of a procedure and the guidelines for performing the procedure were not followed, the employee could be guilty of contributory negligence. On the other hand, following the procedures manual conscientiously could absolve the employee and/or the physician of any fault, particularly if it is shown that equipment used was faulty. In a lawsuit to recover damages under these circumstances, the patient would probably press a cause of action for product liability against the manufacturer of the equipment or medication.

The importance of a procedures manual is illustrated in the following Georgia case involving a nurse at a Kaiser call center working without written protocol. Medical call centers are identified as nurse-triage lines, demand management call centers, or nurse-on-call centers and function twenty-four hours a day to allow patients an opportunity to make informed, cost-effective health care choices.

A nurse received a call from a family with an infant with a 104 degree fever. She recommended that the child be driven to a network hospital forty-five minutes from home. The parents drove part way and circled back to the nearest hospital emergency room. The infant suffered circulatory collapse and lost both hands and most of both legs. The family sued alleging that the nurse's bad advice caused delay in treatment which in turn caused circulatory collapse and loss of limbs. On February 2, 1995, a Fulton County jury found Kaiser negligent and awarded the family in excess of $45,000,000 in damages. . . .

Kearney, Kerry A., "Legal Liability and Risk
Considerations for a Medical Call Center,"
The Health Lawyer 9(3):20 (1996)

Kerry A. Kearney, in an article for *The Health Lawyer* published by the American Bar Association (Vol. 9, No. 3), analyzed the case and suggested the following to reduce the risks of catastrophic damages:

1. Hire experienced and appropriately trained nursing personnel. Telephone nursing is different from hospital or even clinic based nursing. Most national call centers hire nurses with eight to ten years experience then train for six additional weeks.
2. Medical call center (MCC) nurses should tell callers the limitations of advice. . . .
3. Nurses must work from written protocols.
4. MCC should document the care and any options discussed.
5. Patient calls and records must be kept confidential. . . .
6. The MCC should provide options, not advice, to the patient. . . .
7. The MCC should describe the limitations of phone advice in plan booklets given to patients, employers and subscribers. . . .

Kearney, Kerry A., "Legal Liability and Risk
Considerations for a Medical Call Center,"
The Health Lawyer 9(3):20 (1996)

The Handbook

The handbook, often referred to as a personnel manual, usually provides personnel policies and related instructions under one cover. It imparts information to the employee concerning work hours, sick leave, pension benefits, evaluation procedures, and so on. If the company is unionized, the handbook cannot be changed without negotiating with the union, whereas if the employees are not protected by a union, handbook changes are usually placed in a prominent place to put employees on notice prior to company policy change. Some courts consider the handbook an extension of the employment contract while other courts hold the opposite. It either situation, the handbook is an important document whose contents should be reviewed and understood early in the employer-employee relationship. On the following page is a map of the United States. Those states with court decisions that support the contractual nature of employee handbooks are marked with state abbreviations.

COLLECTIONS

Overdue Accounts

Every business has overdue accounts. Some patients do not pay because they do not have the money, but others are habitual delinquents. Office staff members who are on top of collection problems keep in contact with patients and update addresses and phone numbers.

The first step in collection is to contact the individual and determine whether there is a valid reason for failure to pay. The second step is to set up a pay schedule. If a patient owes the doctor, that patient probably owes many others as well.

Some physicians prefer to handle all collections through the mail and make use of colored stickers that are available to place on an overdue bill to emphasize the matter. Because the debt is "incurred primarily for family or household purposes," attempting to collect the due amount is subject to a number of federal and state regulations. If a doctor's staff members or their agents engage in overly vigorous collection activity, they risk being sued for defamation, invasion of privacy, intentional infliction of emotion distress, or other torts.

The federal Fair Debt Collection Practices Act (*United States Code* section 1692 *et seq.*) prohibits many different collections practices, for example, threats of violence, use of abusive language when trying to collect the debt, harassment by means of phone calls, and deception and unfair methods of collection such as threatening to deposit a postdated check before the date of the check and intentionally causing the debtor's other checks to be dishonored.

The FDCPA regulates all collection of debts and prohibits all false, deceptive, misleading, and unfair or harassing collection policies. A physician should be certain that the provisions of the FDCPA are followed by the office staff, attorneys, and collection agencies.

Collection Practice

A typical collection suit begins with the filing of a small claims action in civil court. If uncontested, a judgment will be entered for the plaintiff (creditor). If contested, the judge makes a ruling on the facts as presented by the parties before the court. In either case, after the judgment, an execution

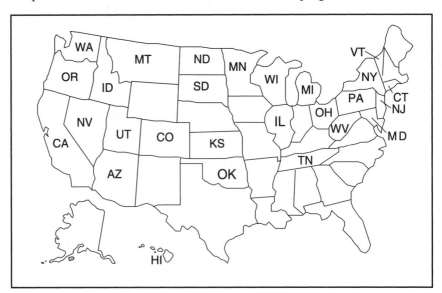

will be issued. An execution is a document that contains the judgment obtained in a civil action and commands payment. With an execution, **levy** can be made on specific property owned by the debtor to receive payment.

Where the debt owed is relatively small, the execution is filed as evidence of debt in a supplementary process proceeding in district court. A summons issues for the debtor to appear in court to be "examined" by the judge as to ability to pay.

Bad Checks

A check **tendered** for services rendered that is returned unpaid by the bank, for whatever reason, is grounds for a criminal complaint. In some states, creditors are allowed to simultaneously pursue both criminal and civil actions to secure payment; in others, the creditor must choose the **venue.** A criminal suit cannot be used to settle a civil action.

Collection of physicians' fees is complicated because of third-party reimbursement. Regardless of the insurance coverage, the patient is responsible for the payment of the fee unless the physician has entered into an agreement to accept the insurers' rate of payment as payment in full.

Bankruptcy

Bankruptcy is the process by which a financially troubled individual is declared by a bankruptcy court to be incapable of paying his or her debts, the debtor's available assets are distributed to creditors as required by bankruptcy law, and the debtor is granted a discharge from liability for most of the remaining unpaid debts.

There are three major kinds of bankruptcy proceedings: liquidation, business reorganization, and repayment plans for debtors with regular income.

Once an individual initiates bankruptcy proceedings, the physician's office can only comply with the requests of the court-appointed receiver within the stated time limits and should not contact the patient for further payment of the bill.

Letter to Terminate Delinquent Patients

When a patient refuses or is unable to pay a medical bill, the physician must make a decision about whether to continue to treat that patient. If the doctor decides to terminate the patient, the following procedures should be followed in order to avoid abandoning the individual:

1. Write a letter to the patient stating that the bill is overdue and has been overdue for a defined period of time.
2. Check the contents and form of the letter with the doctor's attorney in order to make certain that the procedure complies with all local and federal laws.

3. Allow the patient a reasonable amount of time during which payment will be accepted (thirty days). After that date, inform the patient that the doctor-patient relationship will be terminated.
4. Mail the letter first-class, certified mail, return receipt requested. In addition, send another copy of the letter regular first-class mail. Many times patients will not pick up certified mail at the post office but will open or at least accept a first-class letter at the door. First-class mail is not returned to the office unless the person is no longer at the address.
5. The return of the certified mail with notification of the first-class mailing on the bottom of the letter will document that the letter has been mailed.
6. Keep records of the letter and the return postal receipt on the patient's chart.

SUMMARY

Health care is big business. Between 1986 and 1990, total health care expenditures in the United States increased from $425 billion dollars to $666.2 billion dollars. The organizations through which this money was channeled, in addition to the federal government, included proprietorships, partnerships, and corporations.

A proprietorship is the simplest form of business organization. A partnership is two or more individuals engaged in business for the purpose of making a profit. A corporation is a more complicated business structure. Corporations, partnerships, and individual practitioners are responsible to the public for their offices, laboratories, buildings, and equipment. Managed care organizations usually fall under the umbrella of a corporation.

Different standards of responsibility are required for trespassers, licenses, and invitees. Business owners are responsible to the public for equipment used in the business.

The relationship between employer and employee is contractual in nature. As the health care industry has increased in size and the treatment has become more technological, hiring patterns in hospitals and other facilities have changed. The union movement has infiltrated large hospitals. Clerical workers are still to be unionized. Whether to join a union must be a personal decision.

Discrimination is an issue in the hiring and promotion of employees. Sexual harassment is defined as discrimination in the courts and is a serious problem for women in the workforce.

The business aspect of health care is highly regulated. The Americans with Disabilities Act (ADA) regulates the hiring and promotion of physically and mentally disabled individuals. The Federal Age Discrimination Act (FADA) protects the rights of older workers. The Equal Pay Act prevents the practice of paying women less than men for the same job. The Fair Labor Standards Act (FLSA) establishes a federal minimum wage, mandates extra pay for overtime work, and regulates the employment of children. The Employee Retirement

Income Security Act (ERISA) has to do with pensions. The Occupational Health and Safety Act (OSHA) affects health care workers, particularly with regulations involving right-to-know laws and blood-borne pathogens. The Medical Waste Tracking Act regulates the disposal of waste from health care facilities.

Procedures manuals, job descriptions, and employee handbooks are all part of the business side of a medical practice, as are laws affecting collection processes. Workers' compensation and social security affect every employer and employee.

Government regulations affecting the health care practitioner include medical practice acts, boards of regulation, and mandatory reporting of births, deaths, and communicable diseases. Controlled substances acts restrict the distribution, classification, sale, and use of certain drugs. Physicians, nurses, and other health care personnel are mandated in most states to report abuse of children, elderly, and patients.

SUGGESTED ACTIVITY

Sexual harassment is a problem in almost every workplace. In order to determine your sophistication about harassing behaviors, answer the following questionnaire. Discuss your answers with your classmates.

		AGREE	DISAGREE
1.	What percentage of the female workforce is affected by sexual harassment? _____%		
2.	Only young and attractive women are harassed by men.	❑	❑
3.	Every race experiences the same sexual harassment.	❑	❑
4.	Bosses are the only ones who have the power to sexually harass.	❑	❑
5.	The way a woman dresses influences whether or not she is harassed.	❑	❑
6.	Sexual harassment is only a problem between people.	❑	❑
7.	We have laws to protect people against sexual harassment.	❑	❑
8.	There is an equal amount of sexual harassment of men as of women.	❑	❑
9.	Ignoring sexual harassment is the best way to handle it.	❑	❑
10.	Sexual comments and advances should only be considered as sexual harassment if they are repeated more than once.	❑	❑

Modification of Sexual Harassment Survey
by the Massachusetts State Department of Education

STUDY QUESTIONS

1. Identify the major disadvantage of a sole proprietorship or a partnership.
2. A corporation differs from a partnership in many ways. Identify five differences.
3. Identify three alternative delivery systems.
4. Every day a postal employee delivers mail to the office. The mail carrier always comes inside and chats with the staff. Is this person a trespasser, licensee, or invitee?
5. A woman brings an elderly patient to the office. The patient tells you he is being abused by the family. What would you do?
6. During a routine examination, a medical assistant notices cigarette burns on the bottom of a child's foot. What should the medical assistant do?
7. Construct a hiring interview for a woman you suspect is pregnant.
8. An office nurse smells of alcohol when she arrives at work. She is your boss. How would you handle the situation?
9. One of the medical assistants receives a needle stick. As office manager, what would you do?
10. A union is organizing in your hospital. You are interested in speaking to the union representative during lunch. Your supervisor informs you that no one in "this office" will become a member of the union. What are your rights?
11. Write a letter requesting payment on an overdue account from a friend of the doctor's husband.

CASES FOR DISCUSSION

1. Dr. Webber joined the Gelder Medical Group, which was a medical partnership. Part of the agreement was that if for any reason his association with the group ended, he would not for five years practice medicine within thirty miles of the Village of Sidney, where the partnership was located. The agreement also provided that any member could be required to withdraw from the partnership upon a majority vote of the other members. Dr. Webber's work with the group turned out to be unsatisfactory to his partners, who felt he was an embarrassment to the group. He was characterized as being "a perfectionist who was a rather idealistic, sincere, direct, frank individual who quite possibly could be perceived at times as being somewhat blunt." Dr. Webber refused to withdraw from the association after he was terminated by the other physicians. Two months later, despite his earlier agreement, Dr. Webber opened a medical office in Sidney. The partnership brought

suit to prevent him from carrying on his practice. Could they do this successfully?

2. A British television medical expert called for nurses to wear short skirts, black stockings, and sexy garter belts to improve the morale of male patients. Dr. Vernon Coleman, an author and television medical commentator, said sexy garb on nurses would make male patients more cheerful, take their minds off their pains, and ultimately help their recoveries. "The sight of a pretty nurse dressed like that would make any man's heart miss a beat or two and make him feel happier and more cheerful," he said. "It's a proven fact that cheerful people get better quicker." What did the Royal College of Nursing have to say about this matter?

3. In December 1978, a local of the retail clerks' union was certified as the collective bargaining representative of the East Chicago Rehabilitation Center service and maintenance employees. During contract negotiations, the labor negotiator noted that employees had the right to leave the nursing home premises. The negotiators stated that the employees could not do this because contract settlement was close at hand. In June 1979, a memorandum was issued stating that all employees must remain on the premises during lunchtime. The day-shift employees became upset. As a result, seventeen nurses' aides decided to walk out and protest the change. The union asked the striking workers to return to work because the union could not legally sanction the walkout. The center refused to reinstate the employees who walked out and initiated firing proceedings. The seventeen employees were fired after contract negotiations concluded. The contract package had a clause that allowed employees a half-hour unpaid lunchtime during which they could leave the premises. Did the center have to reinstate the seventeen nurses' aides?

4. Joan Leikvold was hired by Valley View Community Hospital as an operating room supervisor in 1972. She did not have a contract for a specific duration, nor was she told that the hospital would discharge her except for cause. She was provided with a policy manual and told that the policies were to be followed in her employment relationship with the hospital. In 1978, she became the director of nursing. In October 1979, she requested a transfer back to her former position in the operating room. The chief executive officer (CEO) felt that it was inadvisable for someone who had been in a managerial position to take a subordinate position. Leikvold withdrew the transfer request but was subsequently fired. Her personnel record indicated "insubordination" as the reason for discharge.

   Leikvold was an at-will employee. At-will means that there is a contract made for an indefinite duration and either party, employer or employee, may terminate the contract at any time for any reason, or without reason. Can the CEO fire Leikvold? (*Leikvold v. Valley View Community Hospital*, 688 P.2d 170 (Ariz. 1984).

5. Plaintiff Raymond Vadnais alleged that in 1986, he visited [a doctor] at Beth Israel Hospital's ear, nose, and throat clinic complaining of ear pain. After antibiotics failed to relieve the pain, [the doctor] recommended surgery. However, after [the doctor] learned that the plaintiff was infected with HIV, he refused to perform the operation (*Vadnais v. Beth Israel,* 19 M.L.W. 965 (1991)). Should the doctor be required to perform the operation?

Chapter 7

The Medical Record: The Medical Assistant's Responsibility

"Speck in cornea, 50 cents."

Sir William Osler

OBJECTIVES:

One hundred years ago, the great Canadian physician, Sir William Osler, adequately and accurately recorded in the medical record the happenings during an office visit with the above medical record entry. Record keeping was very simple. Since then, the medical record has evolved from an uncomplicated statement of treatment to a highly valued document important to the patient, essential to the physician, and necessary to various other parties. The medical assistant is the **custodian** of the medical office record and all the information it contains. After reading this chapter, you should be able to:

1. identify the owner of a medical record.
2. list different types of medical records.
3. determine who has legitimate access to patient information.
4. recognize new dimensions of confidentiality with the use of computers for medical records.
5. identify the procedures necessary for release of information from the medical record.
6. identify the concerns associated with faxing medical information.
7. respond properly to a subpoena duces tecum.
8. determine who has access to a medical record.
9. appreciate the importance of medical record credibility.
10. follow an acceptable method for making corrections to a medical record.

BUILDING YOUR LEGAL VOCABULARY

codify	forum	statutes
conspiring	integrated	subpoena
custodian	premises	subpoena duces tecum
data	property right	
Federal Rules of Evidence	settlement	

Basically, a medical record is a recorded collection of **data** on a patient. It includes past history, a statement of the current problem and diagnosis, and the treatment procedures used to solve the problem. Medical records are created for the following reasons: licensing authorities require record keeping; records are essential for communicating important data to all those who participate in a patient's care; records create a legal document to record and substantiate a standard of care for medico-legal and other services; and physicians' liability insurance may require specific guidelines for development of the record.

The Harvard Risk Management Foundation indicates that a medical record should be:

1.   a viable record of patient care that coordinates the efforts of all the members of the health care team;
2.   a tool to support reimbursement;
3.   a useful defense tool (if necessary); and
4.   legible.

In addition to diagnostic tests and results, information related to prescriptions and patients' allergies and sensitivities, informed consent, patient compliance (notes regarding "no-shows") and documentation regarding physician follow-up and attempts to arrange care by another provider, if necessary, should be included. . . . Telephone calls should be treated as patient encounters, and documentation should be made in the patient record.

Cox, Thomas, "A Risk Management Approach to
Computerizing a Physician's Office," *Forum*
(Harvard Risk Management Foundation)

The medical record is increasingly being used to determine the necessity for and quality of health care. This is reflected in the greater use of the medical record by HMO peer review teams and insurance company audits. In addition to the fact that reimbursement from parties may depend upon adequate documentation of services provided, the medical record is the standard by which the practice is judged.

OWNERSHIP OF THE MEDICAL RECORD

A hospital owns all of its records. The records of a physician, made in the course of professional office practice, are in the same category as hospital records; these are owned by the physician, corporation, or managed care organization. While the physician and others as owners have a **property right** to the record and can restrict its removal from the **premises,** the patient's interest in the information is protected by law.

Ownership usually carries with it the right and power to exercise authority and control over the use of the property. In the case of the medical record, control cannot be exclusively exercised. The fact that a hospital or physician owns the piece of paper on which the record is written does not prevent other individuals, professionals, corporations, and courts from claiming a right to see and copy the information. There are competing interests in and claims upon the contents of a medical record. For example, a physician is ethically obligated to furnish office records to another physician who assumes responsibility for the care of a patient. The following case involves ownership of a medical record:

CASE STUDY   A dispute occurred between a physician who was employed by a clinic and the estate of a deceased physician, owner of a medical clinic. Following the death of the owner, the employee removed from the clinic the Daily Reference Book, which disclosed the identity of all the persons treated . . ., the receipt book, which contained a statement of funds, and all current patient records. The estate accused the physician employee of wrongfully removing the records from the clinic.

The court held that the employee had wrongfully removed the records from the clinic but the importance of the rights and the interests of the patients who elected to receive [the physician employee's] professional services required that he be allowed to retain such of the medical records of these patients as might be found necessary in order to enable him to render them proper care and treatment.

Jones v. Fakehany,
67 Cal. Rptr. 810 (1968)

Another example of the physician's inability to absolutely control medical records occurs in the disbursement of property at death. Following the death of a doctor, the records, which are owned by the physician, cannot be dispensed with or distributed in the same manner as other property. For example:

CASE STUDY   The doctor's will directed his executor to burn and destroy all of his office records and files without opening them. The court held that this was against public policy and ordered the executor to make available records and notes pertaining to patients to succeeding physicians upon authorized request.

In re Culbertson's Will,
292 N.Y.S.2d 806 (1968)

X-rays, MRIs, electrocardiograms, and the results of other diagnostic tests are a form of medical record and belong to the physician or the hospital where they are taken. Access to X-rays depends upon the policy of the owner. Policy is affected by **statutes** that may require the owner to give the films to another physician selected by the patient, but may not require the owner to give them to a patient for personal viewing. When a physician refers a patient to a radiologist for X-ray studies, the films usually belong to the radiologist, and not to the referring physician who receives the radiologist's report.

TYPES OF MEDICAL RECORDS

In large outpatient clinics associated with teaching hospitals, the **integrated** medical record is often seen. With an integrated medical record, the patient is represented by a single record that includes all outpatient and inpatient activity. Under the current organization of American health care, this is not usually the case. Hospitals, HMOs, or private physicians' offices are totally separate and distinct organizational and legal entities. Cross-indexing of the hospital and outside office records is very limited and usually represented by a copy of the discharge summary from the hospital chart in the office record of the attending physician. The hospital record seldom carries any direct report of medical office visits.

The medical record of the nonhospital situation, identified as a record of medical care given in a facility that does not retain the patient bodily overnight, has unique qualities, depending on the specialty of the physicians and the requirements of the state. The more the outpatient facility resembles a hospital, the more the record resembles a hospital record. For example, a surgical center requires detailed intake charts, operating room notes, and postoperative care forms, while an office record of some highly specialized physicians may be limited to entries on one side of a three-by-five card. The care of the medical record by the medical assistant requires the same attention to detail and confidentiality whether it is in a hospital setting or a specialist's private office.

Managed care plans, over the past few years, have accumulated large amounts of patient care information.

As medical record systems have become automated and health plans have begun to comprehensively review patient care services and utilization information in detail, managed care plans have engaged in a systematic accumulation and assessment from physicians' office practices, a domain formerly outside any external organized evaluation process.

> "Health Care Facility Records: Confidentiality,
> Computerization and Security," *Forum of Health Law*
> (American Bar Association, July 1995)

Technology has entered into the storing of medical information:

> Medical records for each of the 7,000 athletes competing in the 1995 Special Olympics starting in Connecticut this weekend will be stored on bar codes attached to credentials.
>
> "Medical Records," *The Wall Street Journal,* p. B1 (1996)

This type of storing of medical information is available to the rest of the population through the E.M.X. card, a form of electronic medical identification.

> When the card is passed through a device similar to a credit card reader, emergency medical workers or doctors can, in minutes, get vital information, like the name of the patient's primary care doctor, chronic illness or allergies, medications being taken and even an image of the latest electrocardiogram.
>
> Some companies are developing smart cards, which contains such information on computer chips that can be read with special software. . . . For now, most medical records exist either on paper or in computer data bases in doctors' offices and hospitals. But doctors predict that in the next few years, electronic medical identification will be carried, along with credit cards and driver's licenses, by most people with chronic conditions like heart disease, high blood pressure, diabetes and allergies. "It's not a matter of if," says Dr. Barthall, an emergency room physician in Milwaukee, "It's a matter of when."
>
> Gilbert, Susan, "Life Saving Medical History . . ."
> *New York Times,* p. 1 (August 21, 1996)

PRIVACY AND PRIVILEGED COMMUNICATION

Professional confidentiality goes back to the time of Hippocrates:

> Whatever in connection with my professional practice, or not in connection with it, I see or hear in the life of men which ought not be spoken abroad, I will not divulge as recommending that all should be kept secret.
>
> Hippocrates

Privacy, in the medical setting, involves at least two different kinds of interests. One is individual interest in avoiding disclosure of personal matters; the second is interest in independent decision making.

There is no federal law that protects the confidentiality of medical records. Instead a patchwork quilt of state laws and regulations governs the use of medical information, but these rules are so inconsistent that lawyers say it's hard to tell which ones apply to specific situations.

Compounding the problem is that patient records—which are rapidly making their way from file folder to the computer screen—can now cross state lines with the press of a button.

Harvard Health Letter 20(11):1 (September 1995)

Avoiding Disclosure of Personal Matters

Over the years the issue of privacy in the maintenance of medical records has undergone change. During the Middle Ages, patients' medical information was public information, but during the nineteenth century, secrecy became the practice. Currently, because of the number of professionals involved in an individual patient's care, absolute privacy cannot be expected by a patient, but a high standard of professional confidentiality is expected. Health law is evolving, and most states have enacted comprehensive medical records statutes.

Communication between a physician and a patient is private and is legally recognized as privileged. Privileged communication is a legal label put on information passing from one person to another that cannot be submitted into evidence in a courtroom because of the relationship. For example, communication between a husband and wife in the privacy of their home is privileged and cannot be admitted into evidence unless certain criteria are met; communication between a priest and penitent is also private and cannot be admitted into evidence. In addition to the physician-patient privilege, some states have social worker and psychotherapist privileged communication statutes.

In the typical physician-patient privilege, a physician is prevented from revealing, in court, confidential information obtained during the treatment of the patient unless the patient waives his or her privilege against disclosure. This right is conditional and may be overruled, as in the following case:

CASE STUDY Poddar was undergoing treatment as a voluntary outpatient. He had become obsessed with Tatiana Tarasoff, a student he had met at a dance. He had tape-recorded conversations with her and spent hours replaying the tapes in order to determine her feelings for him. A friend became concerned and suggested that he seek professional help.

Poddar was seen by a psychiatrist, who did not believe that Poddar required hospitalization, but did prescribe medication and arranged weekly outpatient psychotherapy with a staff psychologist. During therapy, Poddar revealed his fantasies of harming, and perhaps even killing, Tarasoff. The friend told the psychologist that Poddar planned to purchase a gun. Poddar stopped therapy. The doctors believed that Poddar should be evaluated for hospitalization and requested help from the campus police.

The campus police went to Poddar's apartment and questioned him about his plans but then left when he denied any intention of harming Tarasoff. Two months later Poddar stabbed Tarasoff to death. He was convicted of second-degree murder, the conviction was overturned on the basis of improper jury instruction, and Poddar returned home to India.

Later, in a civil suit, the Tarasoff family sued the university, including both therapists and the campus police, for negligence. The court held that the therapists had a duty to warn Tarasoff.

Tarasoff v. Regents of University of California,
118 Cal. Rptr. 129 (1974)

The Supreme Judicial Court of Massachusetts handed down an important decision concerning the liability of physicians. It involved the liability of physicians who disclosed medical information provided to them by their patients and of those who requested such information:

CASE STUDY   The plaintiff, Alberts, was a Methodist minister who failed to be reappointed to his position as minister of the Old West Church in Boston. Alberts alleged that two of his supervisors induced his psychiatrist, Dr. Devine, to disclose information about his mental condition, which they then used to cause him not to be reappointed. Alberts brought suit against Dr. Devine and the two supervisors, alleging that Dr. Devine had breached his expressed and implied promise not to disclose any information, observations, or opinions relating to the diagnosis, condition, behavior, or treatment of Alberts that Dr. Devine gained in his professional capacity.

The court held that physicians have a duty not to disclose medical information provided to them by their patients unless they are faced with a serious danger to the patient or to others, and that they may be held liable for all the damages resulting from any violation of this duty. In addition, the court held that a third party who induces a physician to violate the duty of confidentiality may also be held liable to the patient for any resulting damages.

Alberts v. Devine,
395 Mass. 59 (1985)

An individual has the right to be left alone under certain circumstances. The court calls these circumstances events that occur within a zone of privacy. Such events are illustrated by the following:

CASE STUDY

The deceased was suffering from cancer of his larynx. The defendant, an otolaryngologist, had treated him twice surgically. A laryngectomy was performed; and later, because of a tumor that had appeared in the patient's neck, a radical neck dissection on one side was done. Many photographs had been taken by the defendant or under his direction. It was stated that these pictures were taken solely to be placed in the deceased's medical record.

Shortly before the deceased died, the defendant and a nurse appeared in his hospital room. In the presence of the deceased's wife and a visitor of the patient in the next bed, the defendant, or the nurse under the defendant's direction, raised the dying man's head and placed blue operating room toweling under his head. The dying man raised a clenched fist and attempted to move his head unsuccessfully from the camera's range. The pictures were taken.

The appeals court, concerned only with a claimed intrusion upon . . . physical and mental solitude or seclusion, recognized a "right to privacy" . . . and stated that the jury should have been instructed . . . that the taking of pictures without the decedent's consent or over his objections was an invasion of his legally protected right to privacy.

Estate of Berthiaume v. Pratt,
365 A.2d 792 (Me. 1976)

Privacy also includes the right to make personal decisions. At the core of this right is the concept of personal autonomy—the notion that the Constitution reserves to the individual, free from government intrusion, certain fundamental decisions about how he or she will conduct his or her life. This is not absolute and depends upon the impact of the decisions.

ACCESS TO THE MEDICAL RECORD

A hospital or physician may impose strict or lenient rules with regard to giving information from a medical record. If a lenient policy is adopted, it means that requests will be scrutinized, but allowed. If a strict policy is adopted, it means that the burden of decision is shifted onto the courts. If this is the situation, the person seeking the information will have to obtain a court order directing the hospital to release the information. In either event, hospitals and physicians should have a written policy on file detailing staff procedures for release of patient information.

The policy must reflect local statutes. In certain states, legislators have given the patient, the patient's physician, and/or the authorized agent the right to examine or copy the medical record. The policy must take this into consideration. In other states, judicial precedence has been set for those who base the right to examine the record on the patient's rights.

There is general authorization for the physician or hospital to release information to insurance companies about patients submitting third-party payment claims. In addition, office records, as well as hospital records, are subject to inspection by an attorney authorized by the patient to examine them for use in possible litigation against either the physician or a third party. When a patient submits a claim to litigation, the authorization is not clear-cut and must be determined on an individual basis, but a patient cannot use the privilege as a sword and a shield. When a patient submits a medical malpractice claim against a physician, he or she releases the physician from the requirement of confidentiality.

Patients are often required to submit to a physical examination before receiving benefits such as life insurance or welfare, participating in school athletics, obtaining a marriage license, or employment. In these situations, the patient implicitly consents to the sending of a truthful record to the third party. For example:

CASE STUDY   Following a physical examination, the physician disclosed to a patient's employer that the patient had a long-standing nervous condition, despite the patient's express orders not to release such information. The disclosure caused the patient's dismissal. The court found that the duty for the physician to maintain confidentiality was qualified and depended upon the context of the physician-patient relations. The physician was authorized to release the information.

Horne v. Patton,
287 So. 2d 824 (1973)

On the other hand, all insurance company requests for information need not be honored.

CASE STUDY   At least one court has denied the right of inspection to an insurance company where the company sought a review of the records of all its policyholders who were confined to the hospital. The court would not allow any "fishing expeditions" even though all the patient policyholders had signed authorizations.

Cannell v. Medical and Surgical Clinic,
315 N.E.2d 278 (Ill. 1974)

Confidentiality and Computer Records

Maintaining confidentiality is a serious security issue for institutions changing to computerized records. In order to protect the information within computerized records, staff should be trained, and computer passwords should be utilized, not shared, and changed on a regular basis. Restrictions should be placed on the availability of information.

Health Insurance Portability and Accountability Act of 1996

In order to improve efficiency in transferring information about patients within the health care system, the Health Insurance and Portability Act of 1996 directs Health and Human Services (HHS) to adopt standard "data elements" and "code sets" for electronic coding throughout the entire health care industry. All providers of health care are required to participate in these provisions. The initial standards were scheduled to be available February 21, 1998. Health plans have two years following the publication of HHS standards to comply and use the standard data elements and code sets. Under the present schedule, health plans have until February 2000 to implement them.

Facsimile (FAX) Transmission of Medical Information

Society is increasingly dependent on the use of the FAX to transmit information. However, there are times when a FAXED message goes astray, either because of error on the part of the sender or imprecise handling by the receiver. In the health care industry, this may cause a breach in the confidential relationship between physician and patient. Because of the importance of the timely receipt of information about patients in emergency circumstances, a FAX may be an appropriate mode for the delivery of medical information. Under other circumstances, either because of the content of the information or the lack of urgency, another method of transferring sensitive information may be more appropriate.

The American Health Information Management Association (AHIMA) recommends facsimile transmission of health information only when the original record or mail-delivered copies will not meet the needs of immediate patient care. The sensitive information contained in health records should be transmitted via facsimile only when: (1) urgent need for patient care or (2) required by a third-party payer for ongoing certification of payment for a hospitalized patient. The information transmitted should be limited to that necessary to meet the requestor's needs. Routine disclosure of information to insurance companies, attorneys, or other legitimate users should be made through regular mail or messenger service. . . .

Unless otherwise prohibited by state law, information transmitted via facsimile is acceptable for inclusion in the patient's health record. If the document is on thermal paper, a photocopy of the document should be placed in the record to avoid the fading that may occur over time with thermal paper. (The facsimile copy should be destroyed after the photocopy is made.)

> American Health Information Management Association
> (AHIMA) Position Statement: "Issue: Facsimile
> Transmission of Health Information," pp. 1, 2 (May 1994)

Patient's Access to Own Record

An issue of chronic aggravation between the public, their representatives (lawyers), and the medical establishment is the cost of gaining access to medical records. Kentucky handled the issue by passing an access to record law that allows patients to receive one free copy of their medical records from a health care provider. The law was passed because consumers complained about having problems when they tried to gain access to their own medical records.

Nancy Galvani, a researcher for the Kentucky Hospital Association, said lawyers are apparently requesting the free copies on behalf of patients, then using them to see whether there are grounds for possible lawsuits against providers. "Patients usually don't ask for copies of their medical records, so the volume never was very high," Galvani said. "What we see now is almost all records are going out free and most requests are coming from attorneys. . . ."

The director of the Kentucky Association of Trial Lawyers says the provision actually reduces lawsuits. "I think what it does is facilitate people getting their cases investigated. . . . If someone comes into your office and says such and such has happened to me, a good lawyer is going to need to look at that person's medical records and see just what happened. The records may show there is no case."

> "Groups Spar over Outcome of Kentucky Medical Record Law,"
> *American Medical News*, p. 29 (January 23/30, 1995)

In Massachusetts, forty hospitals resolved a class action complaint against them by placing caps on charges for photocopies of medical records:

According to Lubin and Meyer, a medical malpractice law firm, patients and lawyers were charged as much as $18.50 per request plus 75 cents a page. Because lawsuits can require hundreds of pages of hospital records, the charges sometimes ran into many hundreds of dollars per patient.

> Now after 2 1/2 years of negotiation, the parties have reached a five year agreement. In the first year of the pact, the maximum that can be charged would be $9 per request plus 50 cents a page for the first 100 pages and 25 cents a page thereafter, plus postage and sales tax.
>
> Shao, Maria, "Hospitals, Patients Settle Suit on
> Photocopy Charges," *The Boston Globe*

Physicians disagree about whether patients should have access to their own records. Some feel that there is the possibility of misinterpretation by the patient; others are of the opinion that a little knowledge can be more dangerous than no knowledge at all. Legal commentators view patients' access to their own records cynically, observing that almost everyone except the subject of the records can know what is in them. Some physicians are considering placing their patients' records on the internet.

The federal government, through the Privacy Protection Act of 1974, allows patients in federal hospitals to inspect their records. As a result, patients in veterans' hospitals have found many errors in their records. Most states allow patients to receive information from their records but do not allow direct access to the record itself. In Burlington, Vermont, a group of physicians routinely gives patients copies of their medical records. The physicians' group reports that the practice stimulates cooperation, does not harm patients, and reduces their anxiety. A family practitioner in San Jose, California, hands the patient his or her folder when leaving and expects the patient to bring it along on the next visit. The physician claims that this radical system works; saves time for him; saves time, money, and trouble for patients; and makes each patient more of a participant in personal care. The patient is made to sign a printed form that reads: "I accept responsibility as custodian of the medical records for _____." In some countries, patients are encouraged to be the sole keepers of their records.

Physicians who do not support a patient's direct access to medical records comment that there may be information in the records that the patient or members of the family should not see; for example, confidential information on past pregnancies, abortions, sexually transmitted diseases, or mental illness. Artificial insemination presents ethical dilemmas in that the availability of the record to the family affects the woman's privacy concerning conception; on the other hand, there is the responsibility of the doctor to maintain an accurate record as well as to preserve information for the future benefit of the child.

Patients' access to their own records may profoundly affect a physician's record-keeping practices, as can be seen in the following:

> A female patient was being professionally treated by a young physician when the doctor was suddenly called away from his office and left her medical record

open on his desk. The patient read the first sentence: "This woman is a crock." Needless to say, she became very distraught and angry.

> "Personal Comments in Medical Records May Cause Trouble,"
> *Medical World News,* p. 128 (January 12, 1976)

In another situation, a patient had a very upsetting experience following review of her medical record:

While waiting to see a physician, a patient had been given her own record. Curious, she took out the notes and read them only to find that the doctor had written at the heading of the page, "Beware, hysterical and manipulative, determined to be unwell." She left immediately.

> "Case Conference: Fain Would I Change That Note,"
> *Journal of Medical Ethics* 4:207–209 (1978)

The courts have recognized that certain medical information may be damaging to a patient, as can be seen in the following case:

A former mental patient and her husband brought action to have medical records made available for copying and inspection by the woman, who had contracted to write a book about her experiences. The court held that the Fourteenth Amendment does not support the claim that "former mental patients have a constitutionally protected unrestricted property right directly to inspect and copy their hospital records" and refused the patient access to her medical records.

> *Gotkin v. Miller,* 379 F. Supp. 859, 866–867
> (E.D.N.Y. 1974), *aff'd,* 514 F.2d 125 (2d Cir. 1975)

Innocent Party in the Medical Record

In the case of the mentally ill patient, medical records may contain sensitive and private information concerning the patient's family, friends, employers, and associates. A therapist frequently will record intimate aspects of relatives' and associates' lives. This information may contain a number of falsehoods and inaccuracies based on the patient's delusions and misconceptions. The patient's record may also contain the therapist's assessment of the patient's interaction with family members and other patients.

Release of information concerning other persons contained in the patient's medical record is potentially harmful to all parties involved. Disclosure may damage reputations within the community, affect employment opportunities, cause severe emotional distress, and infringe upon the individual privacy of others. If the patient obtains access to the medical record and learns about others' opinions, an adverse clinical reaction may occur, and family and social relationships may be severely and permanently disrupted. Information in the medical record may be used against persons other than the patient in legal proceedings, for example, divorce, child custody, and competency hearings.

At least three courts have held that when family members participate in counseling sessions along with the patient, the medical records of the patient may not be disclosed without the consent of the patient and family members. Another potentially troublesome area is the maintenance of confidentiality in group psychotherapy settings.

Release of Information

When working in a physician's office, the best rule to follow, unless instructed otherwise, is to refuse to disclose information—even to the point of acknowledging whether the individual is a patient. It is always possible that an enterprising sleuth could figure out the nature of a patient's illness from the specialty of the doctor.

Six basic principles are suggested for preventing unauthorized disclosure of information:

1. When in doubt, err by not disclosing rather than by disclosing. There are exceptions to this principle but a mistaken refusal to disclose confidential data is, at least, reversible.
2. Remember that the owner of the privilege to keep information confidential is the patient, not the doctor. If the patient is willing to release the data, the physician may not ethically decide to withhold it even "for the patient's own good."
3. Apply the concept of confidentiality equally to all patients despite the physician's assessment of their goals, mores, and lifestyles. A physician cannot ethically inform an insurer of suspicions that a patient is trying to defraud an insurer or that a young man is trying to use a medical excuse to evade the draft.
4. Be familiar with the local statutes including federal, state, and local law plus ordinances, rules, regulations, and administrative decrees of various agencies such as public health departments.
5. When required to divulge a confidence, discuss the situation with the patient. When obligations to society conflict with those of the patient, the physician should discuss the conflict with the patient. When legal guidelines are absent or vague, the criteria of decision are the immediacy and degree of danger to either the patient or society.
6. Get written authorization from the patient before divulging information. To meet standard situations such as requests from third parties, have the patient sign a blanket authorization in advance to release pertinent data to specific third parties.

Beck, Leif C., "Patient Information—When and When Not to Divulge,"
Patient Care 72:60 (April 15, 1972)

Information should not be released unless the request is specific. The request should have time limits, identify the purposes for which the records will be used, and identify the particular information requested. When records are sent to another party, making an extra copy of the information released and marking it in the record with the note of authorization documents the matter. It is important to check the credentials of the person and/or organization requesting information from the record.

Capacity to Consent to Release of Information

Any patient who has reached the age of majority can consent to the release of medical records. If a former patient is dead, the executor, administrator, or personal representative may release the record. If an adult patient is temporarily unable to consent, a court-appointed guardian has authorization. If an attorney is authorized by a patient to view a record, the patient need not be of sound mind at the time the decision to consent is made. In an emergency, a record may be released to the extent necessary without consent, because the emergency creates the power to act.

Minors have particular problems with regard to the release of medical information. In a drug abuse or sexually transmitted disease diagnosis, only the minor involved can release the record, even to his or her parents or guardians. Normally, a parent or guardian can release the minor's records until the minor reaches majority. If one parent has been awarded custody of the minor, it is preferable to get that parent to release the medical information. The mature minor doctrine allows minors to release their records under certain circumstances: when they are living away from home, self-supporting, or married. Under certain conditions, when a minor knows the nature, quality, and consequences of his or her act, a medical record can be released on the minor's authorization.

Release of Information to the Legal Profession

Attorneys need information from medical records under many circumstances. If there is likelihood that medical malpractice charges will be brought against a physician, an attorney will usually ask to examine the records prior to going to court. By responding indifferently to a lawyer's request for records, a physician frequently causes problems. The attorney may find that it is cheaper to file the lawsuit and engage in formal discovery than to pay exorbitant fees for photocopying records or having the physician prepare a medical report. This attitude hardens feelings between attorneys and physicians. Attorneys expect that a physician will charge for a report based on the time spent in preparing it, as well as office and secretarial time. A report cannot be withheld pending payment of the patient's bill to a physician or a hospital.

> Caution is advised in the handling of record which contain information concerning:
>
> - illegitimacy of birth
> - sexually transmitted diseases
> - mental illness or retardation
> - alcoholism/alcohol tests
> - drug dependence, addiction, or abuse
> - AIDS/HIV testing
> - sexual assaults
> - abortion
> - communications to social workers, psychotherapists, psychologists, family or marriage counselors, or other mental health advisors
> - other information that would tend to embarrass a patient.
>
> Wagg, Dorothy, "Medical Records Basic," p. 17.
> Massachusetts Hospital Association (August 24, 1995)

Release Forms

A simple oral request or telephone call is insufficient to properly bring about the release of medical records. The request must be in writing. When the information requested is disclosed, it must be accompanied by a note forbidding redisclosure. The following are suggested forms authorizing the release of medical information:

APPROVAL FOR RELEASE OF MEDICAL INFORMATION

Date:

I hereby authorize Dr/Hospital/HMO/other (identify) _____
_____ to release
the following information for the following purpose: (indicate any limitations)

1. Medical Records including history and diagnosis.
2. Records of Outpatient treatment. (Inclusive dates)
3. Records of Inpatient treatment. (Inclusive dates)
4. Medical records including psychiatric records. (Inclusive dates)
5. Psychiatric records limited as follows:

I understand that I have a right to inspect and copy any information for release by me. I also have the right to revoke approval of release of information at any time.

This is a (   ) one time release or a (   ) continuing release. Please check.

Please send this information to the following:

Name _____

Address _____

_____

Signature: _____

Address: _____

TO: FROM:

1. You are hereby granted my permission to release oral and written reports from the records of the above named individual to:

2. It is my understanding that this record may contain information about my diagnosis and treatment of any physical or mental illness or reference pertaining to alcohol and/or drug abuse.

3. This authorization is for the purpose of preparing ————————— report and is limited to disclosure for that purpose only.

4. This authorization is to expire two months from the date of signing and is subject to revocation at any time by a notice in writing before that time unless action on it has already begun.

5. A photocopy of this authorization shall be valid as the original.

Signature: _____
          (patient)

Date: _____

Signature: _____
          (parent or guardian)

Address of patient: _____

_____

Telephone Number: _____ Witness: _____

Date: _____

To compel the production of documents, both a court order and a **subpoena** are necessary. A subpoena is a command to appear at a certain time and place to give testimony upon a certain matter. The particular type of subpoena used for documents is called a **subpoena duces tecum.** It identifies the records that are requested in court. Legal subpoenas and court orders do not require the release of all requested medical information. When sensitive information about patients and other persons has been requested without consent of the parties, the issues can be discussed with the judge and attorneys. The judge may then make the decision to review the material privately to determine whether it should be allowed into evidence.

CREDIBILITY OF THE MEDICAL RECORD

Credibility of a medical record refers to whether the information recorded in the record is believable. An article written for lawyers informing them how to recognize a good medical malpractice case (one they can win) stated the following:

> If you take on a case where the doctor or the hospital changes something in the records, you will need less than the usual quantum of fault to prevail before a jury. The same is true if a record or x-ray is missing. Even a change that the doctor argues was made for a good faith reason or a record lost with the explanation, "fire," "flood" or "robbery," will suggest to the jury that there was a guilty motive afoot—and there probably was.
>
> Gage, S.M., "Alteration, Falsification and Fabrication of Medical Records in Medical Malpractice Actions," *Medical Trial Quarterly* 27:476 (Spring 1981)

> Inadequate, missing or improper documentation can be red flags to a plaintiff's attorney. They are likely to look for (1) holes [a break in the information], (2) missing pieces, (3) conclusory statements and (4) contradictory statements.
>
> Ryan, John, "Dispelling Common Myths about Documentation: Advice from a Defense Attorney," *Forum* (Harvard Risk Management Foundation)

The credibility of the medical record is crucial in the defense of a physician, medical facility, or employee. Medical information is needed to try cases in nearly every area of law. The **Federal Rules of Evidence** allow the medical record to be introduced into evidence under the Uniform Business Records Act.

When a client comes to an attorney with a complaint about medical care, the lawyer obtains any medical records available and has them reviewed by an independent physician. The second physician's evaluation may prompt the attorney to further investigate the potential malpractice claim or to convince the client that malpractice did not occur. Sometimes attorneys find that they can settle with a potential defendant or the insurance company before filing a malpractice suit if the evidence is in their client's favor.

The credibility of the record-keeping procedure is subject to question when investigation reveals delayed filing of laboratory test results, incomplete files, illegible records, altered or fabricated records, or the loss or concealment of information. On the other hand, the search is satisfied if the potential doctor is "let off the hook" and the client is informed that there is no basis for a case. The following are office procedures that have caused problems for defendant-doctors.

Delayed Filing of Laboratory Tests

Sixty-seven closed claims with a diagnosis of melanoma were reviewed by the Aetna Life and Casualty Company. Failure to diagnose was the most common allegation in the claims, and the doctor's office was the setting most often identified as the site of the alleged malpractice. The study suggested that the flow of medical reports, such as X-ray readings, may be a factor in malpractice suits involving malignancy. In four cases, the doctor who ordered an X-ray study did not see the final positive radiology report—the one that probably would have led to earlier diagnosis and treatment. For example:

> A 78-year-old woman was evaluated by an internist for recurrent indigestion. The radiologist's report suggested the presence of a small soft tissue mass below the left diaphragm, but the patient did not call the physician's office to ask about the result as she had been told to. The physician did not see the results until approximately eight weeks later. An upper G.I. series confirmed the diagnosis. Surgical exploration and biopsy disclosed the unresectable reticulum cell sarcoma of the stomach. The patient died within six weeks. The original report may have been placed in the patient's file during the physician's vacation.
>
> Mittleman, Michael, "What Are the Chances When
> Malignancy Leads to a Malpractice Suit?"
> *Legal Aspects of Medical Practice,* p. 42 (February 1980)

Incomplete Files

> A 48-year-old woman, by self-examination, discovered a mass in the right breast. In an office visit, the physician noted the mass was olive sized and just above the nipple. At the recheck examination, two weeks later, the primary

complaint of the patient was a headache. The breast was unchanged. Because of financial problems, the physician advised the patient to attend a free clinic. At the next office visit, the breast was not examined. Two months later, another physician performed a radical mastectomy because of infiltrating ductal carcinoma with axillary metastases. The original medical records from the doctor's office were difficult to read and incomplete.

Mittleman, Michael, "What Are the Chances When
Malignancy Leads to a Malpractice Suit?"
Legal Aspects of Medical Practice, p. 42 (February 1980)

Illegible Records

It's rumored that there is a secret course in most medical schools called, "Scribbling for Beginners," and word has it that most students score an A+.

Graedon, J., *The People's Pharmacy,* p. 2 (1980)

Although the handwriting of physicians is the butt of many jokes, it is a potentially serious hazard to patients. Drs. Karen B. White and John F. Beany, III, of Georgetown University Hospital in Washington, D.C., screened the handwriting of fifty physicians in patient charts and concluded that "a considerable portion of most handwritten medical records are illegible, which confirms the common but unpublished wisdom on this subject." They found that sixteen percent of the words in reports were illegible, as were eighty percent of the doctors' signatures. Because of poor penmanship, forty-two percent of the patient reports could not be fully understood. Every month *Pharmacy Times* reproduces examples of illegible prescriptions, and the editors caution readers to phone physicians if there is the slightest doubt about what is being prescribed.

Altered Medical Records

If a record damns a doctor, he or she may be strongly tempted to change it. For the change to stand up, all other people involved—doctors, nurses, administrators—have to go along with it. Somewhere along the line the chain is almost bound to snap. Altered records demostrate the defendant's consciousness of wrongdoing and strongly establish liability. If a jury learns that a doctor has intentionally altered a record, they will award much larger damages. The insurance companies are well aware of this. It is no coincidence that when lawyers discover that a doctor has tampered with records, they immediately move to settle, as in the first case presented on the following page.

Another case was settled when a different diagnosis was written over an existing one in a hospital record. When this was brought to the attention of the doctor, he claimed that the nurse had made an error and that he had promptly corrected it. It was an easy task for experts to determine when ink met paper, and while the analyzing process was going on, the case was settled. The record was fifteen years old.

A 23-year-old woman was admitted for delivery of her first child and was administered a spinal anesthetic by the obstetrician. Her chart indicated that her blood pressure was normal when the anesthesia was given and no change was indicated until the "moment her infant delivered." At that time a "heart stat" emergency was called, and artificial respiration and other resuscitative efforts were promptly instituted to restore breathing and heart rhythm.

Photocopies of the mother's hospital record showed close monitoring of the patient—consistent with the defendant's claim of no malpractice. As the litigation continued, plaintiff's counsel sent out a photocopy service to obtain the baby's chart. The record contained a carbon copy of the delivery room record from the mother's chart. Although these records were duplicates of the originals, comparing the two revealed that significant alterations had been made in the mother's chart. The carbon copy revealed these alterations and demonstrated that the defendants were guilty of malpractice.

Gage, S.M., "Alteration, Falsification and Fabrication of
Medical Records in Medical Malpractice Actions,"
Medical Trial Quarterly 27:476 (Spring 1981)

Fabricating Medical Records

Altering medical records modifies the content of the record, while fabricating records means inventing a story. The motive is faking or forging a document or signature. What follows are true examples of fabrication:

In a situation where a patient suffered gross deformity of a leg and loss of joint function at the knee following treatment by an orthopedic surgeon, the physician attempted to construct a record. During discovery, the doctor chose to answer written interrogatories by allegedly attaching his medical records and continually referring to those records as his answer to questions. There were no office records accompanying the answers and this matter was pursued on deposition. At the deposition, he produced medical records, including a medical chart that appeared fresh and unused in relation to the length of time since the accident and the number of office visits. The chart was date-stamped for each patient visit, and written in three different kinds of ink to give the appearance of preparation on each date listed. The doctor did not produce the original office records at the deposition, stating that they were lost or misplaced. During the proceeding, the doctor physically grabbed the records from the plaintiff's attorney, removed them from the custody of the court reporter, and left. Needless to say, the case was settled out of court.

Gage, S.M., "Alteration, Falsification and Fabrication of
Medical Records in Medical Malpractice Actions,"
Medical Trial Quarterly 27:476 (Spring 1981)

> A physician claimed he had given a drug sensitivity test to a child and commented that his office record would so indicate. Because the plaintiff was a child, the suit had been delayed for five years. At the time the doctor's deposition was taken, the attorney asked for the right to examine the case from the patient's file because he wanted to find out when the paper had been manufactured. At times it has been determined that the paper was not in existence on the date shown on the entry. In this case the defense decided to settle.
>
> Preiser, S.E., "The High Cost of Tampering with Medical Records,"
> *Medical Economics,* p. 85 (October 4, 1976)

Loss and Concealment of Records

Related to the alteration of medical records is the destruction, unavailability, or loss of relevant X-rays, laboratory test results, and other physical evidence. To give an example, counsel for the plaintiff in the following case decided that the original patient's chart was needed after careful review of a photocopy of the records revealed evidence of modifications and inserts in the original reports:

> Spacing, wording and other factors indicated that a handwriting expert would be in order to examine the original records. On the day of the deposition, the original records were produced, but in a totally obliterated fashion. Defense counsel reported that the night before the deposition his youngster had taken the records and dropped them into a puddle of mud. By the time they could be retrieved, he reported, they were completely spoiled, unintelligible and obviously unsuitable for a documentation expert to review. The case was settled out of court since such conduct is in violation of law and criminal in nature.
>
> Gage, S.M., "Alteration, Falsification and Fabrication of
> Medical Records in Medical Malpractice Actions,"
> *Medical Trial Quarterly* 27:476 (Spring 1981)

Medical records may also be summoned in fraud situations where a physician claims excessive amounts from insurance companies or welfare agencies, as in the following:

> Dr. Emanuel Stolman, a diplomat of the Academy of Family Physicians, had practiced for over twenty-five years when he was indicted in 1976 on twenty-three felony counts of illegally receiving state funds from the Medi-Cal program. Dr. Stolman's method of treatment was a folksy sort of approach, and did not match the rigid bookkeeping methods required by the state. The main question was whether or not Dr. Stolman was present in hospitals and nursing homes on the

dates he claimed he had examined patients. At issue was whether Dr. Stolman altered his records when he discovered the state was investigating him.

Dr. Stolman followed the motto, "Patients, not Paper," and had been writing pulse counts and blood pressure measurements from memory as long as a week later. He stated that he had a good memory, and would write prescriptions for patients from memory within a week's time after a visit. Dr. Stolman's memory became difficult for nurses, ward clerks and medical records clerks to verify during the ten-week trial. The entire medical community went on trial with Dr. Stolman as discrepancies surfaced in records in nursing homes, extended care facilities, hospitals and within the doctor's office.

C. Jean Poulos, "A Case of Fraud,"
The Professional Medical Assistant, p. 14 (May/June 1987)

Legal Implications of Record Tampering

The medical record is the doctor's only **forum** for defense. The medical record gives the physician the opportunity to say accurately what occurred and why. Changing this document after the fact infers that the doctor knew the patient suffered because of negligent acts previously recorded in the medical record. Changing a record will usually result in a **settlement** prior to trial. If not, and the incident is made known to the judge or jury, the awards of money damages are higher, and there may be an additional cause of action for the recovery of punitive damages.

Acceptable Method of Making Changes in Medical Records

Altered records are likely to be the object of disparaging innuendo by a skilled lawyer. Consider what a jury might conclude from the following questions and answers:

Lawyer: "Please read your first entry from January 2 at 10 A.M."
Defendant: "I'm sorry, but I can't."
Lawyer: "You can't?"
Defendant: "No."
Lawyer: "Why is that?"
Defendant: "Well, I crossed that part out."
Lawyer: "You did more than cross it out. You completely obliterated it, didn't you?"
Defendant: "Yes."
Lawyer: "And will you tell us why you obliterated your own notes?"
Defendant: "Well, I think I'd made a mistaken entry."
Lawyer: "You think? You mean you're not sure? Could it be that rather than a mistaken entry, you instead made a medical error, charted it, and then, in anticipation of this lawsuit, decided to obliterate the evidence?"

Defendant: "No. I just wanted to correct a mistaken entry."
Lawyer: "But you did completely obliterate the entry, didn't you?"
Defendant: "Yes, but . . ."
Lawyer: "And it isn't readable at all, is it?"
Defendant: "No . . ."
Lawyer: "If it was merely a mistaken entry, as you would have the jury believe, why did you have to totally obliterate it?"
Defendant: "Well, I suppose I didn't have to."

To avoid even the possibility of such an attack, accompany any alteration with an explanation and date of change and leave the previous entry legible. And don't throw any records away.

Bergerson, Stephen R., "Charting with a Jury in Mind," *Nursing*, p. 5 (1984)

There are occasions when making a change in a patient's records is necessary. If the changes are made while the patient is under treatment, they may be accepted as rewritten. But if the changes are made beyond a reasonable period of time following discharge, particularly after a physician or hospital is on notice of a potential lawsuit, changes in the medical record are almost always serious.

If correction is necessary to achieve accuracy, the following procedure is recommended:

The best way to indicate an entry correction is to leave the original recordation intact with a single line drawn through the entry being corrected. An initialed notation with date and time should be made in the side margin indicating that the entry was in error. The correction should be entered in the record chronologically.

Hirsh, H.L., "Tampering with Medical Records," *Medical Trial Quarterly* 24:450 (Spring 1978)

It is the responsibility of individuals charged with keeping medical records to be accurate. They must bring any error in record keeping to the attention of the physician at the time it is discovered, as well as any ambiguous section that may affect the reader's understanding. It is the physician's responsibility to correct his or her own error. Keeping good notes is as important to the doctor as the diagnosis. If the keeper of the record is in dispute with a physician, the facts should be recorded and, it is suggested, reviewed by a neutral third professional. The doctor is ultimately responsible; the assistant is responsible only if negligent in the performance or omission of assigned duties, or if **conspiring** to defraud.

SUMMARY

The owner of a medical record is the facility that generates the record; a hospital record is owned by a hospital, and an office record by the physician or corporation that owns the medical practice. Each facility has a medical record that is adequate to meet its own needs.

Medical records and information concerning patients are subject to the laws of privacy. The physician-patient relationship is one protected from disclosure by privileged communication. Whatever privilege or privacy requirement is made of a physician is also extended to the office personnel and other delegated employees.

Patients often wish to see their records. The medical profession is split as to whether a patient should have access to his or her medical record. In some states, legislatures have enacted laws requiring hospitals and other health care facilities to allow patients to see their records. Permission to see medical records is not absolute and depends upon the reason behind the patient's request. Physicians are required to transfer medical information to other physicians engaged by their patients and to allow attorneys access to records of their clients. Contents of a medical record should not be transferred without a release of information by the patient.

Records are often required in court and are demanded by the issuance of a subpoena duces tecum. The subpoena must be accompanied by a court order with the information required clearly spelled out.

Medical records must be credible. This means that there can be no alterations, fabrications, or concealments in a record. If a change must be made, a single line should be drawn through the error with the date of the change and the initials of the person making it. A medical record is a legal document. Tampering with the record will bring legal sanctions. Sanctions are designed to secure enforcement of the law by imposing a penalty for violation of the law.

SUGGESTED ACTIVITY

Draft a letter for a fictitious patient who has requested a copy of her medical records. Include a copy of an appropriate release form. Type the letter.

STUDY QUESTIONS

1. List the content of a medical record.
2. Discuss the difference between ownership of a medical record and ownership of other property.

3. A patient requests his X-rays to take home and show to the family. Role play how you would handle this matter.

4. Privacy means many different things in a medical setting. Distinguish between the patient's right to physical privacy and privacy under privileged communication.

5. As a medical assistant, privileged communication extends to your knowledge of the patient. Your office has a famous celebrity as a patient. A well-known newspaper reporter calls and asks you to go to lunch with her. How will you handle this matter?

6. Your office has a strict policy with regard to release of information in medical records, and despite a state statute allowing patients access to their records, the physicians you work for will not give patients their records. An obnoxious attorney storms into the office and demands access to your files. The patient has signed a release form. You are at the front desk and the office is full of patients. What do you do?

7. Your office has a relaxed policy with regard to the release of information in medical records. A patient asks to see his record. You know that there is information in the record concerning telephone calls from the patient's relatives that would interfere with the family relationship. The physician is away for a week. How would you handle the matter?

8. A record has been subpoenaed and a court order accompanies it. The doctor has removed important parts of the record. You know that this information is missing. The office sends you to court as the keeper of the record. You must testify about the completeness of the record. What are you going to say?

9. There is an error in a medical record that has been subpoenaed. This is a good-faith error and should be corrected. It has to do with the information the plaintiff is interested in and could be damaging to the defendant-doctor if changed, but also damaging if unchanged. The doctor asks you to blot out the error, write in the correct information and put the paper, with surrounding papers, through the copy machine. What do you do?

CASES FOR DISCUSSION

1. The plaintiff's physician received a release of information from the plaintiff to an insurance company following the plaintiff's application for major medical insurance. The physician released the following information:

> Enclosed is a summary of Mr. Millsaps's recent hospitalization. Physically the man has no notable problems; emotionally, the patient is quite mercurial in his moods. He is a strong-willed man obsessed with faults of others in his family, for which there has been no objective basis. He has completely resisted any

constructive advice by his wife, family, minister, or myself. The man needs psychiatric help for his severe obsessions and depressions, some of which have suicidal overtones. He is an extremely poor insurance risk.

The application for major medical insurance was rejected. Did the physician have a right to release this information to the insurance company?

2. The plaintiff was committed to the Hastings State Hospital by order of the Probate Court, which found him to be "mentally ill—inebriate." The commitment petition was brought by the plaintiff's mother, apparently in order to secure treatment for him for a developing drug and alcohol problem. Several attempts at voluntary treatment, prior to the commitment proceedings, had proved unsuccessful. Shortly after admission, the plaintiff allegedly attempted to strangle a member of the hospital staff and was transferred to the Security Hospital. Upon admission to the Security Hospital, the plaintiff was diagnosed with simple schizophrenia. He was treated with tranquilizing and anti-depressant medications but apparently failed to improve. Consent was sought from the plaintiff's mother to administer electroshock treatment. Consent was not given, but the mother did request the consultation of a second psychiatrist, who concurred with the doctors at Security Hospital. Without the consent of the plaintiff or his mother, electroshock treatment was begun. Did this treatment without consent invade the patient's privacy?

3. The defendant was executive director of Planned Parenthood. A second defendant was the physician who served as medical director for Planned Parenthood. Both gave information, instruction, and medical advice to married persons about how to prevent conception. The defendants were arrested and found guilty of violating a statute that forbade the use of contraceptives. They then appealed, contending that the statute as applied violated the Fourteenth Amendment. Does a law forbidding the use of contraceptives invade the zone of privacy in violation of the due process clause of the Fourteenth Amendment?

4. The patient alleged that the defendant physician fraudulently and negligently advised her that she had a brain tumor that required immediate surgery, that the doctor negligently performed an unneeded craniotomy on her at the hospital, and that the doctor had held staff surgical privileges at the hospital on a continuing basis. The plaintiff patient further alleged several theories against the hospital. Underlying these was the contention that the hospital had sufficient prior information to be put on notice that the defendant physician was an incompetent, overaggressive neurosurgeon with a history of performing unnecessary operations, particularly elective craniotomies. The court ordered the hospital to produce copies of all preoperative consultations, operative notes, interpretations of preoperative X-rays, and brain tissue analyses obtained on 140 patients. Included in the order were provisions to ensure the privacy

of the patients. The hospital refused the records on the grounds that consent had not been obtained from any of the 140 patients and the production order was in violation of the physician-patient privilege statute. Should the appeals court agree with the hospital?

5. Following a visit to a physician's office, the doctor wrote the patient a letter informing her that she had a sexually transmitted disease. The patient showed the letter to two or three friends. When the physician came to her home to talk with her about it, a friend was visiting her, and the patient discussed the matter in the presence of the physician and the friend. The patient then sued the physician for breach of confidentiality. Did the doctor breach her confidentiality?

6. The plaintiff was seen by a physician for a blocked tear duct. During the treatment, an instrument brushed her cornea with resulting abrasions. Following the incident, the plaintiff's daughter, who was a nurse, requested permission to review the physician's records. After seeing the records, the plaintiff filed against the physician. At the trial, the daughter testified that her mother's records, which she had seen in the physician's office, had been materially altered by the time they were admitted into evidence. It was also noted that a visit that the patient made after the accident was not documented in the record. Should the court presume from this testimony that there was negligence?

7. A patient came to the emergency room of the hospital complaining of nausea and chest pains. The nurse on duty refused to call a physician, determining that there was no need at that time. The patient died of a myocardial infarction minutes after leaving the hospital. The widow's attorney attempted to review the records during discovery but found that they had been destroyed. Could the court presume from this information that there was negligence?

Chapter 8

Introduction to Ethics

There is no country in the world in which everything can be provided for by the laws, or in which political institutions can prove a substitute for common sense and public morality.

Alexis de Tocqueville

OBJECTIVES:

After reading this chapter, you should be able to:

1. distinguish between law, morals, ethics, and etiquette.
2. appraise the impact of economics in the making of ethical decisions.
3. analyze conflict between personal and professional ethics.
4. discuss the importance of studying ethics.
5. develop a thought process for making ethical decisions.

BUILDING YOUR LEGAL VOCABULARY

amoral	etiquette	shibboleths
bioethics	immoral	teleological
deontological	philosophy	values
ethics	politics	virtue

Ethical dilemmas are found in every aspect of health care delivery. The study of law in the last few chapters has introduced the process of thinking legally as well as applying legal doctrine to real life situations in a health care setting. The study of **ethics** is related to, yet distinguished from, the study of law. For example, consider the following editorial published in *The Baltimore Sun* on June 6, 1987:

We are appalled that Baltimore City firefighters who tried to save the life of a wounded, pregnant woman they rushed to the Johns Hopkins Emergency Room were exposed to the AIDS virus—and no one let them know. Only through the compassion of one nurse at Hopkins, where the woman [patient] was also receiving obstetrical care, did the message finally get to the firefighters.

The men returned home that night—back to their wives and their children—and might never have known. Might never have been tested. Might have exposed the virus to someone else.

Hopkins authorities explain that doctor-patient confidentiality laws tied the hospital's hands. Dandy! What kind of ludicrous system have we created where confidentiality protections for a dead person carry greater weight than society's concern for the living?

One can sympathize with the plight of the firefighters, the concerns of the nurse, and the implications of the men returning to their families without the knowledge that they had been exposed to AIDS, but the legal issue embedded in the firefighters' story is confidentiality. First, even though the woman died, the nurse breached the confidentiality of the patient. Death does not dissolve legal obligation. Second, society imposed sanctions for breaking the law. The consequences may be loss of job, possible suspension of license to practice, certainly a letter of reprimand in an employment file, and/or the possibility of litigation or payment of damages if the victim or survivors decide to sue.

The story also illustrates an ethical dilemma, the conflict between a nurse's concern for the public's health and her professional code of ethics. Conflict surfaces, for example, if the nurse applies the personal ethic of the Golden Rule: "Do unto others what you would have them do to you." It may be argued that under the Golden Rule, the nurse has an ethical obligation to inform the firefighters of their exposure to the infectious disease, AIDS. It may also be argued that the nurse had an obligation to her patient to keep her secret.

The law allows exceptions to confidentiality. For example, statutes exist that require physicians to report certain contagious diseases such as syphilis, measles, meningitis, and AIDS. A physician must report gunshot wounds, child abuse, and other victim abuses. Does mandated reporting of the disease to authorities include informing other involved parties? What is the nurse's ethical obligation to the public's health? Does obligation to the public overshadow obligation to a single patient? These questions represent only a few of the issues raised by the situation described above.

ETHICS

The study of ethics is grounded theoretically in **philosophy,** which can be defined broadly as the pursuit of wisdom. The word is derived from the Greek term *ethos,* meaning custom, usage, or character. Ethics referred traditionally to a custom of a particular community and evolved to include standards of good or bad and questions of moral duty and obligation.

There are two major classifications of ethical theories: **deontological** and **teleological.** The term *deontological* comes from the Greek term *deonotos,* which means duty or obligation. Two major deontological ethical theories are the divine command theory and Kant's "categorical imperative." Within this ethical system, decisions are based on the intrinsic right or wrong of an action rather than on the consequences of an action. The term *teleological* originates from the Greek words *telos,* which means end, and *logos,* which means words or sayings. Teleological theories of ethics concern themselves with outcomes—whether the results of an action produce greater good in the world. Today ethical studies frequently involve both personal understanding of what is right and wrong and appropriate behavior.

The study of **bioethics** deals with ethical implications of biological research and applications, especially in medicine (medical ethics). Medical ethics applies both deontological and teleological ideas to daily medical practices, to conflicts between theories and positions, to questions involving traditional ethical positions and threats posed by modern medical technology, and to the interaction between ethical constraints and the law.

Distinguishing between legal and ethical issues is difficult. Ethical dilemmas in medicine occur when the enforcement of law does not appear to bring about justice, where there is no obvious right or wrong behavior, when right behavior appears to have the wrong effect, or when personal sacrifice is the consequence of following ideals. Studying ethics involves examining emotions, reasoning, and constitutional issues of freedom and personal responsibility.

Some people may perceive being ill as a degrading and dehumanizing experience and may view themselves to be at the mercy of the physician. Because of the perceived unequal status of physician and patient, ethical constraints are necessary. In the United States, individual privacy and an individual's right to make decisions is highly valued. As a result, ethical codes restrain a physician's right to take action without informing and receiving consent from the patient. To touch a patient without permission changes the physician's action from ethical misbehavior to a legal claim of battery and/or negligence. Breaking ethical codes results in the disapproval of at least a segment of society, but breaking legal codes results in penalties enforced by the law.

MORALS

Morals are recognized as principles of "right" conduct. Right moral conduct is based on traditional religious teachings found in Judeo-Christian, Buddhist, Islamic, and other traditions and cannot be separated from these thought systems without distorting its meaning. The term *moral* is sometimes used as a word of praise, as in "she is a very moral person," but on other occasions it has a much broader meaning, taking into consideration the

virtues of courage, wisdom, balance, or fairness. Morally bad actions are characterized by opposite qualities. Behavior that goes against morals is known as **immoral;** behavior that does not take moral principles into consideration is known as **amoral.**

In 1992, the Lakeberg twins, who shared a defective heart, were separated at the parents' request despite the fact that doing so would inevitably result in one child's death. The family followed Islamic religious traditions.

In an Islamic society, religious traditions and values guide such decisions. Although the desires of the parents and the advice of medical experts are considered, powerful cultural influences ultimately determine the course of events. In Saudi Arabia, sharia law, shaped by the Koran, governs everyday life. Making the unique decision about whether Nura and Sarah [the twins] should be separated required the opinions of religious leaders and scholars at various judicial levels in Saudi Arabia. They were asked to interpret and apply the precepts and guidance of the Koran to this case and make an appropriate judgment.

The twins' primary physician first contacted the Islamic Opinion Committee (IOC), a religious advisory group established to handle cases such as this one. The IOC instructed the doctor to complete all the feasibility studies on the separation and to form a medical committee that would make a final recommendation. If the medical findings indicated that the twins could be viably separated, the surgery could take place under Islamic law. But if the medical committee decided that one or both of the twins were likely to die as a result of separation, the IOC would review the case further in light of Islamic religious beliefs. It could well have ruled against surgery.

"The Lakeberg Siamese Twins: Were Risks,
Costs of Separation Justified?,"
Medical Ethics Advisor 9(10):121

Right conduct for a person practicing in the Islamic tradition follows Islamic Law and is a matter requiring a moral decision. Determining whether an operation will be conducted to separate the twins, and which twin will live if a decision has to be made terminating the life of one of the two individuals, is moral in its substance. Unless the consequence of practicing within sharia law is in conflict with the law of the United States Constitution or the state in which the situation occurs, it is moral to follow the practice advocated by those affected by the decision. It would be immoral for the parents to go against the tenets of their religion if religion is a stronghold in their life. It is difficult to make an argument for or against amorality in this matter because the morality of the clinical decision makers would have to be taken into consideration along with that of the parents. A situation like the separation of the Lakeberg Siamese twins might end up in court and be subject to the decision of the judge if the parties cannot agree on a course of action.

In United States society, because it is a "melting pot," ideas about right moral conduct may differ widely and cause the terms *moral* and *ethical* to have several different meanings. In general, ethics provides a framework within which right and wrong can be studied. When one group attempts to enforce its concept of right conduct on others, a **political process** occurs. In contrast, an ethical solution to moral differences occurs when the conscience, or that "still small voice within," activates a sense of moral obligation within an individual.

ETIQUETTE

Etiquette is the socially accepted procedure for interacting in society and changes with the times and the community. It does not require moral understanding or ethical reasoning even though it is based on societal laws, morals, customs, and beliefs. Etiquette requires that one behave in a specific manner in a given situation. For example, Emily Post's *Book of Etiquette* spells out the etiquette for preparing a family wedding. Each military branch has highly developed customs and rituals requiring strict adherence to their codes of etiquette.

A less structured code of medical etiquette and protocol exists for those working in the health care community. Politeness, proper dress, and courtesy are at its core. Etiquette extends privileges to other medical professionals. For example, a physician will usually instruct staff to put through all calls immediately from other physicians. A physician will rarely bill another physician for more than an amount covered by insurance. In addition, individual medical offices have their own etiquette for staff to follow.

Telephone etiquette is at the core of medical office management. Failure to adhere to a patient-centered telephone ethic results in dissatisfied patients and families who express negative comments and who can affect the entire health-delivery process.

ETHICAL ENVIRONMENT OF MANAGED CARE

In the past, our economic system, based on supply and demand, has operated to regulate the health care system. When demand exceeded supply, the cost determined who could afford access to what services. In 1946, the Hill-Burton Act provided millions of dollars for the construction of hospitals. Hospitals built with Hill-Burton money were required to provide a "reasonable volume of services . . . to persons unable to pay." Although a universal health insurance bill was never passed, in the 1960s, Medicare and Medicaid amendments to the social security legislation were enacted with the intent of ensuring access to health care for all the elderly and poor. The 1983 report of the President's Commission, "Securing Access to Health Care," concluded that society has a moral obligation to ensure equitable medical care. Equitable health care infers that medical care is a right. This requires adjustment in thinking and practice from treating the poor only in emergency situations to treating them as normal, fee-paying patients. It also leads to an overall increase in the cost of health care.

If you promise everyone broad access to medical care you will enormously increase the total amount the nation spends on health care. . . . Most economists agree that the need to contain medical costs is absolute and urgent. The questions that divide us involve how it should be done. So far, the experts and policy makers in Washington have been focusing on the deficiencies and failures of modern medicine; greedy pharmaceutical and insurance companies (not to mention physicians); unnecessary procedures and bureaucratic inefficiency; expensive technologies, etc. . . . The **shibboleths** that identify their approach include managed care, health maintenance organizations and managed competition. Implicit in their recommendations is the assumption that the elimination of waste will obviate the need for rationing health care. It will not.

Gaylin, Willard, "Faulty Diagnosis,"
New York Times, sec. 4A, p. 1 (June 12, 1994)

Managed care is synonymous with managing costs. In order to manage costs, managed care organizations must participate in making patient care decisions. Key to making decisions is the identification of what is to be decided. One problem fundamental to the financing of health care is the definition of health care.

Health Care versus Medical Care

Defining health care is a fundamental problem that affects decisions about financing health care. The World Health Organization (WHO) defines health as "a state of complete physical, mental, and social well-being, and not merely the absence of disease or infirmity." The WHO definition describes a utopia that may be an unrealistic goal and includes medical care within the broad definition of health care. Being healthy is a subjective state and means different things to different people. Being ill and requiring medical care to function is easier to objectively determine. As Willard Gaylin writes:

We also have to recognize that health today does not mean what it did a hundred years ago. My reading glasses, for example, are paid for by a health insurer, based on the diagnosis of presbyopia (an eye "disease") made by an ophthalmologist. Before the invention of the lens there was no such disease as presbyopia; there were also no ophthalmologists. A decline in faculties was simply part of the aging process; with age, sight would be impaired or lost, as would hearing, potency and fertility.

The vast expansion of the concept of health can be demonstrated in surgery, orthopedics, mental health, gynecology—indeed, in any field of medicine. People do not have operations on their knees or elbows merely to continue to be employable, for example; most of us do not work at jobs requiring physical strength.

> Many such operations are performed strictly so that the patient can continue to lead a "normal" life, to be able to play golf or ski. Are these justifiable medical expenses? If one is free of pain except on the tennis court, is one "ill"?
>
> Gaylin, Willard, "Faulty Diagnosis,"
> *New York Times* sec. 4A, p. 1 (June 12, 1994)

Preventive medicine straddles the dividing line between health care and medical care. Preventing illness with inoculations against communicable disease is important to the whole of society, as well as the individual. It can easily be objectively classified as medical care. It makes sense to allow society to allocate funds and personnel to prevent communicable diseases. However, in matters of prevention of illness by controlling diet, smoking, exercise, driving habits, stress, and the like, there is too much subjective personal preference to allow a clear-cut classification. On the other hand, not caring for these aspects of health may cost society more in the long run because neglect may result in the development of an expensive disease. Also competing for a piece of the health care pie are alternative medical providers such as chiropractors, acupuncturists, herbal healers, massage therapists, and so on.

The American public is interested in health. Newspapers, books, television, and politicians comment on health. This interest in health concerns has led to what some writers call the "medicalization" of American society where all social and personal problems are considered within the realm of physicians' expertise. As a result:

> physicians exercise control over such diverse matters as the dispensation of drugs, pregnancy and childbirth, sexual activity, growing old, the treatment of the dying and determination of death, access to and the use of hospitals, health certification for jobs, absences from work, for insurance and for disability compensation, and so on.
>
> Ladd, John "The Concepts of Health and Disease
> and Their Ethical Implication," in Gruzalski and Nelson (Eds.),
> *Value Conflicts in Healthcare Delivery,* p. 23.
> Ballinger Publishing Company (1982)

Private Choice versus Common Good

Increasing the number of individuals covered by medical insurance and ensuring coverage to a larger number of people requires certain restrictions, including limiting a patient's choice of medical providers. There is usually a short time to choose a primary care physician when entering a plan and few opportunities to change a primary care physician if either the physician or the patient is unhappy with the arrangement. Choice of a specialist, if needed, must be from the confines of a plan's accepted list, with no opportunity provided for evaluation by physicians outside the plan unless prior provisions are written within the managed care contact. These conditions might result in the following scenario:

The doctors at Karin Smith's health maintenance organization kept telling her she was fine. She knew that wasn't true. She was sick and getting sicker. Frustrated and frightened, she went to an independent physician. The news couldn't have been worse. Ms. Smith had advanced cervical cancer. If she had been properly diagnosed when she first sought help, at age 22, her chances of survival would have been 95 percent or better. Now she is 28 and doctors say it is unlikely she will see 30.

"Even though my medical records were fully documented with the classic physical characteristics and symptoms of cervical cancer, no doctor or medical practitioner associated with my HMO or its lab ever made the correct diagnosis." Three Pap smears and three biopsies were performed. "All but the fifth test were misread by the lab my HMO contracted with," Ms. Smith said. "Unfortunately the one Pap smear they did read correctly was dismissed when they misread the biopsy they performed to confirm it. All six tests clearly indicated that I did, in fact, have cervical cancer." . . . Ms. Smith tried for three years to convince her HMO doctors that she was ill. . . .

Herbert, Joe, "Profits Before Patients,"
New York Times, p. E19 (September 11, 1994)

Ms. Smith is an example of a patient suffering because she required a referral to receive another opinion about her condition. This is an example of managed care harming the patient. In the past, doctor's sole responsibility was to take care of the patient, but under managed care, physicians have evolved into "gatekeepers" who manage an HMO's purse strings as well as expenses for patient care and the course of treatment for the duration of the illness. Ms. Smith stayed with the HMO, but Carley Christie's family chose another route:

Carley Christie was eleven years old and lived in Woodside, California. She was diagnosed with Wilms' tumor, a rare childhood kidney cancer. Her parents, Harry and Katherine Christie, found a surgeon with expertise in removing this tumor. But the HMO refused to pay his bills, proposing a less experienced surgeon from its network. The Christies assumed the initial burden of paying their expert, and while nursing their daughter through chemotherapy they battled the bureaucracy for 15 months. The American Arbitration Association sided with the Christies' claim.

Chase, Marilyn, "Can a Doctor Who's a Gatekeeper Give Enough Care?"
New York Times, p. B1 (December 5, 1994)

The American Medical Association Council on Ethical and Judicial Affairs reaffirms the priority of physicians' commitment to patient welfare within a managed care practice.

> The Council identifies two types of ethical conflict facing physicians: (1) balancing the interests of their patients with the interests of other patients; and (2) balancing the needs of patients with the financial interests of their physicians. . . . When physicians are employed or reimbursed by managed care plans using financial incentives to limit care, a serious ethical conflict results. Financial incentives are permissible only if they promote cost effective delivery of quality care—not the withholding of necessary medical services.
>
> "Ethical Issues in Managed Care," *JAMA,*
> pp. 330–335 (January 25, 1995)

IMPORTANCE OF STUDYING ETHICS

Although medical office personnel do not usually make life-and-death decisions for patients, they are involved with patients and the patients' families or significant others. Skilled health care practitioners know the patients, understand the risks involved in certain procedures, are sensitive to the mood swings and caring levels of other professional staff, and internally deal with their own personal questions of ultimate concern.

It is important that medical providers develop their own understanding of ethics. Without some basic recognition of the depth of thinking that goes into ethical decisions, a practitioner has little resource to deal with the conflict that may develop between personal value systems and daily occurrences within the profession of medicine.

These conflicts may potentially lead to either burnout or growth. Knowing that others are dealing and have dealt with many of the same issues encourages interdisciplinary support and understanding. Questioning conflicts may lead to further exploration, education, and the development of different perspectives about an issue. The resolution of conflict may lead to transfer to another job that is more in line with personal beliefs.

In addition, the medical employee's family members, friends, and the community may look to a health care provider for insight into troubling ethical issues facing society. Listening skills and knowledge gained from personal investigation may help others understand. Many ethical questions do not have "right" answers, and acknowledging this also contributes to the education of the community.

SUMMARY

Making an ethical decision may be quite simple or very difficult. It may be easy to get lost in a multitude of factual details or go off on a tangent without addressing the problem. When given a fact pattern containing an ethical dilemma, resolution requires distinguishing between clinical (medical), legal, and ethical issues. Once this analysis has been made, the next step is to further clarify the ethical issue(s).

This chapter introduces the matter of medical ethics, sometimes identified as bioethics. The importance of distinguishing between clinical, legal, and ethical decisions is addressed; the distinctions between ethics, morals, and etiquette have been introduced; but a process for making an ethical decision has not been offered because there is no one way to search for a solution to an ethical dilemma. Each individual approaches an ethical problem from his or her own perspective, which includes cultural **values,** moral upbringing, present circumstances, society's expectations, and a multitude of other variables.

The next four chapters address the ethical issues of confidentiality, allocation of resources, and autonomy versus paternalism under the headings: Privacy, Confidentiality, Privileged Communication: A Nexus of Law and Ethics; Birth and the Beginning of Life; Professional Ethics and the Living; and Ethics: Death and Dying. As each of these sections is addressed, other ethical issues emerge.

Once having identified the issue(s), the questions becomes, "Who owns it (them?)" Is this a problem for the physician, other health care providers, a lawyer, or medical office personnel? Perhaps it is a problem for administration. Often we take on burdens that are not ours, and clearly identifying responsibility may shift the ethical perspective. In dealing with ethical solutions to health care problems, many individuals may have something to say about what is happening, but at some point, "the buck stops here." Where it stops is where the decision is "owned." As managed care becomes the health care of today, responsibility for ethical issues may be changing among providers, but one's personal ethic is always one's personal responsibility.

SUGGESTED ACTIVITY

Review the local newspapers and find reports that deal with medical/legal/ethical issues. Clip these stories and analyze the health, legal, and ethical components. Watch the "Letters to the Editor" columns and collect any letters relating to these matters. After doing this for a month or more, you will begin to sense the variety of ways the public views ethical issues. Document your reaction to the ethics of the article, and review your documentation approximately three months later. If you have changed your mind about any matter, try to determine what personal or societal events caused this change.

STUDY QUESTIONS

1. List three situations that bring about ethical dilemmas in medicine.
2. Why are ethical constraints important in practicing medicine?

3. Define morals and give examples of a personal medical/moral dilemma.

4. Define ethics and identify the ethical problems associated with DRGs and the physician's right to care for a patient.

5. Describe one medical/ethical issue that was raised in your lifetime involving politics. How was political pressure brought on the public?

6. Within the past twenty-four hours, you probably performed an action out of a sense of etiquette. Remember what you did, how you did it, and why. Was this a satisfying experience for you?

7. Give two examples of how AIDS is influencing the economics of health care.

8. Review the latest transplant news and attempt to break down costs. Review the benefits of money being used for the transplant versus other places in society for the common good. Form personal opinions on these issues.

9. Review your local hospital's bill of rights. Find out if it is given to the patient upon admission. Find out if it is explained to the patient. Determine who discusses this with the patient during the hospital stay. If possible, try to interview this person about the success or failure of the process.

10. Try the process for making an ethical decision. Identify something that happened in your life recently that required you to make an ethical decision. Attempt to divide it into its medical (if appropriate), legal, and ethical components. Identify your role and think of all the possible ways you could have handled the situation and their probable results. Weigh each alternative against your personal philosophy. Follow up on the situation and determine whether the outcome was what you expected.

CASES FOR DISCUSSION

1. A premature infant was delivered at Woman's Hospital by the plaintiff. The child died shortly after birth, and the plaintiff was assured by the floor nurse that the hospital would take care of the infant's burial. When the mother went to the obstetrician for an examination six weeks later, she was given her folder to hold while waiting for the physician. She found in it a note from the pathologist about disposal of the baby's body. When the plaintiff asked the physician about the disposal of the body, he instructed his nurse to take her to the hospital across the street to see someone who would tell her what had been done with the baby. When the woman and the nurse found the person, the plaintiff was handed a large jar with the baby's body inside. As a result, the plaintiff suffered nightmares, could not sleep, was depressed when she was around children, had surgery for a pseudopregnancy, and required psychiatric treatment. Should a doctor-patient relationship include the contract to dispose of a dead body?

2. The plaintiff's eighteen-year-old son died suddenly at home. His body was taken to the hospital where the cause of death could not be found without an autopsy. The deputy medical examiner ordered a post-mortem examination. The plaintiff was a member of the Jewish Orthodox faith and refused the postmortem examination of his son on the basis that religious conviction prohibited any molestation of the body after death. Is freedom of religion curtailed by a law that has a compelling state interest?

3. The plaintiff was a fifty-nine-year-old woman who had been a practicing Christian Scientist for approximately ten years. She was unmarried and on welfare. She was involuntarily admitted to Bellevue Hospital by the police when she would not leave her hotel room. Upon admission, she was examined by two psychiatrists and certified according to New York law for commitment for sixty days. The plaintiff informed the hospital staff of her religious preference and that, based on these beliefs, she was unwilling to receive medical treatment. Over her objections she was given tranquilizers. She was never adjudicated mentally ill or incompetent prior to the treatment.

    The plaintiff brought an action under federal civil rights statutes, claiming damages for violation of her right to freedom of religion under the First Amendment. Can an individual be determined mentally ill and treatment initiated without an adjudication of incompetence?

4. The plaintiff, a Jehovah's Witness, was injured in an automobile accident and was taken to the hospital where it was determined that she would die unless operated upon. The operation required blood transfusions. A tenet of the Jehovah's Witness faith forbids blood transfusions. The plaintiff was accompanied by her mother. The plaintiff was in shock, and evidence was presented that she was incoherent. Her mother signed a release of the hospital for all liability, but the hospital went to the court for the appointment of a guardian who would consent to the transfusions. A guardian was appointed, and the operation, with transfusions, was successfully performed. Does a state have the right to authorize the use of force to prevent an individual's death?

5. The plaintiff was injured when a tree fell on him. At the hospital, he refused to consent to blood transfusions because of religious beliefs. The plaintiff's wife agreed that he should not be transfused. The hospital petitioned the court for the appointment of a guardian for the plaintiff. The court decided that the plaintiff understood the consequences of refusing the transfusion, that the plaintiff's wife and children would be taken care of, and refused to grant the petition. Should a patient refuse treatment?

6. The physician plaintiff was licensed to practice medicine in Maine and, as a licensed physician, was a member of the Maine Medical Association. Following an informal meeting with the plaintiff, the association's ethics and discipline committee, in a report, charged him with submitting invoices to the Maine Department of Health and Welfare

that showed "gross overutilization, malpractice, and unethical practice." The plaintiff was not informed of the charges against him before the meeting. The committee placed into evidence confidential documents used against the plaintiff without his consent. In charging the plaintiff, the association went against procedures established in its own bylaws, which required that ethical complaints be disposed of at the county society level. Should this report be withheld from disclosure?

7. The New York Legislature passed the New York State Controlled Substances Act of 1971 because of concern about the illegal use of drugs in the state. The act requires that records concerning the use of certain prescription drugs be filed by physicians with the New York State Department of Health. These records are kept on computers and include the name and address of patients using the drugs. The concern of the physicians and patients who were plaintiffs was that patients in need of treatment with these drugs would decline treatment for fear of being labeled drug addicts. Was the collection of these records by the state a violation of the patients' Fourteenth Amendment rights?

8. The plaintiff was arrested in Denver and charged with solicitation and prostitution and held in the city jail. She had the choice of remaining in jail for forty-eight hours for examination and treatment for sexually transmitted disease or of taking penicillin without examination and being released from jail immediately. She chose to take the penicillin. In Denver, any person arrested for vagrancy, prostitution, rape, or any other sexual offense must be examined and treated for sexually transmitted disease. The plaintiff brought suit against the city and county of Denver, claiming that her civil rights under the Fourth and Fourteenth amendments had been violated. Is the arrest, involuntary detention, and treatment of individuals suspected to have sexually transmitted disease a valid exercise of the state's police power?

9. The defendants, Griswold and Buxton, were arrested for violating a statute that forbade the use of contraceptives. Griswold, executive director of Planned Parenthood, and Buxton, a licensed physician and medical director for Planned Parenthood, gave information, instruction, and medical advice to married persons regarding the prevention of conception. Griswold and Buxton charged that the statute violated the due process clause of the Fourteenth Amendment. Did the United States Supreme Court find that the statute violated the due process clause?

10. An unmarried female, Jane Roe, brought an action against the District Attorney in Texas, charging that the Texas criminal abortion statutes were unconstitutional. The plaintiff stated that she was unmarried and pregnant and that she wished to end the pregnancy in safe clinical conditions but that she was unable to get a legal abortion in Texas because she was not in a life-threatening situation. She claimed that the statutes abridged her right of personal privacy protected by the First, Fourth, Fifth, Ninth, and Fourteenth amendments. Should her right of personal privacy include the right to have an abortion?

Chapter 9

Privacy, Confidentiality, Privileged Communication: A Nexus of Law and Ethics

In six weeks I was going to die if I did not have a transplant. The best place for a transplant is Massachusetts General Hospital. I had it in Maryland because in Massachusetts the press would have put me on the front page. My life was on the line. I took the press and confidentiality into consideration.

Joseph Mokley, United States Congressman for
the Ninth Congressional District, Commonwealth of Massachusetts

OBJECTIVES:

After reading this chapter, you should be able to:

1. distinguish between privacy, confidentiality, and privileged communication.
2. recognize the role that every member of the health care community plays in maintaining confidentiality.
3. identify the challenge that the media presents to maintaining confidentiality.
4. discuss the importance of confidentiality of the medical record.
5. begin to develop your personal philosophy for dealing with confidentiality dilemmas within an ethical framework.

BUILDING YOUR LEGAL VOCABULARY

privileged communication   slander   waives

To tell or not to tell, that is the question. Privacy and confidentiality in the medical setting address both legal and ethical issues and contain at least two areas of conflicting interests. One area is the individual's interest in avoiding disclosure of personal matters versus society's need to know. The second area is the individual's interest in making an independent decision versus being forced to accept a predesignated outcome. The first conflict involves secrecy; the second conflict involves a constitutional right.

DISCLOSURE OF PERSONAL MATTERS

History

The expectation of privacy between physician and patient was first documented in 1134 B.C., when Greek physicians recorded case histories on columns in their temples. These primitive recordings included patient names, medical histories, and treatments. Patient privacy was protected by restricting temple access to authorized persons. During the Middle Ages, medical information was public, and during the nineteenth century, medical information was secret. Contemporary physicians' promise to honor a patient's confidentiality originated with Hippocrates:

> Whatsoever in my practice or not in my practice, I shall see or hear amid the lives of men which ought not be noised abroad, as to this I will keep silence holding such things unfit to be spoken.

A patient's expectation of privacy, known as confidentiality in the doctor-patient relationship, and the doctrine of **privileged communication** in the legal arena, has evolved from Hippocrates's fundamental concept. Because of the many professionals involved in patient care in the nineties, absolute privacy cannot be realistically anticipated. High standards of professional confidentiality appear to be contradicted if a physician decides to place his patients' medical records on the internet. The doctor-patient relationship extends to others employed in the health care field. Medical office personnel must maintain the same standards of confidentiality as a physician.

In the United States, the confidentiality of medical information is not included within constitutional rights of privacy. Until October 21, 1996, when the Kennedy-Kassenbaum bill was signed into law by President Clinton, there was no Federal Privacy Act for medical records. Some commentators believe that provisions in the Kennedy-Kassenbaum bill for a computerized databank and the requirement that all Americans have a health care ID number will make it virtually impossible for patients to get confidential medical care. Others believe that having one's entire health care history on a computerized databank could save lives due to the growing needs of emergency medical care is an increasingly mobile population. Under the Kennedy-Kassenbaum bill, those found guilty of wrongfully disclosing private health information face ten years in jail and a $250,000 fine.

There is tradition and a history of precedence set by common law for maintaining the confidentiality of medical records. The following article provides an example of the strength of this tradition:

A state panel suspended a therapist's license for speaking publicly about her counseling sessions with Nicole Brown Simpson. Susan J. Forward, who was among the first to reveal Nicole Simpson's history of abuse at the hands of O.J. Simpson after Nicole Simpson's death, is barred from seeing patients for three months and placed on three years' probation for violating Nicole Simpson's confidentiality.

Deputy Attorney General Anne Le Mendoza, who represents the state Board of Behavioral Science Examiners, stated: "Therapy is based on privacy and secrecy, and a breach of confidentiality . . . destroys the therapeutic relationship."

Susan Forward, who is the author of the best selling *Men Who Hate Women and the Women Who Love Them,* acknowledged that she spoke to ten reporters about Nicole Simpson.

"Therapist Punished for Simpson Revelations,"
The Boston Globe, p. 19 (November 24, 1995)

Privileged Communication

Privileged communication is a label placed on information passing between people that cannot be submitted into evidence in a court of law because of the relationship between the individuals. For example, communication between a husband and wife in the privacy of their home is privileged and cannot be admitted into evidence unless certain criteria are met. Communication between a physician and patient is legally recognized as privileged, and in some states this extends to social workers and psychotherapists. Communication between a priest and penitent is also private and under most circumstances cannot be admitted into evidence.

In the typical physician-patient privilege, a physician cannot reveal in court confidential information obtained during treatment unless the patient voluntarily **waives** (gives up) his or her privilege against disclosure. This right is conditional. When an individual or family files a medical malpractice cause of action, for example, the right may be overruled.

"The 'gloves are coming off,' " reads the headlines for an article about Lewis' doctor. Dr. Gilbert H. Mudge, Jr. intends to aggressively defend himself in the medical malpractice lawsuit filed against him Tuesday by the widow of [former] Celtics captain Reggie Lewis, telling associates that Donna Harris-Lewis as well as Celtics team officials will be interrogated about their actions in the case. . . . Lewis, who collapsed while casually shooting hoops at a Brandeis University gym in 1993, apparently "died under no greater cardiovascular strain than if he brought in groceries from the car," said [the family's malpractice attorney]. The critical question then becomes, "Was his death preventable?" . . . Among the main factors that Mudge and his attorney will focus on will be statements that Donna Harris-Lewis allegedly made in calls to Mudge following her husband's death that implied that he had used drugs.

Kurkjian, Stephen, "Gloves Are Coming Off,"
The Boston Globe, p. 1 (May 2, 1996)

Confidentiality

According to Kirk B. Johnson, an attorney for the American Medical Association, "Confidentiality used to be a sacred principle in medicine, but this is changing":

Growing concern about the cost and quality of health care is prompting changes that are eroding confidentiality rules that have long protected hospitals, patients and doctors. Hospital records are increasingly available to outside reviewers. Employers, and insurers, who ultimately pay many medical bills insist that their representatives need to see information that used to be closely guarded.

Freudenheim, M., "Guarding Medical Confidentiality,"
New York Times, p. 1 (January 1, 1991)

Each state approaches protecting citizens' privacy through its legislature. When contested decisions reach the United States Supreme Court, the Court uses a balancing test to weigh the interests of the community and the person against the expectation of privacy. When studying confidentiality and privacy in the medical office, it is difficult to analyze isolated ethical issues. The ethical questions concern whether the legal solution promotes justice for the individual and society.

THE MEDICAL OFFICE

The High Profile Client

The media is interested in gathering medical information on public figures. Former Senator Paul E. Tsongas of Massachusetts suffered non-Hodgkins lymphoma, and his survival of cancer became an issue in the presidential campaign. His doctors said that Mr. Tsongas had been cancer-free since a bone marrow transplant. The *New York Times* reported that the cancer had recurred. The senator and Dana-Farber Cancer Hospital became involved in a dispute with the media over the withholding of key details about the senator's case. As a result of his experiences, Tsongas called on President-elect Clinton to establish a commission to determine what medical information candidates must disclose.

Although a presidential candidate has rights to privacy, review of presidents' past medical data has shown that health of a president may influence the course of history and be a proper subject for publication in the media. For example:

> A link exists between Woodrow Wilson's debilitating stroke in 1919 and his subsequent inability to persuade Congress to ratify the Treaty of Versailles, thus keeping the United States out of the League of Nations.
>
> The questionable performance of Franklin D. Roosevelt was severely weakened by congestive heart failure during the historic Yalta Conference in February 1945, just two months before he died.
>
> The suggestion [is] that Ronald Reagan was under the influence of prescribed medication in July 1985, when he allegedly authorized the shipment of arms to Iran just two days after cancer surgery.
>
> Hearn, Wayne, "When the President Is the Patient,"
> *American Medical News,* p. 13 (October 21, 1996)

In New York, the congressional campaign of Nydia M. Velazquez stumbled when New York newspapers reported that she had sought hospital emergency treatment after a suicide attempt. Despite the revelation, Velezquez won the election and later sued a Manhattan hospital for $10 million for failing to protect her privacy.

The health of another political candidate became public when a billing supervisor leaked information that led *The Boston Globe* to print the following medical commentary:

> Massachusetts General Hospital (MGH) officials had built a strong circumstantial case that an employee was the source of confidential medical data leaked about gubernatorial candidate Francis X. Bellotti. . . . [It was determined that] TB, a billing supervisor at MGH for two and one half years, had signed out billing and admissions records from Bellotti's April 30 visit less than a week before the information appeared in the *Boston Herald.* She resigned under fire. . . .
>
> Mooney, Brian C., *The Boston Globe,*
> p. 23 (September 5, 1990)

Consequences for those committing confidentiality violations may result in employee resignation, as in the preceding example, or the initiation of a lawsuit, as follows:

> A person who suffered emotional distress and loss of reputation as a result of a false rumor that he had AIDS can collect damages for **slander,** says the Nebraska Supreme Court. This ruling is believed to be the first in the country in which a false allegation of AIDS has been found to be defamation although false allegations of other disease have been held to be ground for such suits in the past.

In this case, a resident of the plaintiff's small hometown told her family and a home nursing aide that the man had AIDS and was in the hospital. He did not have AIDS, and as a result of this rumor he suffered from stress, began drinking heavily, was unable to work and eventually lost his job. A jury awarded him $23,000.

McCune v. Neitzel, No. 88-552 (Neb. July 13, 1990),
Lawyer's Alert No. 215-13

Medical Office Personnel

The medical office offers many opportunities for privacy to be violated, for example, the simple clerical matter of sending a "checkup reminder":

A month after the death of a woman in a hospital, the family physician's office sent a notice to her home for a periodic checkup. Her husband and children were upset by the notice and informed the office in writing of her death and their distress.

Her husband subsequently filed a malpractice action against the doctor for wrongful death, apparently for failure to diagnose her illness. Two more "checkup" reminders were received by the family, the second being sent to the daughter.

In its decision, the Court held that sending the first notice would not have constituted an action for invasion of privacy since it would have been mailed by mistake, but sending two more after the commencement of a malpractice lawsuit was grounds for a cause of action for invasion of privacy.

McCormick v. Haley, 307 N.E.2d 34 (Ohio 1973)

Harry T. Paxton, in an article entitled "Today's Guidelines for Patient Confidentiality," writes:

The other day I was in an office where a secretary yelled across a room to another secretary "Mr. Jones needs a vasectomy scheduled with Dr. Smith." There were a number of people in that room and they all heard that Mr. Jones was going to have a vasectomy. Matters like that are very personal. There's a potential lawsuit when something like this happens. . . .

Harry T. Paxton, "Today's Guidelines for Patient Confidentiality,"
Medical Economics, p. 198 (February 1, 1988)

Violations of privacy occurring in the medical office are not restricted solely to the actions of medical office personnel. Following is an old case that is still good law:

A sales representative was trying to persuade a physician to purchase a cauterization machine. While the salesman was in the office, a patient was seen who had a growth on her uterus which required cauterization. The doctor allowed the salesman

> to cauterize the woman in order to demonstrate the equipment. Unfortunately, there were disastrous results and the woman sued not only for negligence in allowing the salesman to perform the procedure, but also for invasion of privacy. She won and collected damages.
>
> *Carr v. Shippolette,* 82 F.2d 874 (D.C. Cir. 1936)

Reminders to employees, physicians, and other professionals that someone may be listening to their conversations are posted in most hospitals. Confidentiality of symptoms and treatment is essential to preserve a patient's privacy and to prevent others from recalling bits and pieces of information that can lead to wrong conclusions. Breaching confidentiality is not only unethical but may cause legal problems.

> A woman who was employed by a caterer had a condition which raised false positives on Wasserman tests. Her physician knew she did not have syphilis. The office nurse attended a social affair catered by the employer of the patient. The nurse told the hostess that the patient was being treated by her employer for syphilis. The information affected the patient's employment and the employer's business. The Court held that there was a good cause for slander against the nurse.
>
> *Schlesser v. Keck,* 271 P.2d 588 (Cal. 1954)

The preceding is an example of confidentiality violation that might be called gossip. The following letter from a "Dear Abby" column reveals how deeply disclosure of confidential information may affect a patient:

> When I was twenty I had an abortion. Seven years later, when I was pregnant with my first child, my doctor asked if this was my first pregnancy, so I told him about the abortion. At one of my early prenatal visits, his nurse walked into the examining room, looked me straight in the eye, and said, "So, you've decided to keep this one?" . . . Never again will I disclose this information on my medical history.
>
> *The Patriot Ledger,* p. 26 (March 30, 1988)

Medical Records

Although the "walls are crushing in" on privileged communication, it is still in effect in most instances. The patient owns the privilege and can prevent a doctor from disclosure.

> The plaintiff, the biological mother of a child years before placed for adoption, brought an action against a physician who had assisted the daughter in her search for the mother.

The daughter, at twenty-one years of age, became interested in finding her biological mother. She was unable to gain access to the confidential court file of her adoption, but did locate the mother's obstetrician who agreed to help her find her biological mother. In order to gain access to the confidential records concerning the daughter's birth and adoption, the doctor/defendant fabricated a letter stating that although he could not find his records, he remembered giving the mother diethylstilbesterol (DES).

Hospital personnel, relying on the physician's letter, allowed the daughter to make copies of her mother's medical records, therefore making it possible for the daughter to find her mother. The Supreme Court of Oregon determined that the mother had a valid cause of action against the physician for breach of a confidential relationship and further stated that the duty of confidentiality could not be disregarded solely to satisfy the curiosity of a person who sought her biological mother.

Humphrey v. First Interstate Bank of Oregon,
696 P.2d 527 (1985)

Placing patient information in a hospital computer system can be like publishing an article in the local newspaper.

Beverly Woodward tells of a friend, a physician who gave birth at a hospital—and soon found that ten of her colleagues had looked up her medical record on the hospital's computer system, eager to check on the status of mother and baby. "She has an extensive medical record, and she was appalled to realize her colleagues had instant access to everything in it," said Woodward, a sociology researcher at Brandeis University who has studied the problem of patient privacy. "When a medical record is on paper, a lot fewer people have access to it."

Bass, Alison, "Computerized Medical Data
Put Privacy on the Line," *The Boston Globe,*
p. 5 (February 22, 1995)

The Privacy Protection Study Commission set up by Congress in 1974 to study individual privacy rights and record-keeping practices revealed that medical records now contain more information and are available to more users than ever before. Further, the control of health care providers over these records has diminished, and restoration of this control is not possible. Often the only person who does not known what is in the record is the patient. Some believe that the federal regulation of medical databases is necessary due to the large health care networks that maintain computer files. There are concerns that information from these databases will be released to employers, insurers, universities, police and courts, state and federal agencies, health researchers, and others.

An example of a bizarre incidence that violated confidentiality in computerized medical records occurred in Florida when a teenage girls called former hospital patients and told them they had tested positive for AIDS:

> The 13-year-old's mother, an employee at University Medical Center, took her daughter to work because she could not find anyone to watch her. Getting telephone numbers of former emergency room patients from a computer, the child called seven people and told them they had tested positive for H.I.V. One of the victims tried to commit suicide. A call to one patient was traced to the child's home because the patient had Caller ID, a device that records the telephone number of incoming calls.
>
> "Girl Accused of Making False AIDS Calls,"
> *New York Times* (March 1, 1995)

In Massachusetts, a convicted child rapist used a former employee's computer password to invade nearly one thousand confidential hospital files of patients and then used the telephone numbers to make obscene calls to girls. He was charged under a statute that makes it a criminal offense to use another person's password to gain access to a computer system.

> Dr. Denise Nagel, president of the Massachusetts chapter of the Coalition for Patient Rights, reacted by saying, "People are being assured privacy as their medical records are being computerized and this is a sad example that there is no privacy once records are computerized."
>
> Brelis, Matthew, "Patients' Files Allegedly Used for
> Obscene Calls," *The Boston Globe*, p. 1 (April 11, 1995)

LIMITS OF CONFIDENTIALITY

Keeping medical information confidential can breed conflict. The following is a situation that demonstrates ethical dimensions involving a diagnosis of herpes:

> The K's are prominent members of the community. Mrs. K is pregnant and Dr. O'Brien, her obstetrician, has been following the pregnancy. Mrs. K had an appointment with Dr. O'Brien in her office and upon examination Dr. O'Brien found an open lesion in her genital area. Dr. O'Brien diagnosed it as a genital herpes lesion and Mrs. K requested that the information not be entered into her medical record. Dr. O'Brien explained that if Mrs. K has open lesions at the time of delivery, a C-section would have to be performed to prevent infection to the child. Mrs. K pleaded with Dr. O'Brien to keep this information confidential, appealing as a friend and a trusted physician.
>
> Purtile, Ruth, and Sorrell, James, "The Ethical Dilemmas of a
> Rural Physician," *The Hastings Report*, p. 25 (August 1986)

The incident took place in a community where "everyone knew everyone else." The receptionist was Mrs. K's sister-in-law. The county public health clerk to which this sexually transmitted disease should be reported was Mrs. K's cousin. Other relatives worked as nurses' aides in the hospital where she would deliver. In this case, the physician did not record the information about the lesion in the patient's medical record. She did record the information in a second set of records she kept in a locked place accessible only to her and her partner.

An ambulatory care unit is often the scene of similar conflicts in confidentiality.

A teen-ager who's just been raped rushes in to the ED, requesting a pelvic exam and a morning-after pill but insisting that no one call the police. What do you do? In every state, rape is a reportable offense, one of a number of instances in which public welfare takes precedence over a patient's right to privacy. . . .

AIDS, more than any other diagnosis, confuses issues of privacy and confidentiality. That's because disclosure has meant the loss of jobs, medical insurance, and even housing for many patients. . . . HIV infection presents an additional dilemma: what to do when you know your patient has not informed his sexual partner of his diagnosis. Here, as in a case of child abuse, the welfare of a third party take precedence over the patient's desire not to have this information disclosed.

Greve, Paul A., "Keep Quiet or Speak Up?
Issues in Patient Confidentiality," *RN*, p. 53 (December 1990)

A landmark case involving conflict between the disclosure of information to a third party and doctor-patient confidentiality follows:

Poddar was undergoing treatment as a voluntary outpatient. He had become obsessed with Tatiana Tarasoff, a student he had met at a dance. He had tape-recorded conversations with her and spent hours replaying the tapes in order to determine her feelings for him. A friend became concerned and suggested that he seek professional help.

Poddar was seen by a psychiatrist, who did not believe that Poddar required hospitalization, but did prescribe medication and arranged weekly outpatient psychotherapy with a staff psychologist. During therapy, Poddar revealed his fantasies of harming, and perhaps even killing, Tarasoff. The friend told the psychologist that Poddar planned to purchase a gun. Poddar stopped therapy. The doctors believed that Poddar should be evaluated for hospitalization and requested help from the campus police.

The campus police went to Poddar's apartment and questioned him about his plans but then left when he denied any intention of harming Tarasoff. Two months later Poddar stabbed Tarasoff to death. He was convicted of second degree murder, the conviction was overturned on the basis of improper jury instruction, and Poddar returned home to India.

Later, in a civil suit the Tarasoff family sued the university, including both therapists and the campus police, for negligence. The court held that the therapists had a duty to warn Tarasoff.

Tarasoff v. Regents of University of California,
17 Cal. 3d 342, 131 Cal. Rptr. 14 (1976)

CONFIDENTIALITY AS AN ETHICAL DILEMMA

Breaking confidences in the medical office enters into what is right and wrong given the subject matter of the information. For example, is it right or wrong to keep a patient's AIDS diagnosis confidential? The law plays an important part in the decision-making process about revealing private information because confidentiality and privacy are regulated. Failure to adhere to regulations brings about personal consequences for the violator. For individuals who believe that it is ethical to follow the rules at any cost, regulations about confidentiality solve the dilemma. For individuals who are motivated by other values or ethical thought systems, regulations only add conflict to the dilemma.

THE RIGHT TO BE LEFT ALONE

Privacy conveys the right to be left alone to make personal choices. In the Tarasoff matter described above, the patient forfeited the right to be left alone because he demonstrated an intent to harm a third party. In *Griswold v. Connecticut* (1965), *Katz v. United States* (1967), and *Roe v. Wade* (1973), the United States Supreme Court cited several constitutional amendments that imply the right to privacy.

For example, the well-known abortion decision of the United States Supreme Court, *Roe v. Wade,* protects a woman's right to privacy in a first-trimester abortion. This right to privacy allows the woman to communicate solely with her physician concerning an abortion. Although this decision has been attacked by those believing that having an abortion is tantamount to killing a child, the decision still stands as law.

The human right to privacy is grounded in the basic moral tenet that each individual has an incalculable worth. This right is a core issued of the abortion conflict. One side holds that an individual's incalculable worth extends to the fetus; the other side holds that the woman's worth is a high priority. At issue, also, is the privacy of the physician-patient relationship. Alasdair MacIntyre, in "Moral Disagreements," formats three arguments as follows:

A. Everybody has certain rights over their own person, including their own body. It follows from the nature of these rights that at the stage when the embryo is essentially part of the mother's body, the mother has a right to make her own uncoerced decision on whether she will have an abortion or not. Therefore each pregnant woman ought to decide and ought to be allowed to decide for herself what she will do in the light of her own moral views.

B. I cannot, if I will to be alive, consistently will that my mother should have had an abortion when she was pregnant with me, except if it had been certain that the embryo was dead or gravely damaged. But if I cannot consistently will this in my own case, how can I consistently deny to others the right to life that I claim for myself? I would break the so-called Golden Rule unless I denied that a mother has in general a right on abortion. I am not of course thereby committed to the view that abortion ought to be legally prohibited.

C. Murder is wrong, prohibited by natural and divine law. Murder is the taking of innocent life. An embryo is an identifiable individual, differing from a newborn infant only in being at an earlier stage on the long road to adult capacities. If infanticide is murder, as it is, then abortion is murder. So abortion is not only morally wrong, but ought to be legally prohibited.

"The Belmont Report: Ethical Principles and Guidelines for the Protection of Human Subjects of Research," Appendix I. DHEW Publications (OS) 78-0013 (Washington, D.C.: Government Printing Office)

DEVELOPING AN ETHICAL DECISION-MAKING PROCESS

To develop an ethical decision-making process for dealing with problems of confidentiality and privacy, distinguish between what is clinical, what is legal, and what is ethical in a fact pattern. Having identified the ethical issues, the next question becomes, who owns the problem? If you own the problem, how do you respond?

You can respond to the dilemma by refusing to disclose anything at any time except to those to whom you are immediately responsible. You can choose to adhere to existing regulations about the breaking of the confidential relationship with a patient. If you choose to follow another line of reasoning, the consequences of your action must be accepted by your peers, your bosses, and society or you risk losing your job and the possibility of being sued. You must then balance the risk against personal internal conflict. Refer to the case of the Baltimore firefighters in the preceding chapter, and again address the issue of breaking a regulation.

SUMMARY

Privacy, confidentiality, and *privileged communication* are terms used to define the relationship between medical professionals and their patients and between legal professionals and their clients. The terms refer to the tradition and precedence requiring the maintenance of silence by medical and legal personnel. Maintaining confidences often involves ethical conflict.

Included in matters of privacy is the right to be left alone, to make personal choices. All factors must be reviewed when making decisions about breaking patient confidentiality. What is right for one individual may be wrong for another.

SUGGESTED ACTIVITY

Play the game of rumors. You may be familiar with this game from your childhood years. The game began when a player "started a rumor" by secretly telling the person next to him or her a story; the second person passed the rumor on by secretly telling the next person, and so on. When the rumor had traveled around the entire circle of players, the last player repeated what he or she heard. The first player then disclosed the content of the original sentence or story. A comparison of the resulting story with the original version usually lead to gales of laughter.

Members of the class should arrange themselves around the perimeter of the room. The instructor will begin the "rumor" by telling something to the next person (*e.g.,* giving directions for taking medication). As the rumor travels around the circle, each student should remember and pass along what he or she has heard. The last person to receive the rumor should repeat aloud what he or she has heard; the teacher then will disclose the content of the original. In comparing the resulting version with the original, students will understand how medical terms imparted to a patient during an office visit can be confused and misunderstood.

STUDY QUESTIONS

1. Research your local hospital's methods of maintaining the confidentiality of their medical records.
2. Attempt to obtain a copy of your own medical record from your family or primary care physician. Document the process required to receive a copy of the record.
3. Apply quality of life concerns to issues of the confidentiality of medical information.
4. Apply sanctity of life concerns to issues of the confidentiality of medical information.

CASES FOR DISCUSSION

1. "Gregg Wiatt was stunned. On his 28th birthday—six months before the death of the man he had thought was his natural father—his mother told him the truth. She told him he was the offspring of a semen donor. Long before, though, Wiatt had felt somehow different. 'It was like there was always this secret I could never put my fingers on,' says the 37-year-old Denver sales and marketing executive. 'When I finally

learned the truth, it felt like I was living between Disneyland and the Twilight Zone.' Bill Cordray, 47, also felt odd. 'It was something that kept edging into my consciousness,' says the Salt Lake City architect. He and his dad were 'so different. My interests were artistic—music, building, creative. So different from everyone else. I felt like a stranger in my family.' Wiatt and Cordray are among tens of thousands of people literally born out of the high-tech merger of egg and sperm. And, like most of the others, they're still in the dark—because records are confidential." ("When Dad's a Sperm Donor," *USA Weekend* (January 15–17, 1993). Develop arguments on both sides of the question: Should sperm donor records be confidential?

2. "A $10,000 judgment was entered against a plastic surgeon for performing an illegal HIV test on a patient. Douglas W. Wooldridge agreed to pay Jason Gavann the money in an offer of judgment. . . . The complaint, filed earlier, alleged that during surgery Dr. Wooldridge took a sample of Gavann's blood and sent it to a laboratory for an HIV test. Gavann stated that he was unconscious during surgery and that his blood had been tested for HIV without his knowledge. Gavann said he inadvertently discovered the HIV test result in his medical file during a follow-up visit at Wooldridge's office several weeks later. The HIV test was negative. Wooldridge claimed, in a deposition, that he had stuck himself with a needle and feared HIV." (Peratta, Ed., "Wellesley Doctor Settles Complaint Stemming from Patient's HIV Test," *Wellesley Townsman,* p. 1 (June 6, 1996).) Develop arguments on both sides of the question. Should health care deliverers know the HIV status of their patients prior to invasive procedures?

3. "Madison, Wis. (AP) A used computer sold by the state contained detailed medical records of more than 600 people, a legislator says. State Rep. Marlin D. Schneider, said the Wisconsin Coalition Against Sexual Assault purchased the computer as state surplus property for $20. When the coalition's executive director discovered the records from a clinic, she began erasing them, then decided to make a copy of the rest and turned about 500 names and data over to Schneider. She then erased all the original records. 'I don't want any patients upset or to suffer any distress because their records are public,' he said. 'It could create a [liability] problem for the state. The agency itself needs protection.' . . . [T]here is a law against 'knowing and willful' release of such information, but the statute is weak. You have to have a showing that there was a willing disregard." Was there a willing disregard?

4. "Where a personnel manager at a state transit authority told a supervisor that an employee had AIDS, the employee will collect $125,000 as a result of a jury verdict in federal court in Philadelphia. The transit authority is liable under 42 USC § 1983 for invasion of privacy in violation of the due process under the Fourteenth Amendment. The employee relied on prior case law from the Third Circuit which held that medical information is protected by the Fourteenth Amendment

unless the government establishes a public need for it, according to the plaintiff's attorney, Clifford Boardman of Philadelphia. The personnel manager discovered that the employee had AIDS when she reviewed a report of prescriptions filed under the company health plan and noticed that he had purchased drugs commonly used in connection with the disease. She told the employee's boss and one of her own subordinates, according to Boardman. The employee recovered for his 'emotional distress and humiliation' caused by continuing to work at the agency and fearing that other employees would find out." (*Doe v. Southeastern Pennsylvania Transportation,* No. 93-5988 (U.S. Dist. Ct., E.D. Pa., December 5, 1994), 95 LWUSA 96, p. 8.) What should happen to the personnel manager?

5. "Finding that the confidentiality of psychotherapy serves important public as well as private interests, the Supreme Court ruled, on June 13, 1996, that Federal courts must allow psychotherapists and other mental health professionals to refuse to disclose patient records in judicial proceedings. By a vote of 7 to 2, the Court created a new evidentiary privilege, in both civil and criminal cases, similar to the lawyer-client and marital privileges the Federal courts have recognized for years. The case grew out of an effort by a licensed clinical social worker and her patient, a police officer who received counseling after killing a man in the line of duty, to protect records of the therapy sessions from being disclosed in a Federal civil rights suit brought against the officer by the man's family. 'This case amply demonstrates the importance of allowing individuals to receive confidential counseling,' Justice Stevens said. 'If the privilege were rejected, confidential conversations between psychotherapists and their patients would surely be chilled.' The new privilege applies generally and is not limited to police officers. Justice Stevens said the privilege would apply to clinical social workers as well as to psychiatrists and psychologists because the reasons for having the privilege 'apply with equal force' to all the professions. Judge Antonin Scalia dissented from what he called 'a privilege that is new, vast, and ill defined.' He suggested that people would be better advised to seek advice from their mothers than from psychiatrists, 'yet there is not mother-child privilege.' He said the privilege would interfere with the truthfinding function of the courts and cause the courts 'to become themselves the instruments of wrong.' " ([*Jaffee v. Redmond,* No. 95-266] Greenhouse, Linda, "Justices Uphold Psychotherapy Privacy Rights," *New York Times,* p. A1 (June 14, 1996).) Draft a comment in response to Judge Scalia's dissent.

6. "A Simmons College survey of about 150 people who went to the South Shore Mental Health Center's crisis unit has prompted questions about whether the center violated patient confidentiality. The center gave a college research team the names, addresses and telephone numbers of randomly selected people who sought emergency help in September. The decision to turn over names and other information,

which was used to conduct a 'consumer satisfaction' survey, has drawn complaints from two patients who say the center violated their right to privacy. . . . Simmons did the survey as a student research project. Those who were asked to participate had two chances to decline. Patients could call a telephone number to say 'no' after they got the letter, or they could withdraw when a student called them to conduct the phone interview. If they didn't call 'it was presumed that they were giving their consent' to be interviewed. The two patients felt that they'd lost their privacy. 'If you went to a crisis unit, would you want your name passed around by a bunch of college students?' asked one of the women, who went to the center because she was feeling 'suicidal.' The second woman said she doubted she would ever be able to trust the confidentiality of any counseling agency. 'This ices my going to another counselor anywhere,' she said. 'I don't believe there is any privacy.' " (Lambert, Lane, "Mental Health Survey Criticized," *The Patriot Ledger,* p. 1, (March 4, 1996).) Did giving names, addresses, and telephone numbers violate or not violate the privacy of the patients? Justify your answer.

7. "Warning: What you tell your doctor could hurt you. Just asked the California man who fearfully admitted to his doctor that he had smoked marijuana as a youth. His medical record went into a computer system where an insurance company later used drug abuse as one of the reasons to deny him benefits. As the nation's largest credit report company takes its first steps toward linking millions of medical records in a computerized database, chances are growing that private diagnoses, patient histories, even offhand remarks made in a doctor's office could show up on a computer anywhere." (Davis, Robert, "On Line Medical Records Raise Privacy Fears," *USA Today,* p. 1A (March 22, 1995).) Identify points in the medical office where there could be leakage of information in a computerized system.

8. "In a case that has raised questions about the limits of confidentiality in selfhelp groups, a Larchmont carpenter is on trial again on charges of breaking into his childhood home and murdering the couple who had bought the house from his parents. The first trial of the carpenter, Paul Cox, 27, ended in a mistrial, with jurors deadlocked 11 to 1 in favor of conviction. In that trial more than a half dozen members of Alcoholics Anonymous testified under subpoena that Mr. Cox confessed to them that he thought he had committed the killings during a drunken blackout. As in the first trial, Cox had pleaded not guilty and intends to use a defense of temporary insanity." ("Retrial Begins in Murder Case Tied to Confession to a A.A. Group," *New York Times METRO,* p. B7 (Nov. 3, 1994).) Should privileged communication be extended to self-help groups?

9. "TAMPA Fla.—A copy of a confidential computer disk containing the names of 4,000 AIDS patients was mailed anonymously to a news-

paper after a drunken public health worker showed it to friends and dropped it outside a bar. The *Tampa Tribune* said it gave a copy of the disk and the letter that came with it to the state Department of Health and Rehabilitative Services, which yesterday launched an investigation into the breach of confidentiality. . . . The newspaper said it has no plans to publish or otherwise use the names. Nobody knows how many copies of the disk have been made, or who has them. . . . The worker, one of three people with authorized access to the information at the county agency, was placed on paid administrative leave. . . . Florida is among 26 states with mandatory AIDS reporting rules, and plans to expand its confidential reporting program in January to include people who test positive for HIV, the virus that causes AIDS. . . . Elaine Fulton-Jones, a spokeswoman for the Pinellas County Health Department, said 'security at the county agency is tight, with the confidential information kept under several different lock systems, in a locked room, with a secret password.' " ("AIDS Patients' Names Mailed to Florida Paper," *The Boston Globe* (September 20, 1996).) How will this impact on people's willingness to be tested?

10. "OAK RIDGE, Tenn.—Lockheed Martin researchers in Oak Ridge are fine-tuning a prototype system that will allow global access to medical records via computers and still safeguard privacy. . . . The system, which is designed to link medical records from different sources and at different locations . . . is called Communitywide Secure Information Sharing (CSIS). . . . 'With the CSIS system, authorized persons would be able to quickly access patient records through a desktop, laptop or palmtop computer using a World Wide Web browser interface,' Lockheed Martin stated in a news release. In order to ensure confidentiality, access would be limited by security measures, such as electronic pads that match the signatures of users. The messages passed along publicly accessible computer byways would be encrypted so the information would be unreadable—and thus unusable—without the proper decoding on the receiving end." ("Safeguarding the Privacy of Computer Records," [*Knoxville News-Sentinel*] *The Patriot Ledger*, p. 13 (November 22, 1996).) How do you feel about having your medical history placed on the CSIS?

Chapter 10

Birth and the Beginning of Life

"Life is so terrible; it would be better never to have been conceived." "Yes, but who is so fortunate? Not one in a thousand."

Nozick, Robert, *Anarchy, State and Utopia*,
Basic Books, New York, p. 337 (1974)

OBJECTIVES:

Technology has progressed beyond society's readiness to deal with the ethical and legal issues it presents. The question is often asked whether a moratorium should be placed on further scientific investigation to allow society to catch up. Of course, this is impossible, but regulations may be placed on certain procedures while the scales of justice weigh issues of public policy versus private interest. There are no ethical answers provided, only further questions. After reading this chapter, you should be able to:

1. appreciate the impact of expanding technology on ethical questions involving birth and the beginning of life.
2. identify ethical questions surrounding genetic research and its impact on future generations.
3. recognize problems associated with artificial insemination.
4. appreciate the rights of a fetus.
5. recognize the rights of a newborn.
6. recognize the rights of a child.
7. appreciate the conflicts associated with adolescent autonomy in the medical decision-making process.
8. address issues of allocation of resources for children.

BUILDING YOUR LEGAL VOCABULARY

AIDS	eugenics	pluralistic
amniocentesis	fetus	sanctity
anencephalic	genetic	scientific investigation
chemotherapy	gestation	survival action
cloning	HIV	technology
DNA	parens patriae	wrongful death

Birth and the beginning of life is basic to the essence of life. It is a matter dealt with by every religion, questioned by each individual when working through his or her own personal developmental issues, and politicized by various groups for various reasons. The United States is a **pluralistic** society and has difficulty reaching an ethical consensus. This is highlighted by an editorial on the "Baby M" custody fight, entitled "Vatican's Statement Draws Praise, Criticism":

> WASHINGTON—The Vatican's condemnation Tuesday of test-tube fertilization, artificial insemination, surrogate motherhood, and other reproductive technologies drew mixed reactions Wednesday from ethicists, physicians and religious authorities inside and outside the Roman Catholic Church. . . .
>
> "The Jewish idea about all this is directly opposite to that of the Pope," said Rabbi Seymour Siegal of the Jewish Theological Seminary in New York. "Jews believe we have to use nature to outwit nature . . . use it in order to correct problems, to remove disabilities, to increase human happiness. . . ."
>
> Rev. J. Robert Nelson, a United Methodist clergyman who directs the Institute of Religion at the Texas Medical Center in Houston commended the Vatican for the contents of the "very important document," and for "taking the initiative in dealing with the issues. . . . Protestants simply do not have anything comparable," he said, adding that he hoped "the Catholic statement would spur the National and World Councils of Churches to study the issue."
>
> Hyer, Marjorie, *St. Petersburg Times,*
> p. 21A (March 12, 1987)

The preceding represents views of three major religious groups in America. Ethical issues involving conception arise from fundamental moral positions founded on religious beliefs. Birth and the beginning of life were shrouded in mystery before the advent of **scientific investigation.** There is still an element of the unknown, but the issues have changed as the ability of human beings to control their destiny has changed. Science is now at a point where the very beginning of life can be manipulated by **technology.** Ethical dilemmas surround society's willingness to accept intervention in the conception-birth process.

GENETICS

There are 3,000 to 4,000 human **genetic** diseases, 500 of which are linked to a defect in a single gene. Many of the disorders are extremely rare. They include: cystic fibrosis, a disease that afflicts one in 1,600 Caucasians with often fatal chronic lung problems; sickle cell anemia, a blood disorder found in one of 400 African-Americans; hemophilia, a failure of blood clotting that subjects one in 10,000 boys to abnormal bleeding and bruising; and Tay-Sachs disease, a genetically defective enzyme that causes retardation and early death in one of 3,500 persons of Ashkenazic (Eastern European) Jewish ancestry.

Investigating an individual's genetic makeup may have positive effects on society or may produce negative outcomes. Genetic information can be used to invade all individual's privacy, may result in the changing of a person's self-image, and may damage an entire family's identity. It may tarnish our concept of equality by adversely impacting on opportunities for education, employment, and insurance. On the other hand, genetic information may lead to treatments for diseases before they cause harm. It may advance the engineering of genes to remove harmful influences in the development process.

Testing for genetic information is relatively simple, requiring a **DNA** sample from solid tissues, blood, saliva, or other nucleated cells. Genetic data banks are found in both the public and private sector of society and are usually developed for clinical research and public health programs. A genetic data search can explain causes of morbidity. For example, genetic technologies were used to determine whether Abraham Lincoln had Marfan's disease.

Amniocentesis allows physicians to perform genetic tests for defects prior to birth. Because of the financial cost of certain problems to society and the emotional cost to the child and to parents, women may be required to abort infants with certain genetic abnormalities in the future. Some diseases that produce dysfunction in humans later in life, for example, Alzheimer's disease, have been found to have a genetic basis. Will society mandate abortion when a **fetus** exhibits certain genetic traits? Will society use genetic information to determine who will be educated and to what degree, or who will be treated medically and to what extent?

Science also is investigating how to produce "perfect" specimens by **cloning.** Technology has reached the point where a fertilized egg can be cloned and implanted in the wombs of several females for incubation until birth. Is society willing to allow this to happen? What could be the repercussions of these practices?

Research has been conducted to determine whether there may be genetic determinants of behavior:

[The relationship between violence] and the discovery of the first XYY man was reported in late 1961. Within a year, the leap was made between the extra chromosome and possible criminal behavior.

The impact of the **eugenics** movement on sterilization law, the public policy debate over the genetic basis of intelligence, and the brutal application of theories of racial superiority by the Nazis are vivid enough to warn any researcher to proceed cautiously. . . .

Gaylin, William, "XYY Controversy: Researching Violence and Genetics," *The Hastings Center Special Supplement* (August 1980)

One ethical philosophy of life is its **"sanctity"**; another is its "quality." Keep these and other perspectives in mind as you read the following sections.

RIGHTS OF COUPLES TO HAVE A CHILD

Those who protect and represent children who have been abused often question the right of some individuals to parent. They reason that a person must have a license to drive a car, display a sense of financial responsibility to own a home, display emotional stability and a certain mental status to hold job. Why are people not required to demonstrate an ability to parent before conceiving a child? When the state plans adoptions, potential adoptive parent are placed under intense scrutiny. Should potential biological parents not be subject to similar inquiry? For generations, marriages between relatives have been discouraged and even disallowed in some states to prevent the passing of undesirable traits. Now that we can identify disease predispositions through genetic testing, should we not require premarital gene mapping?

On the other hand, does a couple have the right to have a child? Should the financial expense of a child born with a serious genetic disease be shared through insurance premiums?

About 5.3 million people of childbearing age, or one in six couples, experience infertility problems, and roughly one-third of them seek treatment that costs more than $1 billion annually. But only 10 states mandate insurance coverage for employees, and the coverage requirements for the most expensive treatment, in vitro fertilization, vary widely. Overall, about 16% of insurance plans offer coverage for treatments, which typically costs between a few thousand dollars and $100,000.

Jacobs, Margaret A., "Women Seek Infertility Benefits Under Disabilities Law," *The Wall Street Journal*, P. B7 (June 12, 1996)

Bob and Elise had been married for six years and wanted to enrich their lives by having a child. After several months of trying, they visited a fertility specialist who made the diagnosis that Bob did not have enough active sperm to fertilize an egg. They were offered the following options:

1. Adoption.
2. Homologous artificial insemination. The spermatozoa are those of the woman's husband. This is called AIH, or artificial insemination by the husband.
3. Heterologous artificial insemination. The spermatozoa are taken from a donor who is not the husband of the woman. This is called AID, or artificial insemination by donor.
4. Heterologous artificial insemination. The spermatozoa are taken from a donor who is not the husband and mixed with the husband's.

Now change the facts. The husband is able to donate the sperm, but the wife is unable to conceive. She has healthy eggs. Which of the following is personally preferable?

1. Her sister volunteers to allow an embryo to be implanted and to carry the child to term for the couple.
2. A stranger, a female who will become pregnant with the couple's embryo (sperm and egg), will carry the child to term for a fee.

Let us change the facts again. The husband, at the age of twenty-two years, discovers that he has prostate cancer. He has the option, prior to surgery and **chemotherapy,** to have his sperm frozen. His wife could then be artificially inseminated with the sperm at a later date. The control of the cancer is successful, and the couple plans a child. It is determined that the wife cannot conceive because of scarred fallopian tubes. Eggs are surgically removed from the wife's ovaries and conception takes place in a laboratory petri dish. Some of the embryos are frozen for future implantation. The first attempts to impregnate the wife are unsuccessful. The husband dies. Which of the following seems reasonable?

1. Continue to artificially implant the wife with the remaining embryos.
2. Impregnate a surrogate mother.
3. Throw the embryos away.

RIGHTS OF THE FETUS

In the first decision in New York involving a dispute over frozen embryos, a State Supreme Court justice has ruled that the woman who provides the eggs has the sole right to determine the embryos' fate. . . . Steve and Maureen Kent Kass, who struggled for years to have a baby before divorcing in 1993, as part of their divorce settlement agreed to let the court decide whether Mrs. Kass, who is infertile, could have the eggs implanted in herself in the hope of giving birth. Mr. Kass sought to have the embryos turned over to doctors for medical research. . . . The embryos are being preserved in tanks of liquid nitrogen. . . . Mrs. Kass stated that she intended to have all the embryos implanted in herself within a month. "I feel great," she said. "The eggs can now realize their potential to become human life." Mr. Kass said that he objects to being held responsible for the financial support of children born several years after his divorce. The Kasses were married for five years. The five embryos were fertilized with Mr. Kass's sperm in May 1993, two months before Mrs. Kass filed for divorce.

The ruling contradicts the findings of a Tennessee Supreme Court in a similar case, *Davis v. Davis,* where the court awarded custody of seven embryos to the husband, who destroyed them. The court in that case found that his right not to have children outweighed the rights of his wife, who sought to donate the embryos to an infertile couple.

"Judge Rule Favors Mother," *New York Times,*
p. B5 (January 10, 1995)

The repercussions of the disposition of frozen embryos affect other areas of society. Social security refused to pay benefits to a Louisiana girl conceived from her father's frozen sperm three months after he died of cancer. An administrative law judge ruled that Judith Christine Hart, age four years, was clearly her father's child and was entitled to benefits. The Social Security Administration argued that Judith is not entitled to survivor's benefits because she was never dependent on her father due to the fact that she was conceived after he died. Judith's mother responded to the decision by appealing in federal court and stated:

"My husband and I planned this child and I don't feel government can step in and say how you reproduce, or when. We're not going to get rich off Social Security. It's not the money, it's the principle of the thing. How dare someone step into my private life like this. . . ." Both sides say the case raises questions about whether the rules surrounding Social Security, which dates from the Depression, are keeping up with advances in reproductive medicine.

Dixon, Jennifer, "Agency Remains Firm in Refusal of
Benefits in Frozen-Sperm Birth," *The Patriot Ledger*
(July 29, 1995)

The life of the fetus is an area that is steeped in tradition and folklore. Just decades ago, children were told the "stork brought babies." In the nineties, fetal rights are being defended in court. Again technology has entered human lives, providing options for medical treatment unavailable in the past and thereby redefining ethics and practice. In this area, the courts have taken the lead.

The Pennsylvania Supreme Court held that a stillborn child's estate may seek recovery through a **wrongful death** and **survival action** for injuries sustained while in the womb. The court stated that a stillborn child, like one born alive, is a separate individual while in the womb and has a right to be free from prenatal injury. The facts of the case follow:

CASE STUDY   The plaintiffs were the parents of a full-term stillborn girl. They brought two causes of action against the obstetricians, one in their own right and a second as administrators of their child's estate. Both claimed that the obstetricians' negligence was the cause of the child's death. They sought damages for medical and burial expenses, lost earnings, loss of enjoyment of life, physical pain, and mental anguish.

Both sides agreed that a viable child during gestation is an individual separate from the mother. Previously, the court had decided that a child born alive was able to recover from injuries sustained during gestation. The court based its decision on the reasoning that to deny a stillborn child recovery for fatal injuries during gestation while allowing such recovery for a child born alive would make it "more profitable for the defendant to kill the plaintiff than to scratch him."

Amadio v. Levin,
501 A.2d 1085 (Pa. 1985)

This decision brings Pennsylvania into agreement with twenty-nine other jurisdictions that permit a stillborn child's estate to bring a wrongful death action for injuries sustained during **gestation.** The rights of the fetus prevailed in a decision in San Jose, California. The facts are as follows:

Derrick Poole and Marie Odette Henderson were planning to marry and raise their child, but during the twenty-seventh week of pregnancy, Marie was declared brain dead from a brain tumor. Her parents, as was their right, made the decision to turn off the life-support system. Derrick, who was not yet married to Marie, wanted the life-support to remain on until the baby was born, or at least reached the developmental stage that it could survive. The hospital was caught in the middle because Poole was not legally bound to the mother or the child and had no rights to make a decision. The case went to court.

The parents of Marie agreed to continuing life-support until the birth of the child. Judge John A. Flaherty, of Santa Clara County Superior Court, signed the settlement and gave custody of the fetus to Derrick Poole.

The baby was born, a healthy female, and lives with her father, who is assisted in her care by his sisters.

The Patriot Ledger (June 25, 1986)

In the above case, the judge decided that the fetus had a right to be born. On the other side of the issue are cases for wrongful life, which hold that fetuses have a right not to be born. These cases hold that the physician, by failing to inform the parents fully, is responsible for the birth of a congenitally deformed child who otherwise would not have been born and would not have suffered the pain caused by the deformity. For example:

CASE STUDY

Mrs. Park, the plaintiff, gave birth to a baby who lived for five hours. The cause of death was a hereditary kidney disease that had a high probability that future children of this couple would be born with it. Immediately following the birth, the Parks entered genetic counseling with the intention of determining whether another child born to them would be at risk for the same disease. The defendant, Dr. Chessin, stated that the chances were "practically nil." Mrs. Parks gave birth to another baby who was born with kidney disease and died shortly thereafter. The Parks brought a cause of action against Dr. Chessin alleging that the defendant's advice was the proximate cause of the injury.

The court held that there was a viable cause of action on behalf of an infant for wrongful life. Public policy consideration gives the parents a right not to have a child; the breach of this right may also be tortious to the fundamental right of a child to be born as a whole, functional human being.

Park v. Chassin,
80 App. Div. 2d 60, 400 N.Y.S.2d 110 (1977)

Now that it has been determined that a fetus has rights, can a mother be charged for abuse to the fetus that results in a brain-damaged baby? If fetal neglect becomes a cause of action, would it mean that a pregnant woman is guilty of a crime if she does not eat properly, fails to drink enough milk, smokes, or drinks alcohol? Could this be extended to a cause of action against the state for not providing proper food and environment for indigent pregnant mothers? The following case gives one judge's solution to the problem:

Pamela Rae Steward, twenty-seven years of age from El Cajon, California, was arrested on September 27, 1986, in connection with the death of her son, Thomas, who died on New Year's Day in 1986. She was charged with the misdemeanor of willfully failing to provide necessary care for her child. She was freed on $2,500 bond.

Dr. Paul Zlotnik had advised Pamela that her pregnancy was complicated by a misaligned placenta and that she should avoid street drugs, abstain from sex, and take prescribed medication. When she gave birth to a brain-dead son, the doctor ordered tests that indicated that she neglected all three admonitions.

On February 27, 1987, Municipal Court Judge E. MacAmos threw out the criminal case ruling that prosecutors were wrong to apply a section of the penal code to the case. He said the statute is used to ensure that parents pay child support, not to punish women for conduct during pregnancy that could affect their unborn children.

"California Judge Dismisses Fetal Abuse Charges,"
Associated Press, San Diego, *The Boston Globe* (February 28, 1987)

There has been considerable scientific interest in using the fetus for transplants. Using the following hypothetical situations, think about this issue.

Suppose an elderly patient is suffering from the degenerative progression of Parkinson's disease. There is hope that the ravages of the disease may be stopped or reversed by transplanting neural tissue from the human fetus. Experimentation done with monkeys has shown that symptoms similar to Parkinson's can be controlled by transplanting tissue into the brain of an afflicted adult animal.

1. A neurosurgeon at a large teaching facility wishes to transplant tissues from an aborted fetus into the brain of an elderly statesman.
2. The wife of the statesman wishes to become pregnant by having embryos the couple froze implanted in her uterus. Then she plans to abort the fetus to allow for the best tissue match.
3. The technique has never been performed in a human before.

Let us now change the facts. We find that the viable fetus is stillborn following a third-trimester miscarriage.

1. A cardiac surgeon wishes to transplant the heart of the stillborn child into an infant born prematurely who will not survive with her own deformed heart for more than two days.
2. The preemie has additional deformities of internal organs but no apparent physical deformities.
3. The preemie has additional internal and physical deformities.
4. Because of the stillborn's physical anomalies, the pathologist wishes to preserve the child's body in formaldehyde to use as a teaching specimen.

Again let us change the facts to show that a child is born full-term and **anencephalic,** without a brain but with a brain stem. The accepted definition of brain death requires irreversible cessation of all functions of the entire brain, including brain stem.

1. A surgeon wishes to transfer the liver from the newborn to a child who needs a liver transplant and otherwise appears to be able to survive.
2. A surgeon wishes to keep the child alive on life-support systems to increase the size of the heart before transplant to another child. A larger heart has the potential for a better result for the recipient.
3. A surgeon wishes to transfer the internal organs of the newborn to several children, but the family refuses consent.

RIGHTS OF A NEWBORN

The Anencephalic Child

Eighteen months after declaring it ethically acceptable to take organs from infants who were born anencephalic, the American Medical Association (AMA) changed its policy:

> In changing its policy, the AMA reinstated an earlier one favoring prohibition of the use of such babies as organ donors until they meet the legal criteria for brain death: the complete cessation of brain function. . . . That policy reflected concern about the widely recognized shortage of donor organs, particularly for infants. . . . Although organ donation in such cases, as in any others, was already allowed once brain death occurred, by that time the organs have usually deteriorated too much to be used.
>
> A leading opponent to the policy was Dr. James Bernat, a neurologist at the Dartmouth Medical Center who said that the policy "was a mistake because it broke the dead donor rule," a longtime principle under which organs must never be taken from any patient, anencephalic or not, who is not legally dead. Whatever little benefit might occur from the organs would be more than outweighed by the damage to society. Once you start killing people for their organs people would begin to push the development. We felt it was better to maintain the dead donor rule even if there would be fewer organs around."
>
> A particularly strong objection came from Dr. Michael Williams, a neurologist at Johns Hopkins University, who maintains that although it is certain that anencephalics have "zero potential for normal development," it has not been proved that they will never achieve consciousness. "And, I think most people would agree," he said, "that it's unethical to take organs from any human being who has consciousness."
>
> "AMA Opposes Taking Organs from Brain-
> Malformed Babies," *New York Times,* p. 22 (January 7, 1996)

Baby Jesse needed a heart transplant. No donor hearts were available for the child, but that was not the problem. The Loma Linda University Medical Center had refused to consider the infant as a candidate for a transplant because she did not meet one of the following mandatory requirements for heart transplant candidates: (1) the candidate must present no other serious medical problems and no likelihood of survival with conventional treatment, and (2) the parents must be able to understand and follow a complex treatment program.

The medical center determined that Baby Jesse's parents were unable to understand and follow a complex postsurgical treatment program. The parents, who were unmarried, were Deanna, seventeen, and Jesse, twenty-six. After the parents surrendered the child to the grandparents, the medical center reversed its stand, and the child, at twelve days of age, became a candidate for a heart transplant.

As soon as a child is born, he or she is a minor and under the legal and physical custody of his or her parent(s). The state, under the doctrine of **parens patriae,** has the responsibility of removing the child from the family if the child is found to be at risk for neglect or abuse.

In the spring of 1982, an infant, identified only as Baby Doe, was born in Bloomington, Indiana. The diagnosis at birth was Down's syndrome and an obstruction of the digestive tract that precluded normal feeding but was apparently surgically correctable. The parents refused to give consent to surgery, and the hospital took the matter to the court. The superior court concluded that when, as in this case, the parents were "confronted with two competent medical opinions, one suggesting that corrective surgery may be appropriate and the other suggesting that corrective surgery and extraordinary measures would only be futile acts, it was the parents' responsibility to choose the appropriate action without interference by the government." The child soon died.

The case was heavily covered by the press and appeared on television. The media portrayed the child as one who had been denied routine surgical treatment and allowed to starve to death for no reason other than a mild, unrelated handicap. On April 30, 1982, President Reagan sent a memorandum to officials in the government instructing them to take steps to prevent repetition of such an abuse. On May 18, 1982, a notice was sent to most of the nation's hospitals by the Department of Health and Human Services, explaining that the "discriminatory failure of a federally assisted health-care provider to feed a handicapped infant, or to provide medical treatment essential to correct a life-threatening condition," could be found to violate a federal rehabilitation act. The development of final so-called Baby Doe regulations took several more years and demonstrated the difficulty of legislating medical issues and the complexity of regulating ethical issues.

On April 15, 1985, the Department of Health and Human Services provided a final draft of the Baby Doe regulations for the treatment of handicapped children. Public policy behind these regulations prevents withholding of medical care from an infant with one or more noncongenital anomalies by defining the withholding of medical care as neglect. According to the rules, if there is treatment for the condition, it must be provided. There are three exceptions to the policy:

1. When the infant is chronically and irreversibly comatose.
2. When treatment would merely prolong dying.
3. When the treatment would be futile either because the child would not survive or the treatment would be inhumane.

This federal legislation requires the states to establish programs and/or procedures within their child-protective service system. It requires response to needs for treatment by disabled infants with life-threatening conditions.

RIGHTS OF A CHILD

Does a child have the rights of an adult? The allowance by an insurance company for a transplant procedure for a child provides one answer:

After initially refusing to pay more than $500,000 in medical bills for a Norwich boy's transplant surgery, the Connecticut Medicaid office has worked out an agreement with the hospital. The Medicaid office and Children's Hospital of Pittsburgh disputed whether the hospital had filed the proper legal and financial documents for Joey Rogers' intestine and kidney transplant surgery. Joey, 8, was born without a small intestine and was never able to eat solid food until he received the transplant.

The hospital filed the necessary documents and will be reimbursed for 77.9 percent of any Connecticut patient's bills for its fiscal year.

"Connecticut Boy's Transplant Bill is Settled,"
The Boston Globe, p. A21 (October 10, 1995)

Improved technology offers many advances that can improve quality of life but also presents ethical dilemmas that cannot be anticipated. One promising technology is that of harvesting, freezing, and storing a baby's umbilical cord in case the child ever gets sick and needs it. Can we do this for everyone, or is it just for the rich?

It costs $1,500 for the testing and harvesting, and $95 a year for storage and it's probably money thrown away. But, if somewhere down the road the child needed some type of therapy where this could be used, we'd hate to be in the position of saying, "If only we had his umbilical cord blood."

Using umbilical cord blood to treat fatal diseases is still experimental, and no one yet knows exactly for whom it should be used, how well it works compared with other treatments, like bone marrow transplants, how long the stored blood remains useful or what should be the role of public and private blood banks. . . . [I]t could be a kind of health insurance for the whole family. . . . The majority see this as a choice for parents and doctors to make an investment in the future. It's not just for leukemia. It's potentially for breast cancer, or even AIDS.

Lewin, Tamar, "Blood Banks Starting to Harvest
Umbilical Cords," *New York Times,* p. 12 (January 1, 1996)

Children may be conceived by parents for their assistance in the treatment of a serious illness of another family member. The following is an excerpt from an article in the *New York Times* of June of 1991:

At about 8:00 this morning doctors at the City of Hope Medical Center in Duarte, Calif., plan to transplant bone marrow into Anissa Ayala, a 19-year-old girl who is dying of leukemia. The marrow will come from her baby sister, Marissa. Their parents say they conceived Marissa to provide bone marrow to save Anissa's life.

Doctors and ethicists say this is the first time a family has publicly admitted conceiving a child to serve as an organ donor. But many others have done so privately. . . . In a recent survey of bone marrow transplant centers, 40 cases were uncovered in which families had confided to doctors that they were conceiving babies to serve as donors. . . . Ethicists and doctors are asking whether conceiving a child as a source of donated organs violates the principle that individuals should be brought into the world and cherished for their own sake and no other motive.

Others argue that the children who are conceived to donate organs are deeply loved and that it is unfair to point fingers at parents who have a child to save another person's life.

Kolata, Gina, "More Babies Being Born to Be Donors of Tissue," *New York Times,* p. 1 (June 4, 1991)

AUTONOMY VERSUS PATERNALISM FOR THE CHILD

HIV Testing for Pregnant Women

Following is an ethical dilemma involving children and the **HIV** testing of pregnant women:

Since 1985, the Centers for Disease Control and Prevention (CDC) and other agencies have suggested that pregnant women who are at risk for HIV infection, such as those who use intravenous drugs or whose sexual partners are at high risk for infection, be tested for HIV.

As of December 1994, the CDC had received reports of more than 58,448 AIDS cases among adult and adolescent women and more than 5,000 cases among children who acquired HIV infection perinatally. Nearly all new HIV infections among children in the United States are attributed to perinatal transmission.

An estimated 7,000 HIV-infected women delivered infants in the United States during 1993. Perinatal transmission rates are estimated at between 15% and 30%. Based on these rates, about 1000 to 2000 infants were infected with HIV through their mothers in 1993. . . . A randomized study of more than 500 HIV-infected pregnant women, sponsored by the National Institute of Health (NIH), found that zidovudine (AZT) use could reduce perinatal infections by as much as 67%.

Jones, Laurie, "HIV Tests Urged for Pregnant Women," *AMNEWS,* p. 5 (March 13, 1995)

Most of the HIV-infected babies born in the United States each year have mothers who are unaware of their own infections. Women may refuse to undergo testing for HIV because of the stigma associated with intravenous drug use or interaction with multiple sexual partners. Children infected with the HIV virus at birth may live for years without symptoms and without anyone knowing that they are infected. Doctors may fail to recognize that HIV is the source of children's illnesses. Has this become an ethical dilemma placing a baby's rights to medical care against a mother's rights to privacy?

Teenage Treatment Decisions

Billy Best, sixteen years of age, was a patient at Dana-Farber Cancer Institute in Boston when he was informed that he needed four more months of treatments to wipe out the remaining cancer around his windpipe. He was given an ultimatum by his doctors: continue chemotherapy treatments for Hodgkin's disease or face a painful death. His parents agreed with the doctors and required Billy to continue the treatments at the Dana-Farber Institute. At sixteen, he was considered a minor without the capacity to make this decision for himself.

Billy determined he was no longer going to accept chemotherapy and ran away from home, crossing the United States from Boston to Texas. He claimed that the painful treatments were killing him and chose instead homeopathic drug treatment. His parents, after studying the alternative treatments, agreed with his decision, and Billy returned home. A year later tests revealed that the cancer had disappeared. Legally, Billy was unable to make the treatment decision in Massachusetts. Ethically, is it right that he should be forced to undergo treatment against his will?

ALLOCATION OF RESOURCES

Mothers with AIDS

What does a court do when a mother has **AIDS** and the children are brought to the state's attention due to her neglect and/or drug abuse? When children are removed from a mother, the caseworker prepares a contract between the state agency and the parent to map a route for return of the child to the parent.

> Each case has its own particulars, but many judges and caseworkers say that they always present heartbreaking choices. Should children in a loving foster home be put through a wrenching separation when the parent is likely to die or become ill in the near future? Is time with a parent so precious and important to a child's identity that it should override other considerations? Should attempts to find housing and drug treatment be expedited for parents with a terminal illness like AIDS?
>
> Lee, Felicia R., "Difficult Custody Decisions Being Complicated by AIDS," *New York Times*, p. 22 (March 6, 1993)

Treating Children's Behavior Issues

There are many ethical dilemmas in current practices involving the psychopharmacological treatment of children. One controversy is the use of drugs versus the use of more traditional counseling and support therapy for children with suspected mental illnesses. A second controversy surrounds the acceptability of an apparent experimental use of drugs to treat children. Dr. Connor of the University of Massachusetts Medical School, in an article in *JAMA*, gives parameters to the problem:

> Aggressive and antisocial behavior in the broad sense is a huge problem . . . the most prevalent symptoms presenting to pediatric mental health providers regardless

of the setting, occurring in one third to one half of all cases referred to child and adolescent psychiatric clinics. . . . For patients, managed care has meant more emphasis on drug treatment over counseling. . . . [I]f patients need to talk about their difficulties, doctors must send them on to social workers or to free support groups like Alcoholics Anonymous."

Marwick, Charles, "Childhood Aggression Needs
Definition, Therapy," *JAMA,* 275(2):90 (January 10, 1996)

Because the health care industry is determined to cut costs, managed care organizations emphasize drug treatment over counseling. This policy dictates the care that today's children receive.

When Nancy Hull's son was four, the cheerful little boy suddenly turned silent and unresponsive. After she took him for a psychological evaluation, the reason emerged: a neighbor, the father of one of her son's friends, has sexually molested the boy.

The specialist recommended weekly therapy for the child, but Hull's health insurer refused to pay for it. Hull says she had to quit her part-time job and go on welfare so her son could obtain mental health benefits through Medicaid. "It was one of the hardest things I ever did," said Hull, who asked to use a pseudonym.

But it paid off. Her son, now eight, is doing well and Hull has since returned to work full-time. Still, she remains angry at a health care system that she says forced her to choose between her son's emotional health and her own dignity, and also fails to recognize the value of preventive care.

Bass, Allison, "Children's Mental Health Coverage
Often Falling Short," *The Boston Globe,* p. 1 (May 12, 1995)

It is important to consider the consequences of medicating children with drugs whose psychological effect may harm the body. It may be years before we know the effect of certain medications given to children during different stages of development.

SUMMARY

Ethical considerations involving the rights of a fetus, birth issues, the neonatal period, and the growing child are gaining prominence. Technology makes it possible to exercise more control over birth and the beginning of life by detecting genetic and chromosomal abnormalities and by improving techniques for zygote formation.

New techniques for artificial insemination raise questions of surrogate motherhood and paternal responsibility. Whether women have the right to contract their body for the purpose of carrying another couple's child has involved the courts as well as religious institutions.

Questions about fetal rights and maternal legal obligations during pregnancy take on new importance as technology's ability to intervene during pregnancy advances. Because of the value of fetal tissue in transplants, society takes a new look at the need to protect the fetus. Because of conflicting ethical positions on sanctity versus quality of life, society takes steps to control procedures used to care for handicapped newborn infants.

With the advent of newer methods for prolonging the lives of children with AIDS, pregnant women are under increasing pressure to submit to testing for the HIV virus. There has been a change in the care of mentally ill children, resulting from cost reduction policies of health care organizations.

There are many questions but few answers at this point in time.

SUGGESTED ACTIVITY

Contact a local agency involved in the care of children who have been neglected or abused and request a copy of their guidelines for responding to the medical needs of children in their care. Ask for particulars for children with failure-to-thrive syndrome, fetal-alcohol syndrome, HIV positive status, and those with congenital abnormalities requiring surgery. Discuss the process required by the agency and compare it to what you would do if you were responsible for one of these children. During the discussion, consider the availability of the child for adoption.

STUDY QUESTIONS

1. Three major religions in America have commented on artificial insemination of women. Do research to determine if other religious organizations have moral positions on the matter.
2. If you were pregnant and had a family history of a genetic disease, would you have amniocentesis to determine if the fetus was defective? What factors would you consider when determining whether to abort the fetus?
3. Define sanctity of life and give an example of an ethical decision based on this philosophy.
4. Define quality of life and give an example of an ethical decision based on this philosophy.
5. What restrictions, if any, would you place on pregnant mothers?
6. Do you believe aborted fetal tissue should be used for transplant purposes? Why or why not? Do you believe the government should control this area of medicine? How?
7. Anencephalics will not live for an appreciable period of time. The organs in their bodies are often not large enough to be transplanted. What are your thoughts about keeping the body alive long enough to allow the major organs to reach a size where they can be transplanted to other infants?

8. Children born with certain handicaps are born to a life of suffering and pain. If extraordinary means are used to keep these children alive, they may live for a few weeks but not without continual medical intervention. If allowed to die at birth without intervention, they will live a few hours at most. Try to develop a philosophy for both sides of this issue.

9. Defend and differ with this statement: Parents should be required to cover the cost of medical care for every child born to them.

10. Defend and differ with this statement: The state should be required to cover the cost of medical care for every handicapped child.

CASES FOR DISCUSSION

1. The plaintiff became pregnant and bore a child after undergoing a sterilization operation. She sued the doctor who performed the surgery for negligence, for the pregnancy, and for birth and the costs of rearing a normal, healthy child. Should she win?

2. The plaintiff gave birth to a daughter with Tay-Sachs disease. Children born with this incurable degenerative nerve disease do not live long. The plaintiffs claimed that the defendant doctor was negligent in that he failed to take a proper genealogical history or to properly evaluate their genetic histories. The plaintiffs were Eastern European Jews, a fact that should have put the defendant on notice that there was a high risk the child would suffer from the disease. They also stated that if they had known of the risk involved, they would have taken tests and, if the results were positive, aborted the pregnancy. Both parents claimed that they underwent considerable anguish observing their child suffer prior to her death. Was there a cause of action against the defendant-doctor?

3. A woman who was eight-and-one-half months pregnant was in an automobile accident. During emergency surgery, the fetus was found dead. The mother died shortly afterward. Will a cause of action for wrongful death be allowed because the fetus, although stillborn, was viable at the time of injury?

4. The plaintiff contracted rubella in the first trimester of pregnancy and gave birth to a child with multiple birth defects. The plaintiff was hospitalized at the time of her illness and had asked the physician if her illness was rubella. The physician assured her that it was not. The plaintiff brought a cause of action against the doctor for failure to advise her of the risk. What cause of action does the plaintiff have against the doctor?

5. After seven years of marriage, it was medically determined that the defendant was sterile. His wife desired a child, either by artificial insemination or by adoption. At first, the defendant refused his consent. Approximately fifteen years into the marriage, the defendant agreed to artificial insemination of his wife. His wife became pregnant

and gave birth to a baby boy. The couple separated four years after the child was born. The wife then became ill and applied for public assistance under the Aid to Needy Children program. The defendant refused to pay child support. The municipal court ordered him to pay support through the District Attorney's office. The defendant appealed. Should the defendant have to pay support?

6. During a first marriage, a woman bore a child after consensual artificial insemination. Her husband was listed as the father on the birth certificate. The couple later separated and then divorced. Both the separation agreement and the divorce decree declared the child to be the offspring of the couple. The wife was granted support and the husband visitation rights. The woman remarried and her second husband petitioned to adopt the child. The first husband refused his consent. The second husband then suggested that the first husband's consent was not required because he was not the parent of the child. Should the first husband's consent be necessary?

7. C.C. had a child who was conceived with sperm donated by C.M. C.C. wanted to have a child and wanted C.M. to be the father, but did not want to have intercourse with him before their marriage. He therefore agreed to provide the sperm. C.C. learned, after a conversation with her doctor, of a procedure for artificial insemination using a syringe and a glass jar. After several attempts, C.C. did conceive a child. The relationship between the two parties broke off, and C.M. wanted visitation rights to the baby. C.C. does not wish to allow visitation rights. Should visitation rights be allowed?

8. The plaintiff, at thirty-seven years of age, conceived a child. After conception, the plaintiff and her husband engaged the services of the defendants, specialists in obstetrics and gynecology. The baby was born with Down's syndrome, commonly known as mongolism. The plaintiff contends that they were never advised by the defendants of the increased risk of Down's syndrome in children born to women over thirty-five years of age, nor were they advised of the availability of an amniocentesis test. Do the plaintiffs have an action in wrongful life for their child and in their own right for the various sums of money they will spend for the long-term institutional care of their retarded child? Should they sue as well for the emotional and physical injury suffered by the mother as a result of the birth of her child and the medical expenses stemming from her treatment?

9. Considerable publicity has surrounded the custody battle for Baby M. The woman who carried the child had contracted with a couple, a biochemist and a pediatrician, to bear a child in exchange for money. It was a business agreement, but the carrying female began to have a change of heart after the child began growing within her and wanted to keep the child as her own. Should the court allow her to keep the child? Why or why not?

Chapter 11

Professional Ethics and the Living

There was this patient at the nursing home I used to see. And every time I saw him, he asked me if I had the pills he wanted so that he could end his life. Well, one day I walked into the nursing home and he was singing as he walked his walker down the hall. I went up to him and told him that I had the pills he wanted in my pocket and where did he want me to leave them? He told me he didn't want them anymore. You see, an old friend of his that he grew up with as a child had just become a resident of the nursing home and they were having a great time together, singing, playing cards and reminiscing about the good old days. Of course, I didn't have the pills with me.

Jules Rubin, M.D.
Canton, Massachusetts

OBJECTIVES:

Dr. Rubin was a beloved physician in the town of Canton, Massachusetts. The above comment comes from his wealth of experiences. In the difficult area of medical ethics, talking with professionals who have been over the many roads that these chapters on ethics cover will give you the opportunity to profit by their experiences. After reading this chapter, you should be able to:

1. understand the creed of the American Association of Medical Assistants, the Preamble to the Code of Ethics of the American Medical Association, and provisions of the Uniform Anatomical Gift Act and of the Nuremberg Code.
2. appreciate the relationship between time and power.
3. identify some of the problems faced by medical professionals in allocating resources: transplant organs, money, and intensive care unit (ICU) beds.
4. understand the ethics of medical experimentation.
5. recognize the problems the world faces with AIDS and emerging viruses.
6. question the propriety of drug testing in employment.
7. recognize the importance of balancing autonomy and paternalism in patient care.

BUILDING YOUR LEGAL VOCABULARY

autograft	creed	Nuremberg Code
autonomy	heterograft	paternalism
calibration	homograft	personality traits
commitment		

CREEDS

The **creed** of the American Association of Medical Assistants reads as follows:

I believe in the principles and purposes of the profession of medical assisting.
I endeavor to be more effective.
I aspire to render greater service.
I protect the confidence entrusted to me.
I am dedicated to the care and well-being of all people.
I am loyal to my employer.
I am true to the ethics of my profession.
I am strengthened by compassion, courage, and faith.

American Association of Medical Assistants, Inc.
(Adopted, October 1996)

Collectively this creed was developed to embody the highest ethical standards of the medical office professional. It is narrower in scope than the Principles of Medical Ethics of the American Medical Association but is closely aligned with the AMA ethical philosophy that follows:

PREAMBLE
The medical profession has long subscribed to a body of ethical statements developed primarily for the benefit of the patient. As a member of this profession, a physician must recognize responsibility not only to the patients, but also to society, to other health-care professionals, and to self. The following Principles adopted by the American Medical Association are not laws, but standards of conduct which define the essentials of honorable behavior for the physician.

I.   A physician shall be dedicated to providing competent medical service with compassion and respect for human dignity.

II.   A physician shall deal honestly with patients and colleagues, and strive to expose those physicians deficient in character or competence, or who engage in fraud or deception.

III. A physician shall respect the law and also recognize a responsibility to seek changes in those requirements which are contrary to the best interests of the patient.

IV.   A physician shall respect the rights of patients, of colleagues, and of other health-care professionals, and shall safeguard patient confidences within the constraints of the law.

V. A physician shall continue to study, apply and advance scientific knowledge, make relevant information available to patients, colleagues, and the public, obtain consultation, and use the talents of other health care professionals when indicated.

VI. A physician shall, in the provision of appropriate patient care, except in emergencies, be free to choose whom to serve, and with whom to associate, and the environment in which to provide medical services.

VII. A physician shall recognize a responsibility to participate in activities contributing to an improved community.

American Medical Association Principles of Medical Ethics
(Source: Code of Medical Ethics Current Opinions with Annotations,
American Medical Association. Copyright 1994.)

Developing a code of ethics is difficult, but implementing these ideals in daily life is even more difficult. The role of allied health care professionals, such as medical office employees, does not usually involve making life-and-death ethical decisions. It does involve interpersonal interaction with patients and their families before and after difficult decisions have been made. It also involves support and understanding of the physicians who make these difficult decisions. It is important that each employee find his or her place in the office dynamics during intense, pressure-filled, decision-making moments. For example, someone who is not comfortable with abortion should seek employment in an office that is compatible with that moral perspective. The clinical situation is inappropriate for debates or the airing of one's personal preferences. Working in an environment that is not morally comfortable puts intense stress on everyone and can potentially harm the patient. The internal discomfort of the incompatible employee will eventually result in burnout with its undesirable consequences.

Situations that are ethical in nature and aggravating in practice are frequently met by allied health care professionals. A constant sore spot in the doctor-patient relationship is the time patients spend waiting.

TIME

Health care professionals, like most people, prefer their weekends and evenings free. As health care deliverers are forced to utilized their facilities and equipment more efficiently, weekends and evening hours are becoming available for ambulatory patients. Who must work on evenings and weekends? Is it the chief of staff, the resident, or the intern? Is it the head of a department, or the last one to join the organization? Who is able to change a weekend or evening assignment easily—the head of the department or the last one in? The answer to all these questions is the employee with the most power. Is it ethical to base these decisions on status within the organization?

The relationship between time, power, and ethics is evident in the office or clinic waiting room. Powerful people do not wait. The President of the United States is ushered into his private suite for health care. On the other end of the continuum:

> Even for the same services . . . the line is longer for the less important. People who go to clinics usually wait longer to see a doctor than those who can afford to make appointments with private practitioners.
>
> Levine, Robert, "Waiting Is a Power Game,"
> *Psychology Today,* pp. 24–33 (April 1987)

In many medical offices, the doctor keeps patients waiting. Is it ethical to keep all patients waiting the same amount of time, or do the most influential patients get in first? Are there different standards of care in attending to the needs of waiting patients? Does priority depend upon the urgency of each case, for example, an emergency case? Do office ethics take into consideration the importance of time for everyone waiting?

Time is a limited resource. There are ethical considerations with the allocation of time, as well as other resources.

ALLOCATION OF RESOURCES

Should everyone who needs expensive life-saving procedures, such as open heart surgery and organ transplants, have an equal chance to get them regardless of ability to pay, social status, or other nonmedical factors? Is health care for everyone really possible? Who will pay? If health care for everyone is not possible, who will receive life-saving services? Dr. John Kitzhaber, a physician and the president of the Oregon State Medical Society, comments:

> "It's hard for Americans to admit it, but this country does ration health care. And we do it in ways that are unfair and inefficient. For example, we spend over $50 billion a year on people in the last six months of their lives, while closing pediatric clinics. We spend over $3 billion a year on intensive care for newborn babies, while denying prenatal care to hundreds of thousands of expectant women. Is the human tragedy and personal anguish of death from the lack of an organ transplant any greater than that of an infant dying in an intensive care unit from a preventable problem brought on by the lack of prenatal care?"
>
> Robinson, Donald, "Who Should Receive Medical Aid?,"
> *Parade Magazine,* p. 4 (May 28, 1989)

In a response to the allocation of resources, the country has turned to the concept of managed care.

Managed Care

In the 1990s, the term *managed care* is a household word. With the goal of increased patient access and cost-effective preventive medicine constantly appearing on the television advertisements of managed care organizations (MCOs), ethical questions are surfacing that test the industry's credibility. In 1996, it was estimated that fifty to sixty million Americans were enrolled in managed care through their employers, as Medicare beneficiaries or as private subscribers. Ethical and legal conflicts abound for the individuals who operate the system: the doctors, the nurse practitioners, the triage personnel, the case managers, the MCO administrators, the risk managers, the utilization reviewers, and the corporate executives.

The former fee-for-service system contributed to the rise of health care costs. In an effort to contain these costs, a total system change occurred. As a result of the shift to managed care, the seriously ill patient needing more services became a burden. From the consumer's perspective, the single greatest threat posed by this shift is the potential for managed care systems to cut needed care and to save health care dollars. Managed care often obscures the line separating insurers from providers. In addition, health care providers, paid on a capitation basis, who realize bonuses for fiscal restraint or who have portions of their salary withheld in order to control costs make less money with a seriously ill patient. Inherent in the system is this major conflict:

[P]hysicians who act as gatekeepers for their patients' medical needs will make more money and gain greater job security if they make fewer referrals to specialists, order fewer diagnostic tests, avoid costly procedures, and limit their patient's hospital stays. Physicians who refuse to conform to the system risk termination of their privilege or deselection from the plan. . . .

Also inherent within the managed care system is the use of non-medical personnel acting as case managers or conducting utilization reviews to determine whether a given test, procedure, or referral is covered by the plan or medically necessary. . . . [S]uch personnel can effectively deny to a patient directly, or through the patient's physician, access to specialists, access to diagnostic testing, access to second opinions, and access to emergency care. The patient's ability to maneuver within the system and the doctor's unimpeded clinical decision-making ability are stymied by middle management which often has limited, if any, medical training or expertise.

Ristuben, Karen R., "Implications of Managed Care on Patient Care," *Health Law Section Newsletter,* Massachusetts Bar Association (June 1996)

The Public Advocate for New York City assailed false and deceptive advertising by HMOs, saying that the misinformation made it impossible for consumers, particularly the poor and elderly, to make intelligent choices about health care.

> Mr. Green said that in an investigation conducted by the Public Advocate's office, researchers reviewed 150 pieces of advertising and marketing material from 19 different managed-care plans and found that much of it misrepresented the services that the HMO's offered. . . .
>
> The researchers found, for example, that some HMO's trying to enroll the elderly implied in marketing materials that Medicare patients would pay no premiums, when in fact by law they must still pay some Medicare premiums. At the same time, marketing aimed at poor people implied that Medicaid patients who enrolled would get the same treatment as the plan's paying clients, when HMO's often offer largely separate networks of doctors to their Medicaid and commercial customers.
>
> Rosenthal, Elisabeth, "Public Advocate Says HMO's Often Mislead Poor and Elderly," *New York Times*, p. B4 (November 11, 1995)

There are other ethical problems relating to the allocation of resources, one of which was artfully attacked by Mike Barnicle in an editorial in the *Boston Globe:*

> Yesterday, as morning arrived like an open oven door, Dave Dushane, 44 years old, fought the billowing heat by taking his three daughters grocery shopping. The children are Danielle, 6, Meredith, 3, and Renee, who is 18 months old and will die if left untended for longer than a few minutes. Renee Dushane was born with Pfeiffer's syndrome, a crushing combination of defects affecting one in 60,000 births. She has a huge skull, cannot breathe or swallow on her own, has chronic lung disease, a permanent tracheotomy tube and she cannot talk, cannot even say, "Help." Renee also has no mother. Ellen Dushane died of breast cancer at 37. That was last summer's bad news.
>
> This summer's bad news arrived when Dave Dushane was notified by Blue Cross-Blue Shield and the Commonwealth of Massachusetts that his daughter's nursing benefits are being cut back. The father's options are: Quit his job as a Wakefield police officer and go on welfare to provide round-the-clock care for Renee or let the state put the child in a foster home. "I don't think there are any bad guys here," Dave Dushane was saying, "It's just the system. It's the way the health care system operates. It's crazy."
>
> Right now Renee has 24-hour in-home nursing. Eight of these hours are about to be eliminated. Father makes too much—$38,000 a year—to get Medicaid and not enough to pay a nurse to cover the extra eight hours.
>
> Barnicle, Mike, "Father Battles Insane System," *The Boston Globe*, p. 21 (July 16, 1995)

The pressure brought to bear by the editorial forced the bureaucracy to reevaluate the situation, and nursing care was reinstated.

Transplants

The allocation of resources in transplants is physical and gives rise to many ethical problems. Medical transplants are divided into three categories, depending upon the tissue used. An **autograft** is the transplantation of a person's own tissue from one part of the body to another. This term also describes transplants between identical twins. A **homograft** is a transplant from one person to another, while the transplant of animal tissue into a human is a **heterograft.**

The current wave of transplant operations began in the late 1940s with corneal transplants from dead donors. Kidney transplants began in 1954 and are now commonplace. Liver and lung transplants followed, with the first recorded heart transplant to a human being attempted in 1964 with a chimpanzee's heart. The most common transplant is a blood transfusion.

The rise in transplants has increased competition for organs and blood. In an attempt to control the process, California was the first state to pass statutes allowing a citizen to dispose of his or her own body or to separate parts of it on death through a will or other written document. The Uniform Anatomical Gift Act was passed in 1968. The main provisions of the act are:

1. Any individual of sound mind and eighteen years of age or more may give all or any part of his body . . . the gift to take effect upon death.
2. In the absence of a gift by the deceased, and of any objection by the deceased, his or her relatives, in a stated order of priority (spouse, adult children, parents, adult brothers and sisters, etc.) have the power to give the body or any of its contents.
3. The recipients of a gift are restricted to hospitals, doctors, medical and dental schools, universities, tissue banks, and a specified individual in need of treatment. The purposes are restricted to transplantation, therapy, research, education, and the advancement of medical or dental science.
4. A gift may be made by will (to be effective immediately upon death without waiting for probate), or by a card or other document. If the donor is too sick or incapable of signing, it can be signed for him if two witnesses are present. A gift made by a relative can be made by document, or by telegraph or a recorded telephone message or other recorded message.
5. A gift may be revoked at any time.
6. A donee may accept or reject a gift.

In February 1978, the *New York Times* reported that all states use some system of organ and tissue donor identification in deceased persons. Interest in obtaining organs for transplant is found not only in the United States but also in European, South American, and Asian countries. The use of organs from the dead and, later, from animals presented one set of ethical problems. The use of organs from the living presents even greater ethical dilemmas. Procedures that regulate living donor transplants have been developed through the courts.

Using live donors to obtain organs presents many problems. One is the discomfort of the provider—many physicians will not take skin from a donor because of the pain inflicted. The removal of internal organs for transplant, in addition to the ethics involved with inflicting pain on one person for another's benefit, involves multiple dilemmas. For example:

CASE STUDY

Tommy Strunk, twenty-eight years old, married and employed full-time, was the brother of Jerry Strunk, who was twenty-seven years old, with a mental age of six years, institutionalized and further handicapped by a severe speech defect. Jerry was psychologically and emotionally dependent upon Tommy to the degree that a psychiatrist was of the opinion that Tommy's death would have an extremely traumatic effect upon him. Tommy became ill with glomerulonephritis, was on dialysis and his only hope for survival was a kidney transplant. After exhausting all other donors, it was determined that there was tissue compatibility between the two brothers. The parents made the decision that Jerry would give Tommy a kidney.

Procedurally, a separate guardian ad litem was appointed for Jerry to put all arguments against the removal of his kidney before the court. Jerry and Tommy's mother petitioned the court for an order authorizing the removal of Jerry's kidney. A county court decided that the operation to remove Jerry's kidney was necessary and should take place. The case was appealed to determine whether the court had the legal authority to allow the surgery and, if so, whether the county court had been right to authorize it in this case.

Evidence was presented to the court which indicated that Jerry was aware that he was able to help Tommy and that it was important to prevent Jerry from developing guilt feelings if Tommy should die. Evidence was also presented that Tommy was necessary to Jerry's life and was the only person who would be able to communicate with him after their parents' deaths. Throughout the proceedings the guardian ad litem continually questioned the power of the state to allow the removal of a healthy organ from the body of an incompetent ward of the state.

The Kentucky Court of Appeals determined that the removal of one of Jerry's kidneys for transplant to his brother was in Jerry's best interest and should be allowed to proceed.

Strunk v. Strunk,
445 S.W.2d 145 (Ky. 1969)

As the number and kind of transplants increase, the demand for organs will increase. Worldwide there is consensus that dealing in human organs for profit is illegal, but consensus does not always make law. For centuries, human hair has been used by wig makers and teeth have been implanted into the jaws of wealthy dental patients. In September 1979 in England, heart pacemakers were being taken from corpses, and reused in other patients.

The Sunday Times of London, in a detailed report about worldwide trafficking in human organs, disclosed, in 1977, that between 1970 and 1976 a South Korean medical practitioner had sold twelve thousand pairs of fetal kidneys to an American medical supply corporation at an average price of $15 a pair. They were in great demand because fetal tissue grows more quickly than adult tissue and is therefore more efficient as a medium for developing cultures. The kidneys were taken from aborted fetuses (with written consent from the mothers), packed in ice, and flown out of Seoul the same day. A spokesman for the corporation which bought them said that it acquired fetal tissues from some 250 sources in 12 countries, and that the kidneys, which were in great demand, were resold in the United States to various laboratories and hospitals doing research aimed at producing antivirus vaccines.

Scott, Russell, *The Body as Property,* p. 2.
NY: The Viking Press (1981)

There is concern for the rights of the poor when considering the sale of human organs for transplant. Impoverished Indians are selling their kidneys for transplantation into foreigners. The living donors, who are unrelated to the recipients, receive about $1,000 for a kidney but may get as much as $7,000. Dr. K. H. Chugh, president of the Indian Society of Nephrology, warns, "If this is allowed to continue, most of the poor people in India will learn to survive without one kidney by the year 2000."

Funding

A report of the President's Commission came to the conclusion that it is the duty of society to ensure that everyone have equal access to an adequate level of health care. Financial resources are limited. What is an adequate level of health care? Should everyone have the opportunity to get a transplant if needed, or should everyone have the opportunity to get proper nutrition, exercise, and inoculations to prevent disease?

On one hand, it is costly to fund transplant operations; on the other, it is costly to fund school lunch programs for indigent, undernourished children. Values become involved. The artificial heart, for example, might bring four years each of extended life to 25,000 persons annually at a cost of some $100,000 per life extended. The school lunch program might ensure the improved physical development of hundreds of thousands of children, enabling each to live healthier lives for sixty years or more. The appeal of the artificial heart is that it rescues people from certain death. The school lunch program does not provide that same level of excitement or emotional appeal. Other general health problems include exposure to toxic chemicals, cigarette smoke, and radiation. Adults may be deprived of immunization or adequate nutrition. Would the money spent on the development of better artificial hearts be better spent to upgrade the standard of health for a larger segment of the population? All of these factors contribute to the health of the nation, but because society does not have unlimited funds for health care, ethical choices must be made.

Intensive Care Unit

Where there is shortage of beds in the intensive care unit (ICU), the ethics of health care providers are put to the test. Who gets a bed—an elderly person or a young person? Someone whose prognosis is limited or one who will probably have many good years if properly treated? The patient who can pay or the one who cannot? The family man with five dependent children or the playboy with no responsibilities?

If there is a shortage of ICU beds, patients in the unit usually have a shorter stay than when there is a surplus. This may occur because the patients do not need additional care or because the bed is required for a more seriously ill patient. When patients are kept in the ICU for a long time, it may be because the staff did not wish to decrease the ICU census. Some physicians might find their own workload reduced if a patient received care in the ICU rather than on a regular medical ward.

The use of the ICU is just one example of the day-to-day ethical judgments that are made by medical professionals in the hospital setting. No two physicians will necessarily make the same decision for the same reason.

Diagnostic Related Groups (DRGs)

With the arrival of DRGs, the length of stay in the ICU has financial ramifications for the entire hospital. If the insurer does not pay for the stay, payment must come from the consumer or the reserves of the hospital. A hospital, or long-term care facility, will not remain open if it does not receive payment.

Diagnostic related groups (DRGs) bring the rationing of health care to the doorstep of each person. For example, when insurance companies determined that there would be only twenty-four hours of inpatient time allowed for a mother and child following a vaginal delivery, women rebelled. Congress passed legislation requiring minimal additional time in the hospital for those mothers who needed or desired it, and additional days following a Caesarean section delivery.

We are told that the taxpayer cost of funding Medicare will be prohibitive if Medicare policies do not change. As the over-sixty-five population grows, medical care money will have to stretch farther. In addition, there will be a diminishing number of employed adults to refinance the Medicare Trust. The squeeze from both sides will force a change in policy.

Physicians no longer solely determine how long their patients stay in the hospital. The regulations of the government, the insurance providers, and the managed care organization to which doctors belong regulate the number and kind of diagnostic tests allowed for a condition. Third-party intervention has been disruptive to the doctor-patient relationship, which quality care researchers have determined is a key factor in patient-provider satisfaction.

EXPERIMENTS

Approximately twenty years ago, a public health official objected to the

> morality of an ongoing study being sponsored by the Public Health Service—a study compiling information about the course and effects of syphilis in human beings based upon medical examinations of poor black men in Macon County, Alabama. The men, or more accurately, those still living, had been coming in for annual examinations for forty years. They were not receiving standard therapy for syphilis. . . . [This] has been called the longest running nontherapeutic experiment on human beings in medical history and the most notorious case of prolonged and knowing violation of subjects' rights—the Tuskegee study."
>
> Caplan, Arthur L., "When Evil Intrudes,"
> *Hastings Center Report*, p. 29 (November–December 1992)

Public anger over the immorality of the study spurred Congress to create a panel to review both the Tuskegee study and the adequacy of existing protections for subjects in all federally sponsored research. In 1974, the National Commission for the Protection of Human Subjects of Biomedical and Behavior Research was established.

The artificial heart transplant of William Schroeder addresses another aspect of medical experimentation:

> The death of William Schroeder in Louisville, Kentucky, on August 6, 1986, brought to a close a remarkable chapter in public human experimentation. Artificial heart implants represent the most public experiments in the history of the world. The manner in which they are conducted is a matter of utmost public and professional concern. . . . Unfortunately, the brief history of artificial heart implants is neither a happy nor a proud one. . . . In the United States, ethics and law have taken a distinctly back seat to notions of scientific advance; experimental artificial hearts are being implanted almost in a historic vacuum, with scant regard for existing norms and codes of human experimentation. . . . Human experimentation is an area that crystallizes our view of the rights and welfare of individual humans.
>
> Annas, George J., "Made in the U.S.A.: Legal and Ethical Issues
> in Artificial Heart Experimentation,"
> *Law, Medicine and Health Care* 14(3–4) (September 1986)

Because no two patients are medically identical, some argue that therapeutic medicine is inescapably experimental. Society has developed guidelines, however, to deal with medical experimental research. As a result of the medical atrocities conducted by Nazi German doctors on prisoners during World War II, the **Nuremberg Code** was drafted. Human experiments in the United States should adhere to the terms of the Nuremberg Code and federal regulations. Provisions of the Nuremberg Code follow:

The great weight of the evidence before us is to the effect that certain types of medical experiments on human beings, when kept within reasonably well-defined bounds, conform to the ethics of the medical profession generally. The protagonists of the practice of human experimentation justify their views on the basis that such experiments yield results for the good of society that are unprocurable by other methods or means of study. All agree, however, that certain basic principles must be observed in order to satisfy moral, ethical and legal concepts.

1. The voluntary consent of the human subject is absolutely essential. This means that the person involved should have legal capacity to give consent; should be so situated as to be able to exercise free power of choice, without the intervention of any element of force, fraud, deceit, duress, overreaching, or other ulterior form of constraint or coercion; and should have sufficient knowledge and comprehension of the elements of the subject matter involved as to enable him to make an understanding and enlightened decision. This latter element requires that before the acceptance of an affirmative decision by the experimental subject there should be made known to him the nature, duration, and purpose of the experiment; the method and means by which it is to be conducted; all inconveniences and hazards reasonably expected; and the effects upon his health or person which may possibly come from his participation in the experiment.

   The duty and responsibility for ascertaining the quality of the consent rests upon each individual who initiates, directs, or engages in the experiment. It is a personal duty and responsibility which may not be delegated to another with impunity.

2. The experiment should be such as to yield fruitful results for the good of society, unprocurable by other methods or means of study, and not random and unnecessary in nature.

3. The experiment should be so designed and based on the results of animal experimentation and a knowledge of the natural history of the disease or other problem under study that the anticipated results will justify the performance of the experiment.

4. The experiment should be so conducted as to avoid all unnecessary physical and mental suffering and injury.

5. No experiment should be conducted where there is an *a priori* reason to believe that death or disabling injury will occur; except, perhaps, in those experiments where the experimental physicians also serve as subjects.

Trials of War Criminals Before the Nuremberg Military
Tribunals Under Control Council Law 11(10).
Nuremberg, Germany (October 1946–April 1949)

Following the fifth precept of the Nuremberg Code, a French researcher, Dr. Daniel Zagury, has tested an AIDS vaccine on himself. "I consider this to be the only ethical line of conduct," he stated for an interview with *Newsweek* magazine.

> . . . Last November he gave himself 10 million units of [vaccine] through scratch wounds on the skin of his arm. He suffered no headaches, fever or enlarged lymph nodes immediately after the vaccination, the first good sign. In 30 days, laboratory studies showed that his blood serum was "highly positive" for antibodies against one major strain of the AIDS virus. . . .
>
> Marshall, Ruth, "Aids: The Search for a Vaccine,"
> *Newsweek,* p. 79 (March 30, 1987)

In another issue, *Time* magazine reported that the experimental drug AZT prolonged the life of AIDS patients. The drug was tested in a dozen medical centers where some participants received placebos and others received the drug.

> Robert Windom of the Department of Health and Human Services said the results were so remarkable that tests in a dozen medical centers were being halted so that control groups of AIDS sufferers—who had been receiving only placebos, or dummy drugs—could immediately begin treatment with AZT. Furthermore, Windom has petitioned the Food and Drug Administration for speedy approval to distribute the drug to thousands of other AIDS victims. . . .
>
> Levine, Joseph, "A Ray of Hope in the Fight Against AIDS,"
> *Time,* p. 60 (September 29, 1986)

DRUG TESTING ON THE JOB

In December 5, 1986, issue of the *Journal of the American Medical Association,* there was an editorial denouncing random drug testing as "Chemical McCarthyism." In *Newsweek* magazine, the article "Can You Pass the Job Test?" presented the following case history:

> Last year [John] Sexton, then a $30,000-a-year dispatcher at Federal Express Corp. in Atlanta, was one of a group of employees ordered to submit urine samples for a drug test. Sexton tested positive; he says he had smoked marijuana at a party two weeks earlier, but he didn't appear impaired at the time of the test. Next he was ordered to take a lie-detector test or face suspension—but when he denied using drugs on the job or knowing anyone who did, the polygrapher running the test concluded he was holding something back. Fired last May, the 29-year-old college graduate hasn't been able to land another job since.
>
> Dentzer, Susan, et al., "Can You Pass the Job Test?"
> *Newsweek,* p. 46 (May 5, 1986)

Screening the public for medical reasons is a part of our society. Within the medical community, certain testing procedures are recommended for mass screening: hypertension, cervical cancer, diabetes, and so on. The armed services have instituted mass screening for antibodies to the human immunodeficiency virus (HIV). The test results may contribute to medical research of the variables inherent in the disease process, or may indicate latent disease in an unsuspecting individual. These results, used for the good of society, may justify the infringement of testing on our privacy.

There are other uses of medical testing that invade privacy but contribute less to the public good. One example is the Breathalyzer test administered to alleged drunk drivers. There are many inherent problems with the use of these machines: improper **calibration,** untrained personnel, the time span between ingestion and testing, broken machines, and false-positive tests.

Another example is the highly publicized drug testing of professional athletes. Inaccurate results may affect lives and careers. The NCAA's drug testing program for college athletes has been found to violate California's right-to-privacy statute. At least seven other state constitutions provide protection for "privacy."

To what degree can you justify tests that invade rights of privacy in the following situations:

1. Psychological testing for employment:
    a. to assess **personality traits**
    b. to determine who will perform a given job well
    c. to generally screen all employees
    d. to assess for promotion

2. Random lie detector tests on the job to discover employee theft

3. Drug tests for employees:
    a. after they have been warned about their behavior
    b. prior to employment
    c. prior to promotion

4. Drug tests to all high school athletes:
    a. prior to championship games
    b. randomly throughout the school year
    c. on a regular schedule throughout the season

5. Genetic testing to screen high-risk employees for disease:
    a. cystic fibrosis
    b. Alzheimer's disease
    c. sickle-cell trait

AUTONOMY VERSUS PATERNALISM

Being a patient puts one in a role of dependence upon a professional. Both the doctor and the patient have the same goal, but perhaps different

perspectives on how to reach that goal. One of the major issues that generates conflict between persons with different perspectives or different roles is
the tension between **autonomy** and **paternalism.**

Our culture values highly the autonomy of persons—their independence and self-reliance. Paternalism can be interpreted as interference with a
person's independence in order to benefit that individual. The principal goal
of obtaining health care is to benefit from the caretakers' offerings. It is
argued that those administering health care are obligated to take actions that
benefit patients, even if those actions interfere with or neglect the patient's
autonomy. On the other hand, it is argued, according to John Stuart Mill, that
"over himself, over his own body and mind, the individual is sovereign."
These conflicting positions produce ethical dilemma. Following is the way
one judge decided a case:

Mrs. Jones, 25 years old and mother of a seven-month-old child, was brought to
the hospital by her husband for emergency care, having lost two thirds of her
body's blood supply from a ruptured ulcer. She was without a personal physician
and relied solely on the hospital staff. She and her husband were Jehovah's
Witnesses. When death without blood became imminent, the hospital sought the
advice of counsel who applied to the court for permission to administer the blood.
The case proceeded from District Court to the Court of Appeals.

"I called the hospital by telephone and spoke with Dr. Westura, Chief Medical
Resident, who confirmed the representations made by counsel. I thereupon proceeded with counsel to the hospital, where I spoke to Mr. Jones, the husband of the
patient. He advised me that, on religious grounds, he would not approve a blood
transfusion for his wife. He said, however, that if the court ordered the transfusion,
the responsibility was not his. I advised Mr. Jones to obtain counsel immediately.
He thereupon went to the telephone and returned in 10 or 15 minutes to advise that
he had taken the matter up with his church and that he had decided that he did not
want counsel.

I asked permission of Mr. Jones to see his wife. This he readily granted. Prior to
going into the patient's room, I again conferred with Dr. Westura and several other
doctors assigned to the case. All confirmed that the patient would die without blood
and that there was a better than 50 percent chance of saving her life with it.
Unanimously they strongly recommended it. I then went inside the patient's room.
Her appearance confirmed the urgency which had been represented to me. I tried to
communicate with her, advising her again as to what the doctors had said. The only
audible reply I could hear was "Against my will." It was obvious that the woman
was not in a mental condition to make a decision. I was reluctant to press her
because of the seriousness of her condition and because I felt that to suggest repeatedly the imminence of death without blood might place a strain on her religious
convictions. I asked her whether she would oppose the blood transfusion if the
court allowed it. She indicated, as best I could make out, that it would not then be
her responsibility. . . . I signed the order allowing the hospital to administer such
transfusions as the doctors should determine were necessary to save her life. . . .

Before proceeding with this inquiry, it may be useful to state what this case does
not involve. This case does not involve a person who, for religious or other reasons,
has refused to seek medical attention. It does not involve a disputed medical

judgment or a dangerous or crippling operation. Nor does it involve the delicate question of saving the newborn in preference to the mother. Mrs. Jones sought medical attention and placed on the hospital the legal responsibility for her proper care. In its dilemma, not of its own making, the hospital sought judicial direction. . . .

[M]rs. Jones did not want to die. Her voluntary presence in the hospital as a patient seeking medical help testified to this. Death, to Mrs. Jones, was not a religiously commanded goal, but an unwanted side effect of a religious scruple. . . . Nor are we faced with the question of whether the state should intervene to reweigh the relative values of life and death, after the individual has weighed them for himself and found life wanting. Mrs. Jones wanted to live. . . . Her religion merely prevented her consent to a transfusion. If the law undertook the responsibility of authorizing the transfusion without her consent, no problem would be raised with respect to her religious practice. Thus, the effect of the order was to preserve for Mrs. Jones the life she wanted without sacrifice of her religious beliefs.

The final, and compelling, reason for granting the emergency writ was that a life hung in the balance. There was no time for research and reflection. Death could have mooted the cause in a matter of minutes, if action were not taken to preserve the *status quo*. To refuse to act, only to find later that the law required action, was a risk I was unwilling to accept. I determined to act on the side of life.

Excerpted from the decision 331 F.2d 100 (D.C. Cir.), *cert. denied,*
377 U.S. 978 (1964). Reprinted as it appeared in
"Experimentation with Human Beings," Katz, J. (Ed.), pp. 551–552
(NY: Russell Sage Foundation, 1972)

Improved technology makes decisions similar to that in the Jehovah's Witness case a more frequent occurrence. Often the lines between experiment and treatment are blurred as modern technology surges forward and the professional's desire to save life butts the individual's desire to be autonomous and make informed decisions.

To what degree is society responsible for its citizens? Much money has been put into research showing that cigarettes are harmful to health, yet people still smoke. It is estimated that Massachusetts residents pay more than $64 million a year in hospital costs caused by smoking-related diseases. Use of seat belts is mandatory in many states, yet many citizens refuse to wear them. In a related issue, requiring motorcyclists to wear helmets has been the subject of much litigation.

The involvement of the state infringes on the right of privacy when used to regulate personal behavior. Holding the bar serving liquor responsible for a customer's alcoholic indulgence has diminished the responsibility of an individual for his or her own behavior. Mental health law regulates the autonomy of the patient. **Commitment** to mental health facilities, the administration of psychotropic drugs, and release from treatment are matters that involve state regulations and court hearings. Once an individual is adjudicated mentally ill, the ability to make many decisions is taken from his or her hands. Conservators or guardians for the elderly require court appointment and monitoring.

In each of these areas, the autonomy of the individual must be weighed against the danger of the individual to self or to others. In restraining a person's liberty, the need for such restraint must be acceptable to society. When freedom is denied to an individual, the freedom of every individual is endangered.

SUMMARY

Professional organizations have creeds and codes of ethics that proclaim standards the membership strives to maintain. Those outside the organization use those standards to define correct professional conduct. Developing a code of ethics is difficult, but implementing those ideals in daily life is even more difficult. Although medical office personnel do not make the headline ethical decisions, the interplay of power and scheduling of time is ethical in nature and affects both patients and personnel.

One of the most pressing issues in health care is the allocation of resources. Scarcity of organs for transplant, limitation of funds for health care delivery systems, decisions regarding intensive care unit beds, and problems with DRGs all fall under the allocation of resources. The ethics of human and medical experimentation were of particular concern even before the development of the Nuremberg Code.

The threatening global epidemic of AIDS is affecting the ethical fabric of the nation's health care delivery system. The expense of the disease, its etiology, its terminal nature, and the unavailability of a cure require reassessment of priorities in delivery and financing of health care.

Improved technology makes decisions similar to that in the Jehovah's Witness case a more frequent occurrence. Often the lines between experiment and treatment blur as technology improves. A professional's desire to save life sometimes conflicts with an individual's desire to be autonomous and make informed decisions.

The aging of the population affects the thinking of health professionals providing geriatric care. Health care for the elderly includes problems with attempting to maintain the autonomy of the geriatric patient while taking into consideration physical deterioration, family involvement, and degrees of senile dementia.

SUGGESTED ACTIVITY

Visit a local nursing home and listen to what the residents and the staff think about matters involving the autonomy of decision making. Ask the residents what matters they find most difficult to allow someone else to decide. Then talk with the social worker to gain another perspective on issues of autonomy and paternalism with the elderly.

STUDY QUESTIONS

1. In addition to scheduling decisions, list two other instances where ethics enters into the behavior of medical office personnel.

2. You are the office manager. Develop a schedule for three employees, each of whom works a five-day week, sometimes including a Saturday. Two employees must be working at all times. Take into consideration each employee's need to have weekend time free.

3. You feel that the physicians could better schedule patients if they would spend one additional half-hour a day in the office. Write a memorandum to the physician with your suggestion.

4. One of your patients is providing a kidney for transplant to her son. All the tests have been performed, and it has been determined that her tissue is compatible. She confides to you that she is frightened about the operation and living the remainder of her days with only one kidney. How do you handle the situation?

5. You are a medical assistant in a pediatrician's office. One of the patients needs a liver transplant. The matter has been in the newspaper, and additional newspapers are seeking interviews with the doctor, the staff, and the patient. The newspapers will help advertise the need for an organ, but the family is too upset to handle the publicity. The pediatrician has told you to handle the press. What do you do?

6. A person comes into the office and says that he is in a time of financial hardship and wants to sell one of his kidneys. He is not a patient, and you know nothing about him, but one of your patients is waiting for a kidney. Your patient is wealthy and can afford to purchase a kidney. What do you do?

7. A former secretary tells you that she would like to be a surrogate mother. She is a friend of yours and tells you this over coffee. You know of a couple who wants a baby, but the wife is unwilling to carry the child because of her own health. How do you handle this situation?

8. A patient has been taken out of the intensive care unit because the doctors feel he is terminal and the bed is needed for someone who can be helped. The patient's wife comes into the hospital and appears encouraged because her husband is being removed from the intensive care unit. How do you handle the situation?

9. Someone calls on the telephone for an appointment and informs you that she has AIDS. This is your first AIDS patient. Do you make an appointment?

10. The doctor wants everyone in the office to be tested for drugs on a routine basis. Are you in agreement? How will you handle the matter?

CASES FOR DISCUSSION

1. The plaintiff was arrested on August 1, 1973, for driving while intoxicated. A blood test taken shortly after his arrest indicated a blood alcohol level of .12 percent. The Utah statute states that there are two elements necessary to constitute violation of the law: one is that there be a blood-alcohol concentration of .10 percent or more, and the second is that there be concurrent operation or actual physical control of any vehicle. The plaintiff attempted to have this statute declared unconstitutional, the issue being whether a statute that prohibits the operation of a motor vehicle with the presence of a blood alcohol level above a certain percentage is unconstitutional. Is it?

2. The defendant was under indictment for conspiracy to transport, sell, receive, and dispose of goods in interstate commerce. He requested permission to take a polygraph examination at the government's expense. The government opposed the motion on the ground that substantial prejudicial consequences compel denial of the motion. Should the results of polygraph examinations be admitted into evidence?

3. The defendant, as part of his defense in a criminal trial, requested the court to appoint a qualified cytogeneticist to carry out chromosomal testing of his blood at the county's expense. The purpose of the tests would be to determine whether the defendant had the XYY chromosome pattern. If so, the results would be used as part of his insanity defense and would be offered into evidence. Should evidence of chromosome abnormality be admissible as part of the defense of insanity in a criminal trial?

4. The plaintiff was diagnosed as a manic depressive and had been hospitalized and under treatment for many years. The plaintiff's psychiatrist testified that while in the manic phase of his illness, the plaintiff felt euphoric and invincible, and his judgment and behavior were grossly affected. While in such a state, the plaintiff bought from the defendant the privilege of selling a mechanical device to the government under a license that required considerable sales work. The plaintiff's attorney testified that neither he nor the plaintiff's wife intended to let him go through with the deal, but they thought it would be good therapy if he went through with the negotiations. The defendant did not know about the plaintiff's condition. Does a mental disorder that affects a person's judgment, but not the ability to understand, qualify an individual as an incompetent unable to contract?

5. In a civil action, the plaintiff was involuntarily committed as a mental patient for fifteen years. Throughout his confinement, the plaintiff repeatedly demanded his release, claiming that he was dangerous to no one, that he was not mentally ill, and that the hospital was not providing treatment for his illness. Following release, the plaintiff brought

suit against the hospital's superintendent and other members of the hospital staff for intentionally and maliciously depriving him of his constitutional right to liberty. Do patients who are involuntarily committed to a state hospital have a right to treatment?

6. A California law made drug addiction a crime. At the close of the trial, the judge instructed the jury that they could convict the plaintiff on either of two grounds: that he had the status of a drug addict, or that he had actually used drugs. The plaintiff was convicted and sentenced to ninety days imprisonment. Does a state statute that makes drug addiction a criminal offense inflict cruel and unusual punishment in violation of the Fourteenth Amendment?

7. A prisoner in Florida was sentenced to die. A young child in Denver needed a kidney, and the prisoner asked to be taken to Denver to be tested to determine whether he was a suitable donor. Should the court allow him to go to Denver?

8. A man arranged to donate his body to a medical school. His mother, carrying out his directive, employed a funeral home to transport the body by ambulance to the medical school. She wished to ride in the vehicle with the body. The funeral home made an error, and the body was shipped by train. The railroad lost the body, and it took three days to trace it. The mother sued the funeral home for damages for mental anguish. Should she recover?

9. A wife told her husband that she wanted a divorce. The following day, a psychiatrist whom she had never met before arrived at her home but did not tell her that he was there to examine her. A few days later, the psychiatrist and another physician signed commitment papers for her and she was forcibly removed from her home and taken to the hospital. She refused food and medication for six days and was refused permission to mail letters, use the telephone, or call her attorney. She finally was able to contact her relatives by telephone. Should she be released?

10. The defendant was an unmarried mentally competent twenty-four-year-old male who had been serving concurrent seven- to ten-year sentences in Massachusetts correctional institutions. While in prison, the defendant developed a life-threatening kidney condition that required hemodialysis three times a week as well as additional medication to sustain his life. The prisoner refused to submit to treatment. Should he be required to submit to treatment?

Chapter 12

Ethics: Death and Dying

Our moral response to the imminence of death demands that we rescue the doomed. We throw a rope to the drowning, rush into burning buildings to snatch the entrapped, dispatch teams to search for the snowbound. This rescue morality spills over into medical care, where our ropes are artificial hearts, our rush is the mobile critical care unit, our teams the transplant services.

Jonsen, Albert R., "Bentham in a Box: Technology, Assessment and Health-Care Allocation," *Law, Medicine and Health Care* 14(3–4):174 (September 1986)

OBJECTIVES:

The questions asked in this chapter are very difficult, and your answers today will be challenged by your experience tomorrow. Death and dying issues question both the sanctity and the quality of life. Nurses, emergency medical technicians, and doctors are confronted with the reality of life-and-death situations, carrying out do-not-resuscitate orders, and removing life support systems. All health employees are affected by their nearness to and interaction with patients. After reading this chapter, you should be able to:

1. define death.
2. recognize the role individuals, families, hospitals, the medical community, courts, legislatures, and others play in dealing with the ethical, legal, medical, social, and political questions that arise from our ability to maintain life.
3. appreciate the need for a do-not-resuscitate order (DNR).
4. weigh both sides of the question in cases removing life support.
5. identify provisions of the Patient Self-Determination Act (PSDA).
6. develop a personal philosophy on euthanasia.

BUILDING YOUR LEGAL VOCABULARY

advanced directive	geriatric	living will
assisted suicide	guardian ad litem	procedural
cardiopulmonary arrest	health care proxy	purist
clear and convincing	insanity	substitute judgment
cognitive	life-sustaining	terminally ill
durable power of attorney		

Your thoughts and feelings about death and dying emerge when a member of your family becomes **terminally ill.** At some point in life, each individual faces death. The manner in which death and dying are handled depends on personal resolution of the importance of sanctity or quality of life. Death and dying are usually associated with the elderly. Society and medical professionals find death of a young person to be the most difficult.

A religious view of death turns to medicine to define death. Today's universally accepted definition of death was developed by an ad hoc committee at Harvard Medical School. The committee gave the following reasons for the need to add brain death to cessation of heart beat and respiration:

> One primary purpose is to define irreversible coma as a new criterion for death. There are two reasons why there is need for a definition: (1) Improvements in resuscitative and supportive measures have led to increased efforts to save those who are desperately injured. Sometimes these efforts have only partial success so that the result is an individual whose heart continues to beat but whose brain is irreversibly damaged. The burden is great on patients who suffer permanent loss of intellect, on their families, on the hospitals, and on those in need of hospital beds already occupied by these comatose patients. (2) Obsolete criteria for the definition of death can lead to controversy in obtaining organs for transplantation.
>
> Report of the Ad Hoc Committee of the Harvard Medical
> School to examine the definition of brain death.
> *JAMA* 205:85 (August 1968)

Resolution of questions about dying are very important for physicians, whose first obligation to a patient is to heal, cure, or postpone death for as long as possible. When a cure is not possible, the physician's obligation is to care for and comfort the dying patient. Dr. C. Everett Koop explains his resolution of the conflict in the following incident:

> There is this unique tumor of childhood called neuroblastoma in which I have been interested for more than thirty years. Because of this I have developed a broad clinical experience with the behavior of this tumor as it affects the lives of my patients. . . . In a given situation I might have as a patient a five-year-old child

whose tumor was diagnosed a year ago and who, in spite of all known treatment, has progressed to a place where although her primary tumor has been removed she now has recurrence. . . . I know her days of life are limited and that the longer she lives the more likely she is to have considerable pain. She might also become both blind and deaf.

If this five-year-old youngster is quite anemic, her ability to understand what is happening to her might be clouded. . . . I can let her exist with a deficient hemoglobin level knowing that it may shorten her life but also knowing that it will be beneficial in the sense that she will not be alert enough to understand all that is happening around her. On the other hand I could be a medical **purist** and give her blood transfusions until her hemoglobin level was up to acceptable standards. . . . . . . [S]he would be more conscious of the things happening around her, she would feel her pain more deeply, and she might live longer. . . . [A]nd then there are the anticancer drugs which I know without any shadow of a doubt will not cure this child. . . . Would it be better to let this little girl slip into death quietly . . . or should we prolong her life. . . . I opt to withhold supportive measures. . . .

Koop, C. Everett, *The Right to Live: The Right to Die,* pp. 98, 99.
Wheaton, IL: Tyndale House Publishers (1976)

DO-NOT-RESUSCITATE ORDERS (DNR)

As a result of the treatment of **cardiopulmonary arrest** with cardiopulmonary resuscitation (CPR), patients may be literally brought back to life after the traditional signs of a death have appeared. Whether CPR should be used on every patient is a question that haunts institutional professionals. It is estimated that approximately eighty percent of the two million people who die in the United States each year die in institutions. Each institution has professionals training to respond to death with CPR. Is it practicing good medicine to require CPR for every patient, or should it be used like every treatment and prescribed on an individual basis? If CPR is not attempted, is the staff medically abandoning the patient? If an agreement is made between the staff and the patient that this particularly invasive procedure will not be utilized, is the patient psychologically abandoned? These are all ethical and legal questions that have to be answered by the practicing professional.

In 1984, in New York, a grand jury recommended state regulation of do-not-resuscitate (DNR) procedures following their mishandling of the same in a health care facility. In a community hospital, the nursing cards of patients designated not to be resuscitated were marked with a purple dot and were kept only until death, a recording procedure that eliminated both appropriate documentation and accountability:

. . . dot-sized purple decals were stuck to the patient's nursing record cards as a signal to the medical and nursing staffs that CPR should not be initiated if the patient arrested. When a patient died . . . the nursing cards were routinely discarded, leaving no record of the order not to resuscitate. . . . [T]he grand jury said that the surgeon . . . tried to shift the blame to nurses when he testified that oral orders given by physicians not to call an emergency code "were nothing more than suggestions to the nurse who is perfectly at liberty to call the code if she desires to call the code." However . . . doctors at [the hospital] did not allow nurses to give an aspirin to a patient without the physician's permission.

Sullivan, Ronald, "Queens Hospital Accused of Denial of Care,"
New York Times, p. 17 (March 24, 1984)

REMOVAL OF LIFE SUPPORT

Prolonging life today is often a treatment decision. The physician may make this decision, but it is the nurse who carries out the day-to-day patient care. The withholding of food and water is an indication that the medical community is no longer going to continue nurturing the patient. It is an intentional act. In the following case, a competent patient desired to have a nasogastric tube removed. It was her intent to do so even though its removal could result in her death. It was the hospital's intent to continue treatment.

CASE STUDY

In California, Elizabeth Bouvia, a severely disabled quadriplegic suffering from cerebral palsy, wanted removal of a nasogastric tube. The hospital determined that removal of the tube would result in her death. Elizabeth Bouvia was in a public institution and the question became whether Bouvia, competent, could refuse treatment overriding the state's interest to protect her life, thereby making the staff a party to the result of her conduct. She was not comatose, in a vegetative state, nor terminally ill. She had previously expressed a desire to die.

The court held . . . Elizabeth Bouvia's decision to forego medical treatment of life support through a mechanical means belongs to her. It is not a medical decision for her physicians to make. Neither is it a legal question whose soundness is to be resolved by lawyers or judges. It is not a conditional right subject to approval by ethics committees or courts of law. It is a moral and philosophical decision that, being a competent adult, is hers alone.

Bouvia v. Superior Court of Los Angeles County,
179 Cal. App. 3d 1172, 225 Cal. Rptr. 297 (Ct. App. 1986)

Kevin O'Rourke, a prominent Catholic ethicist, has published a Catholic view on tube feeding:

. . . Withholding artificial hydration and nutrition from a patient in an irreversible coma does not introduce a new fatal pathology; rather, it allows an already existing fatal pathology to take its natural course. . . . [T]here is no ethical obligation to strive to prolong the life of that human being. There is an ethical obligation to keep the person comfortable. . . .

O'Rourke, Kevin, "Tube Feeding—A Catholic View,"
America (November 22, 1986)

Do-not-resuscitate orders are no longer hidden or camouflaged with purple dots. It has been legally recognized that individuals have the right to make decisions affecting their own death. Procedures are made available to document a dying person's wishes while the person is still considered legally competent. The ethical conflict in these cases is between the obligation to prevent death and the obligation to prevent suffering. When Elizabeth Bouvia was allowed to have the tube removed, hospital physicians cut back on the morphine medication she was receiving for pain on the grounds that morphine is addictive and the size of the dosage was reaching intolerable limits. The courts affirmed the legal obligation of physicians to prevent suffering by ordering the continuation of medication.

Elizabeth Bouvia was a mentally competent patient. Does being incompetent affect the right of the patient to discontinue treatment, or that of the doctor to suggest discontinuing treatment?

Patient Self-Determination Act (PSDA)

On December 1, 1991, the Patient Self-Determination Act (PSDA) took effect in all hospitals, nursing homes, rehabilitation facilities, and hospices. The legislation (P.L. 101-508) is linked to Medicare/Medicaid payment and applies to the above facilities, plus home health agencies and HMOs. Each entity is required to maintain written policies and procedures concerning advanced directives and provide information to patients at the time of admission or enrollment.

Under the legislation, hospitals must:

- provide written information to patients on admission informing them of their rights under state law to executive advanced directives.
- provide written information about policies to carry out these rights.
- document whether an advanced directive exists for each patient.
- educate their staff and community on advanced directives.

Right to Choose

An **advanced directive** asserts an individual's right to accept or refuse treatment and gives direction to relatives, friends, and medical professionals. The directive is necessary, according to Senator John C. Danforth, R-MO, an Episcopal clergyman, because "[m]edical technology has outstripped ethics. For too many thousands of people, the end of life is a nightmare. . . . [It is] turned over to technocrats whose job it is to eke out every last moment. This constitutes playing God by medicine."

Supporting Senator Danforth, and at the same time giving insight into the physician's behavior, James H. Sammons, former Executive Vice President of the American Medical Association (AMA), adds: "From the day [physicians] enter medical school they are taught to cherish and preserve life. . . . While physicians should never directly cause death, they must always act in the best interest of the patients, and that sometimes includes allowing them to die."

The law affecting death and dying reflects how society regards older people, the relationships that exist between and among the generations, society's ambivalence in matters of a patient's autonomy, and the pluralistic background of our religious heritage. Americans unable to reach agreement on substantive issues concerning the appropriateness of treatment of the dying have concentrated instead on **procedural** matters, such as advanced directives. The United States Supreme Court, in *Cruzan,* reinforced this approach by focusing on the state of Missouri's ability to require that **substitute judgment** decisions be reached from **clear and convincing** evidence. The Supreme Court Chief Justice Rehnquist held that:

CASE STUDY

(1) the United States Constitution did not forbid Missouri from requiring clear and convincing evidence of an incompetent's wishes to the withdrawal of life-sustaining treatment

(2) [the] State Supreme Court did not commit constitutional error in concluding that evidence adduced at trial did not amount to clear and convincing evidence of the patient's desire to cease hydration and nutrition

(3) due process did not require the state to accept substitute judgment of close family members absent substantial proof that their views reflected those of the patient.

Cruzan v. Director, Missouri Department of Health,
110 S. Ct. 2841 (Mo. 1990)

The *Cruzan* ruling originated in the ordeal of Nancy Cruzan who had been comatose since a 1983 automobile accident. Her parents brought the matter into the courts after medical professionals refused to remove the feeding tube that kept her alive in a vegetative state. The court upheld the right of an individual to die but also held that the state could refuse that right absent clear and convincing evidence that the individual would have wanted to die. Advanced directives are a result of the need for evidence.

Formats for Advanced Directives

There are three major forms of advanced directives: living will, durable power of attorney, and health care proxy.

LIVING WILLS

Efforts to define policies on withholding or withdrawing life-sustaining procedures from hopelessly ill patients are a relatively recent development. As of 1997, forty-one states had **living will** statutes. These statutes have differing requirements for the contents of living wills. Most living will statutes cover only patients who are terminally ill at the time the treatment choice is to be made and may contain limitations in terms of the treatment directives. During the late 1980s and early 1990s, living wills became accepted by the courts and physicians, but even in 1997, six years after the PSDA took effect, hospitals reported that there appeared to be little use of them in clinical practice.

A living will is executed when the individual is competent. Its intent is to extend the right to refuse artificial life-sustaining procedures into a possible future time of incompetency. The living wills laws, also known as natural-death acts, offer guidelines for the use of living wills when defined medical conditions have been met.

DURABLE POWER OF ATTORNEY

The American Medical Association (AMA) suggests a medical directive as a substitute for the living will and suggests further that these be made available in doctor's offices and hospitals and included as part of the medical record. Assessing the relative merits of the living will and the **durable power of attorney** for health care, the AMA finds that the durable power of attorney can cover a broader range of illnesses than the living will, which is often linked to situations of terminal illness when death is imminent.

In 1997, nineteen states had durable power of attorney statutes. In a durable power of attorney, a person, in writing, designates another as his or her attorney in fact. The document contains the words "this power of attorney shall not be affected by subsequent disability or incapacity of the principal. . . . [T]his power of attorney shall become effective upon the disability or incapacity of the principal," or similar words indicating the principal's intent that the authority conferred continues despite disability or incapacity. The authority differs from a regular power of attorney, which terminates upon disability or death.

Health Care Proxy

After many years of deliberation, the Massachusetts legislature enacted M.G.L. Ch. 201D, "An Act Providing for the Execution of Health Care Proxies by Individuals." Under this legislation, a **health care proxy** shall:

1. identify the principal and the health care agent.
2. express the intention of the principal that the health care agent has authority to make health care decisions on behalf of the principal.
3. describe any limitations on the authority of the health care agent.
4. indicate that the authority of the health care agent to make health care decisions becomes effective upon a determination of incapacity.
5. be revoked by notifying the agent or health care provider orally, in writing, or by any other act evidencing specific intent to revoke; by execution of a subsequent health care proxy; or by divorce or legal separation of the principal and spouse when the spouse is the agent.

The Massachusetts legislation is similar to other state's health care proxy statutes.

Most incompetent patients in need of **life-sustaining** treatment have not executed an advanced directive. In this situation, it has become standard medical practice to seek consent from family members of incompetent patients. The President's Commission suggests the following:

---

1. The family is generally most concerned about the good of the patient.
2. The family will also usually be most knowledgeable about the patient's goals, preferences and values.
3. The family deserves recognition as an important social unit that ought to be treated, within limits, as a responsible decision maker in matters that intimately affect its members.
4. Especially in a society in which many other traditional forms of community have eroded, participation in a family is often an important dimension of personal fulfillment.
5. Since a protected sphere of privacy and autonomy is required for the flourishing of this interpersonal union, institutions and the state should be reluctant to intrude, particularly regarding matters that are personal and on which there is a wide range of opinion in society.

President's Commission, *Deciding for Forego Life-Sustaining Treatment* 127 (1983)

If refusing treatment may be an appropriate choice, just as choosing treatment may be an appropriate choice, then do physicians, with the intent of providing a "death with dignity" have the obligation to inform patients of the various ways of dying that are available to them, or to assist them with dying? Dr. Kevorkian thinks they do.

"Suicide machine," the words blast over the nation's airwaves during the six o'clock news. "Suicide aid sends shock waves through medical and legal fields" headlines the next morning's newspapers. And a few days later: "In Royal Oaks, Michigan, prosecutors today consider filing charges against a doctor who hooked an Alzheimer's patient to a suicide machine...."

The Patriot Ledger (June 6, 1990)

Euthanasia—mercy killing, or actively assisting someone to terminate their life at their request—is not a new subject. As far back as Hippocrates, "the physician is discouraged from invading the atrium of death" and instructed that in certain circumstances, "attempts to cure must yield to attempts to comfort." Hippocrates's treatise *The Art* instructs physicians: "(1) to do away with the sufferings of the sick, (2) to lessen the violence of their diseases, and (3) to refuse to treat those who are over mastered by their diseases realizing that in such cases medicine is powerless."

In the incident described below involving Janet Adkins and the "suicide machine," it appears that the first two Hippocratic guidelines have been upheld. The third, connected to the other two by the word *and,* includes the phrase *mastered by their diseases.* This phrase invites debate.

Janet Adkins was determined to take her own life after having lived with the diagnosis of Alzheimer's disease for approximately one year. She traveled two thousand miles to use a drug-injecting "suicide machine" installed in the back of a van. During the year, she experience some symptoms of the disease but was still able to live a reasonably full life. At the time when she was presumably able to make competent decisions, she chose death because she "did not desire to put herself or her family through the agony of this terrible disease." She was aided by Dr. Jack Kevorkian.

Doctor-Patient Relationship

Dr. Jack Kevorkian is a pathologist who advocates euthanasia and who built the "suicide machine" to assist patients seeking voluntary active euthanasia. The doctor-patient relationship, as reported in the press, consisted of one initial two-hour visit, a meeting with the patient prior to the act, and the twenty-five seconds when Janet was conscious preceding the last five minutes of her life. Dr. Kevorkian stated he "took the action, in part, to force the medical and legal establishment to consider his ideas."

The Adkins-Kevorkian relationship is a doctor-patient relationship, but it deviates from the usual in that it is a contract to kill. A contract to murder is an illegal contract and unenforceable under contract law. Each state has at least one statute that makes killing another person a felony. In some states, it is a crime to attempt to commit suicide, and in others, it is a crime to aid in a suicide.

Members of the families who have killed another family member with the intent of relieving suffering have been confronted by the criminal justice system. In Florida, a man shot his wife who was in advanced stages of Alzheimer's disease, and he was sentenced to life imprisonment. In Massachusetts, under similar circumstances, a husband suffocated his wife by placing her head in a plastic bag and sealing it with duct tape. He was not sentenced to prison but placed on probation.

In the Adkins situation, at the time of death, it does not appear that the disease had "mastered the patient." There is the possibility that the family may have unduly influenced Janet Adkins. The competence of Janet to make the decision has not been shown. Competence to enter into a contract is a legal issue that requires psychiatric evaluation.

The diagnosis of Alzheimer's disease is a verdict against the healthy spouse as well, sentencing him or her to a future life of poverty due to the length of the disease and the cost of treatment. State law requires couples to spend down to a certain level before either one of the parties is eligible for Medicaid. In some states, the family home will be lost to pay the expenses, while in others, a lien will be placed on the property to pay off whatever welfare spends during the time of crisis.

On June 19, 1996, Dr. Kevorkian participated in his thirtieth **assisted suicide.** No court has been able to convict him of murder.

Euthanasia, Greek for "good death," usually refers to an act in which one person kills another, at the request of and for the benefit of the one who dies. Suicide is the taking of one's own life. There is a blurring of the terms *assisted suicide* and *euthanasia*.

There are many arguments made against euthanasia:

1. Mistake in diagnosis.
2. Difficulty in determining if euthanasia is voluntary, for example, where there is an undue influence exerted on the patient by a member of the family and/or beneficiary of a will for financial reasons.
3. Slippery slope, for example, with the growth of managed care there may be more pressure to hasten death for those who are elderly, uneducated, on welfare, or disabled.
4. Altering the role of physicians to include the practice of killing patients would bring about a psychological upheaval in the doctor-patient relationship, and patients would become less trustful of their physician's role as healer.

The durable power of attorney, living will, and health care proxies are legal instruments that ensure personal preferences are known when competence is questioned. The moral implications of euthanasia are still questioned by society.

AIDS

A headline in *The Patriot Ledger* on Friday, May 1, 1987, read, "I'm living with AIDS, not dying with it." The story that followed told of a young man's personal struggle with AIDS. He had informed his family, and they were shocked and saddened, but supportive. In the next column is a story about a young man who was living with AIDS and portrayed himself as a person who was "dying with it." He had not yet informed his family and was afraid to because of his fear of rejection.

> Since he was diagnosed with AIDS just before Christmas, Robert has seen the tight seams of his life pulled apart in ways he never imagined. . . . [H]e was accustomed to strong traditions and familiar patterns of life in the neighborhood . . . he came to know everyone from the family dentist to the family mortician as friends.

A year ago he had a good job . . . a steady girlfriend and the possibility of marriage and children.

Robert, a bisexual who had occasional "one night stands" with men, faced one rejection after another in the wake of his diagnosis. . . Friends he has known from childhood take pains to exclude him. His girlfriend has left him. His dentist of 27 years put away his instruments and removed Robert's bib when he mentioned he had AIDS during a visit to have a wisdom tooth pulled. The family mortician has said he won't give him a proper burial . . . [and] when he told his sister he had AIDS, she screamed that he had disgraced the family and ran from the house. She has since become more supportive, but each time Robert goes to her house, she sends her two children upstairs.

Pappano, Laura, "Tormented by Fear of Rejection,"
The Patriot Ledger (April 30, 1987)

The two articles portray two people facing death and dying in opposite environments. In the first, the patient is supported, and his psychological needs are met; in the second, rejection closes in from all sides. Patients with AIDS are going to be a part of your professional life as a health care worker. How do you view the ethics of this situation?

1. Because the disease is contagious, the patients should be quarantined with all other AIDS patients.
2. The patients are bisexual. Any homosexual experience is sinful, and the patients are being punished for their sins by contracting the disease. The way people treat Robert is appropriate.
3. The patients are ill and, no matter what the diagnosis, deserve to be supported by society and their families.
4. AIDS patients should be treated only by home health agencies.

Now change the facts. The patient is a child, two years of age, who was born to a women who had unknowingly become infected with AIDS by her husband, The child attends a child care center and bites another two-year-old. How do you feel?

1. The baby with AIDS should be isolated and kept at home with the family in order to prevent other children from being infected.
2. The baby should be allowed to attend the child care center because the child needs other children around in order to have as normal a life as possible.
3. The father of the child should be imprisoned because of the harm he has done to his wife and child.
4. Every woman should be tested for AIDS when she becomes pregnant.
5. Every couple should be tested for AIDS before the wedding.

Let us change the facts again. In the preceding case, the husband contracted the AIDS virus through a blood transfusion performed before blood was tested for AIDS. What do you think?

1. The hospital who provided the blood should be responsible for all the expenses the family incurs while dealing with AIDS.
2. The parents of the husband should be responsible because their son was a hemophiliac and required transfusions from others in order to live.

Public school administrators recently argued that teaching children about AIDS should not be part of their curriculum. Now they are deciding where AIDS should be put into the curriculum and how. Viewpoints differ:

1. Children from kindergarten through grade twelve should be taught about AIDS and how to avoid it.
2. The public schools should not teach about AIDS; the matter should be left to
   a. health care workers
   b. doctors and nurses
   c. the church
   d. television
   e. the family
3. Television should advertise condoms and give instructions for their use.

THE GERIATRIC PATIENT

When talking about a particular group of patients, it is questionable whether special ethics apply to that age group, or if ethical considerations are the same but applied to different problems. The problems of the **geriatric** patient are those of an adult who is ending life. The major ethical dilemma becomes paternalism versus autonomy. These ethical considerations are emphasized at this stage of life because some degree of senile dementia is present in a high percentage of the population over sixty-five years of age. Because the varying degrees of dementia and physical disability reduce the elderly's self-sufficiency, society and/or family assume some support functions, and paternalism begins to supersede autonomy. Ethical considerations form a fine line in deciphering when such custodial care is necessary. Once the elderly accept dependence, the dependency increases, ending in institutionalization. How would you handle the following situations?

An elderly male, eighty-five years of age, comes into the office for a medical examination accompanied by a middle-aged daughter. She is escorting her father by holding his elbow and making certain that he moves at her command. At the end of the visit, the daughter writes a check to the doctor and pays for the visit out of her father's checking account. A week later, the check bounces. Do you:

1. call the daughter and tell her the check bounced?
2. called the patient and explain to him that his check came back to the office because of insufficient funds?

3.   send a letter to the patient with a copy to the daughter?

There are problems with the third-party payor in this situation that require further information from the patient, such as social security number, wife's maiden name, and the group policy number. Do you:

1.   call the daughter and attempt to get the information?
2.   attempt to get the information from the patient?

Laboratory tests reveal a condition that requires surgery, and the physician requests that some consent forms be signed. Do you:

1.   contact the daughter and have her come in and talk with the physician and sign the forms?
2.   contact the patient and ask him to come to the office with his daughter to sign some forms?
3.   call the patient and tell him that the doctor wants to see him in the office and allow the patient to determine how he will get to the office and who will bring him there?

You find that the patient's daughter has been appointed conservator of the patient's funds after the patient has signed surgical consent forms. The doctor remarked to you after the patient left the office that the patient was a sharp person for his age and asked appropriate questions. Do you:

1.   make a note in the file that the patient's daughter is his conservator?
2.   inform the doctor that the patient's daughter is his conservator and that the doctor should call her to get her signature on the form?
3.   call the daughter and have her come to the office to co-sign the consent forms?

The elderly, having once been normally functioning adults, are witness to their own mental and physical deterioration and to changes in the attitudes and behavior of others towards them. Even if there is impairment in **cognitive** function, ethically the question is how much the patient should be involved in personal care decisions.

SUICIDE

Suicide is a disaster for the family. Whenever there has been contact with someone who has committed suicide, there is guilt and the feeling that "maybe if I had done just a little bit more it would not have happened." Following a suicide, there is nothing more that can be done to help the patient. The attention of professionals turns to the family to help them deal with their loss. There often is anger, speculation about momentary **insanity,** guilt, and sorrow. Many consider suicide a disgrace to the family. Compassion and understanding will do much to help them through a difficult time. In the words of Immanual Kant, "Act so that you treat humanity, whether in your own person or that of another, always as an end and never as a means only."

SUMMARY

Each human being is faced with questions concerning death and dying. Working as a health care deliverer requires an ability to deal with these matters on a regular basis. The manner in which a professional handles these matters reflects personal philosophies.

Technology has progressed to the point where it does not appear to be always in the patient's best interest to prolong life. Do-not-resuscitate orders are now recorded in nursing notes for patients; removal of life-support systems is allowed by the courts. The durable power of attorney, living will, and health care proxy are legal instruments that ensure personal preferences are known when competence is questioned. The moral implications of euthanasia are still questioned by society.

But technology has not progressed to the point where illness has been totally eradicated. AIDS is projected to become an epidemic that will drain society's resources in the future. Geriatric patients are still afflicted with dementia, and suicide remains one of life's most tragic endings.

SUGGESTED ACTIVITY

Interview a physician and a religious professional. Document the standards each has about life-support systems and whether they should be used on a terminally ill patient. Note the development of their personal philosophies that has led to their current thinking. Ask what incidents might change their present beliefs.

STUDY QUESTIONS

1. Identify the options available to Dr. Koop for treating the five-year-old patient with neuroblastoma.
2. Research the criteria for death in your jurisdiction.
3. Contact a local hospital to see if its ethics committee has a policy for do-not-resuscitate orders. If you can, get a copy.
4. Contact an attorney and request a copy of an unsigned living will.
5. Contact an attorney and request a copy of a durable power of attorney.
6. Contact the local board of health or another data-collecting agency to determine whether a copy of the current statistics concerning communicable diseases in your area is available.
7. Contact your local school department to determine the procedure for educating students about sexually transmitted diseases.
8. Ask for a tour of a local nursing home and talk with the residents with the intent of observing their orientation to the news events of the day.

9. Contact your local bank to find out what is done with checking accounts when the owner dies.

10. Volunteer for work on the local suicide hotline.

CASES FOR DISCUSSION

1. The patient was a man thirty-four years of age. He left a store and walked toward his car. The defendant, a young man of eighteen, tip-toed behind him and hit him on the head with a baseball bat. He then went into a building, changed his clothes, crossed the street, and entered the store where he worked. When asked why he had hit the man, he said, "For kicks." At the hospital, the victim was placed on an artificial respirator. Two days later, the victim's blood pressure, heart-beat, and pulse were not observable; he failed to breathe when taken off the respirator; and an electroencephalogram failed to reveal any cerebral electrical activity. In the opinion of the physician, the patient had reached the stage of irreversible brain death. Two days later, the patient was again taken off the respirator with the same outcome. After consultation with the patient's family, the respirator was removed and his heart stopped. The defendant was found guilty of first-degree mur-der with the requirement of death satisfied by the proof of brain death. The defendant appealed, stating that "death," as required by the law, never occurred. How should the court rule?

2. For reasons still unclear, the patient ceased breathing for at least two fifteen-minute periods. She received some ineffectual mouth-to-mouth resuscitation from friends. She was taken by ambulance to the hospital, where she had a temperature of 100°F and was unresponsive to deep pain. She lapsed into a coma. Medical evidence indicated that she suf-fered severe brain damage, leaving her in a "chronic and persistent vegetative state." The patient was kept alive through the use of respira-tors and other medical life support systems while her body underwent a continuing deteriorative process. There was no known treatment to improve her condition. Her father requested that life-support systems be withdrawn, but the attending physician refused because the patient did not meet the traditional medical standard for death. Her heart had not stopped, nor was she brain dead. If the life-support systems are removed, should the doctor be subject to civil or criminal liability?

3. The patient was sixty-seven years old and had lived for fifty years in a mental institution. He became ill with acute myelogenous leukemia, a blood disease that leads to death within months if it is not treated. The disease process can be slowed by chemotherapy. This treatment has severe side effects and is effective in only thirty to fifty percent of the cases. Even when effective, the treatment prolongs life for little more than one year. Patients over sixty have a particularly difficult time

tolerating the treatment. At a hearing before the probate court, the patient's **guardian ad litem** recommended that he undergo the treatment, since this is what most people elect. Should the court rule against the guardian ad litem and allow this incompetent person the right to refuse medical treatment?

4. The wife and son of a senile, seventy-eight-year-old man tried to stop the hemodialysis treatments that he had undergone for a year. The family and the physician believed that the request was what the patient would have wanted. The family went to probate court, where a guardian ad litem was appointed to represent the patient. An adversarial hearing was conducted, and the court issued an order to terminate the treatment. The guardian ad litem objected, insisting that there had to be some positive evidence of the patient's will, and not merely a "substituted judgment," before a court could order the termination of the treatment. This matter was continued through probate, appeals, and Supreme Court hearings. What should the court decide?

5. An eighty-three-year-old monk entered the hospital for a routine hernia operation. During the course of the surgery, he suffered cardiopulmonary arrest. When resuscitated, it was found that he was in a chronic vegetative condition. The patient, following his religious convictions, agreed with the Catholic Church's teachings that heroic measures to prolong life were unnecessary. He had discussed those issues in conversations concerning other cases and had clearly stated he did not want any extraordinary measures taken to prolong his own life. His guardian asked physicians to remove the respirator that was keeping him alive. They refused. The surgeon asserted that once such a medical procedure was started, it should not be withdrawn. A spokesman for the hospital stated that the hospital's mission was to do all that it could to maintain life. The guardian then went to court. What should the court decide?

6. At approximately midnight, a patient complained to his wife of a severe headache and lapsed into unconsciousness. Angiograms revealed he had an aneurysm at the apex of the basilar artery. The patient underwent a craniotomy following which a clip was inserted across the aneurysm. The patient never regained consciousness. The patient was put on a respirator. Nutrition was provided through a nasogastric feeding tube. He was later diagnosed as being in a semivegetative or vegetative state. Do-not-resuscitate orders were placed in the patient's chart, a gastrostomy tube was inserted, and the nasogastric tube removed. Although the patient's electroencephalogram was abnormal, it did indicate controlled electrical activity generated by millions of cortical nerves, which were normal. Apart from the brain injury, the patient was not terminally ill. The patient's wife, who was also his guardian, requested that the hospital staff remove the gastrostomy tube. They refused, and the matter went to court. Should the court allow removal of the tube?

7. The patient was an eighty-four-year-old bedridden woman with serious and irreversible physical and mental impairment. She was confined to bed and unable to move out of the fetal position. In addition, she suffered from arteriosclerotic heart disease, hypertension, diabetes, and her left leg was gangrenous to the knee. She had several decubitus necrotic ulcers on her feet, legs, and hips, and an eye problem that required irrigation. She was unable to speak, and her ability to swallow was limited. There was a urinary catheter in place and she could not control her bowels. Experts determined that she was not brain dead, comatose, or in a vegetative state. Her nephew and guardian wanted to remove the nasogastric feeding tube. Should the court allow it?

Appendix

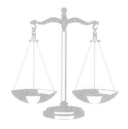

The Civil Case Process

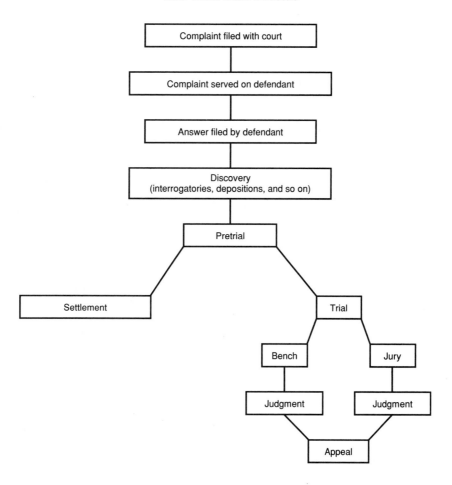

Complaint filed with court

Complaint served on defendant

Answer filed by defendant

Discovery
(interrogatories, depositions, and so on)

Pretrial

Settlement

Trial

Bench

Jury

Judgment

Judgment

Appeal

The Criminal Case Process

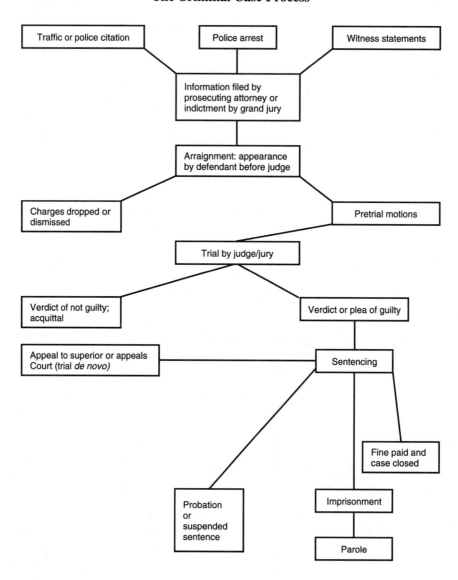

Glossary

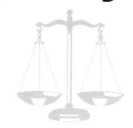

abandon—to give up or cease doing

abandonment—ceasing to take care of someone or something without proper terminating procedure

accepted—admitted to a facility that assumes certain obligations and duties

adjudicated—heard and settled by a judicial process

advanced directive—a document signed and witnessed according to state statute authorizing one person to make a decision for another, allowing treatment or refusal of treatment when the person for whom the document is made becomes incompetent

adversary—opponent

affirmation—a formal declaration that an affidavit is true

affirmative—stating something to be true as represented

affirmative duty—responding to an incident in a predetermined manner

age of majority—the full legal age determined by varying state statutes

agent—someone who has the authority to act for another under specific conditions

aggression—action of the first person to use hostile manner or force

aggressive—behaving in a hostile manner rather than with positive assertiveness

AIDS—Acquired Immune Deficiency Syndrome

amniocentesis—a medical technique used to determine whether a fetus is normal

amoral—without moral sense

anencephalic—a child born without a brain but with a brain stem

appeal—transfer of a case decided in a lower court to a higher court to obtain a new hearing on matters of law

arson—intentional burning of another's building or property or of one's own building or property for either a malicious or illegal purpose

assault—any deliberate attempt or threat to inflict bodily injury upon another person and with apparent ability to do so

assertiveness—taking positive steps to prevent litigation; in a medical setting, this would be the work of improving the physician-patient relationship, with the office staff complementing the doctor's efforts

assets—personal belongings and property owned by a person or, if he or she has died, by his or her estate

assisted suicide—one person making it possible for another person to commit suicide

assumption of risk—voluntary acceptance of a known danger

autograft—the transplanting of a person's own tissue from one part of the body to another. It can also mean transplants between identical twins.

autonomy—the condition of self-government

bargaining unit—the labor union, or group of employees with similar interests, authorized to conduct negotiations on behalf of the employees who are members of the union or group

battery—illegal touching of another person

bench trial—a trial in which a judge serves without a jury and rules on the law as well as the facts

beyond a reasonable doubt—proven in a thoroughly convincing way

bioethics—refers to life and death ethical issues and the implications of the application of biological research

breach—the unlawful violation of an obligation or contract either by commission or omission

Breathalyzer—apparatus used to test the content of alcohol in someone arrested for operating a vehicle under the influence of liquor

burden of proof—the necessity of giving convincing legal proof of any facts in dispute

burglary—breaking and entering for the purpose of committing a crime

burnout—exhaustion from overwork

bylaws—regulations adopted by a corporation or association to govern its internal affairs

calibration—the systematic standardization of quantitative measuring instruments

capacity—ability to understand the possible results of one's actions

capital—the assets in money or property accumulated by individual, partnership, or corporate ownership of a business; net worth

capitalization—a uniform, per person, payment or fee

capitation—payment in a lump sum to physicians, health maintenance organizations, and health care facilities to deliver health care to a segment of the population

cardiopulmonary arrest—cessation of normal functioning of the heart and lungs

cert. denied—when the United States Supreme Court refuses to hear an appeal

chemotherapy—the chemical treatment of disease

citation—references to court decision or legal authorities to support a proposed ruling. The numbers in a citation have special significance; for example, in the citation "484 F.2d 580," the notation "F.2d" refers to the second series of the book entitled Federal Reporter, "484" is the volume number, and "580" is the page number.

cited—mentioned in reference to legal sources that support a proposition of law to be established

civil—pertaining to crimes against a person or persons

clear and convincing—that measure of proof that will produce in the mind of the trier of facts a firm belief or conviction as to allegations sought to be established

cloning—identically duplicating an organism

codify—the process of collecting and arranging systematically, usually by subject, the laws of a state or a country

cognitive—relating to knowledge learned through perception, reasoning, or intuition

collective bargaining—procedural attempt to achieve collective agreements between an employer and accredited representative of a group of employees, to improve the conditions of employment

commitment—the process by which a person is entrusted to a mental health facility or a penal institution

commodity—anything useful or serviceable that can be bought and sold

common law—law deriving its authority from ancient usages and customs affirmed by court judgments and decrees

comparable—the representation of one thing or person similar to another

comparative negligence—negligence measured by percentage, with the determined damages lessened according to the extent of injury or damage committed by the party proven guilty

comprehensive—covering completely or broadly; inclusive

conditional—depending upon a specific condition

confidentiality—the state of being treated as a private matter not intended for public knowledge

conglomerate—a corporation diversifying operations by acquiring varied enterprises

conservator—a court-appointed person given authority to manage the financial affairs of an incompetent person

consideration—something promised that results in making an agreement a lawful contract

conspiracy—an agreement among conspirators

conspiring—secretly planning with another person or persons to perform an illegal act

constable—a public officer with authority to serve writs and warrants and to make arrests

constitutional right—a right guaranteed to citizens by the Constitution and unassailable by law

consumer—one who buys products and services

contingency—something that may occur but is dependent upon an uncertain future event

contract—an agreement, written or unwritten, between two parties that creates an obligation under specific circumstances

contributory negligence—conduct by a plaintiff that is below the standard to which he or she is legally required to conform for his or her own protection

corporation—a means by which a group of people can unite to create an entity to do something impossible for the individual members. The organization is established by filing a certification of corporation in the state where its main place of business is located

credibility—the quality in a witness that makes his or her evidence worth believing

creditors—those to whom money or its equivalent is owed

creed—a statement of belief or principles

criminal—anyone who has committed a criminal offense or who has been proven guilty of such an offense

cross-examination—interrogation of a witness by a party other than the direct examiner

culture—the behavior patterns, customs, beliefs, institutions, and artistic expressions characteristic of a society or class

custodian—one charged with the care of a person or property

damages—monetary compensation for loss or injury

data—the body of information used to form a decision

debts—money, services, or goods owed to some person or persons to whom one is obligated

decision—the authoritative judgment made to settle a controversy

defendant—a person or party against whom a plaintiff's allegations are brought

defensive medicine—a practice by some doctors of ordering every battery of medical tests and procedures known to search out a definite diagnosis so as not to be accused of failing to practice zealously

delegated—authorized to act for another or others

deontological—ethical theory based on duty and obligation

deposition—a prior statement by a witness to be used in court as testimony taken under oath subject to cross-examination

depression—dejection in mood or emotion

deterrence—a means of punishment used to prevent a crime

diagnostic related groups (DRGs)—related medical groups contributing their diagnosis of the nature of a patient's disease upon which standardized fees are based

direct examination—the first interrogation of a witness by the party for whom the witness has been called in behalf of that party's claim

directors—those elected and terminated by stockholders to management responsibility in a corporation

discrimination—failure to treat all persons equally when there is no reasonable distinction between those favored and those unfavored

disparate—a marked difference between two things

disposition—in criminal law, the final settlement of a case

district attorney—the official prosecutor of a judicial district

district court—a division of the trial court (federal or state), serving a specific geographical area, with only one judge usually required to hear and decide a case

dividends—distributed profits of a corporation

DNA—an essential component of all living matter and the basic chromosomal material transmitting the hereditary pattern

documentation—the supplying of written or printed official information that can be used for evidence

domestic violence—abuse, physical or mental, that occurs within the home

due care—the duty to have adequate regard for another person's rights

durable power of attorney—a document allowing the principal (the person writing the durable power of attorney) to delegate to another person the legal authority to act on the principal's behalf

economic—relating to the financial necessities of life

emancipated minor—someone under age eighteen who is completely self-supporting

emergency—an occurrence developing suddenly that calls for immediate action

empathy—comprehensive understanding of another person by vicarious identification with that person's needs

entrepreneur—one who undertakes the financial risks of starting a new business

epidemic—widespread outbreak of contagious diseases

ethical—conforming to professionally proper behavior

ethics—the study of moral choices that conform to professional standards of conduct

etiquette—the prescribed code of courteous social behavior

eugenics—the study of hereditary improvement by controlling genes

euthanasia—an intentional action or lack of action causing the merciful death of someone suffering from a terminal illness or incurable condition

evidence—any type of proof presented by witnesses in a court trial

expert witness—one whose education, profession, or specialized experience qualifies him or her with superior knowledge of a subject

express contract—clear, definitive agreement between two or more parties

facially neutral—on the surface the matter is impartial, or does not take an active part in either side

Federal Rules of Evidence—rules governing evidence allowed in a federal court

fee for service—basis of professional billing, either so much per hour or per identified procedure

felony—a crime more serious than a misdemeanor and punishable by imprisonment for more than one year or death

fertility—the condition of having the capability to reproduce

fetus—an unborn offspring in the postembryonic stage of gestation

fiduciary—holding or held in trust

first-degree murder—premeditated murder or murder committed with extreme cruelty

forum—an assembly place or court for dispensing law

fraud—a deliberate deception intended to produce unlawful gain

genetic—resulting from genes or attributable to them

geriatric—relating to elderly people and their usual problems and afflictions

gestation—the length of time after conception during which developing offspring are carried in the uterus

good faith—honesty of intention

grossly negligent—failing intentionally to perform a necessary duty in extraordinary disregard of the consequences to the person neglected, particularly if it can be proved that there is more than a fifty percent chance the negligence caused an injury

guardian—a person lawfully entrusted to take care of the person, property, and rights of someone incapable of managing his or her own affairs

guardian ad litem—a guardian appointed to prosecute or defend a suit for an incapacitated party

health insurance—a contract obligating the insurer to pay certain benefits to the insured for bodily injuries or illnesses specified by the enumerated risks stated in the policy

health care proxy—document appointing one person to act as a surrogate to make health care decisions for another under certain circumstances

heirs—those who are entitled by law or by designation in a will to inherit the estate or property of another

heterograft—the transplant of animal tissue into a human

HIV—Human Immunodeficiency Virus which causes AIDS

homograft—a transplant from one person to another

idealistic—having high ideals

immoral—not moral

impact—the force of impression of one thing on another

implied contract—not indicated by direct words but evident from the conduct of the parties

incident report—the official statement of an incident

incompetents—those who lack the necessary qualifications to perform a duty

indictment—a written accusation charging a party with committing a crime which is drawn up by the prosecuting attorney and issued by a grand jury

indigent—lacking sufficient means to support oneself or anyone for whom one is responsible

inference—a process of reasoning by which a fact is deduced as a logical consequence of other facts

inflation—abnormal increase in price levels

injunctive relief—remedy provided by a court decision preventing or requiring someone to perform a particular action

insane—sufficiently mentally deranged to affect one's capacity for rational judgment

insanity—unsoundness of mind sufficient to prevent acceptable moral judgment

insurance—a contract binding a company to compensate someone for proven damages or injury caused by the party who has paid premiums in the contract

integrated—all parts brought together to form a unity

intentional—deliberate

interrogatory—written questions about a case addressed to one party by another

interstate—between two or more states

intestate—without making a will

investment—expenditure of capital to secure income or profit

invitee—a person who enters property for business as a result of express or implied invitation

joint ventures—a group of persons together performing some business undertaking

judgment—the court's decision regarding the rights and obligations of the parties in a dispute

judiciary—the branch of government that interprets and applies the law

jurisdiction—geographic area of authority in which courts are empowered to interpret the law

larceny—stealing or removing someone's personal property to convert it illegally or deprive the owner of its possession. Larceny is a felony.

latent defect—a defect not apparent by reasonable inspection

layperson—one who does not have training in a specific profession

legal disability—no legal capacity for mutual assent

levy—to raise or execute a tax

liability insurance—insurance designed to cover a policyholder for acts or omissions for which he or she may be legally obligated

licensee—a person who enters property with implied permission of the owner

life insurance—an insurance policy stipulating that the insurer will pay a specified sum to the designated beneficiary upon the death of the insured

life-sustaining—maintaining or prolonging life in someone not able to do so naturally

litigation—legal proceeding

litigious—prone to engage in lawsuits

living will—a will made by a person in which he or she requests to be allowed to die naturally rather than being kept alive by artificial means in the event there is no probable recovery from mental or physical disability

malfunction—defective performance of a product

malice—an unjust intention to commit an illegal act to injure someone

management—direction or administration of the affairs of a person, business, or organization

mandatory—pertaining to an authoritative command that a person must obey

manslaughter—an unpremeditated taking of a human life

mature minor—a person capable of appreciating the nature, extent, and consequences of his or her (medical) treatment

mayhem—the wanton causing of violent injury to a person or thing

medical malpractice—medical professional misconduct

memorialize—to have a doctor write a letter to a patient who wishes to discharge him or her in which the doctor documents reasons for the patient's desire to change physicians. The letter is sent by certified mail with return receipt requested.

mental incapacity—a condition in which a person lacks reasoning faculties to understand ordinary concerns or to act competently

mental incompetence—lack of reasoning faculties that are needed to enable someone to deal with the ordinary affairs of life

minors—persons who are under the legal adult age

misdemeanor—an offense less serious than a felony and which may be punished by a fine or sentence to a local prison for less than one year

mitigating—make less severe due to considerations of fairness and mercy

morals—rules of conduct based on standards of right and wrong

motion—the application to a court or judge for a ruling in favor of the one applying

murder—an act done with intent to kill the victim

mutual assent—common agreement of both parties

negligence—failure to take reasonable precautions to protect others from the risk of harm

negligent per se—conduct that is against common knowledge that, by its act, without argument, can be declared negligence

negotiate—to meet with another to achieve agreement or compromise on an issue in dispute

negotiated fee schedules—the process of the submission and consideration of offers until an offer is accepted. Fee schedule refers to the amount an insurance company or other third-party payor will reimburse for a medical procedure.

negotiation—exchange and consideration of offers until parties agree on a solution that is acceptable to both

net—that which remains after expenses and taxes are deducted

nonverbal communication—communicating with someone using body language

notice—an announcement, written or displayed, giving pertinent information to those interested in a certain person, place, or event, or in any legal agreement such as a partnership

Nuremberg Code—the code stating that certain types of medical experiments on human beings be kept within reasonably well-defined bounds that observe basic principles of moral, ethical, and legal concepts

oath—an affirmation that a statement is correct and the witness will tell the truth

offer—a proposal to perform a certain action or pay a specified amount

officers—persons holding formal positions of trust in an organization, especially those involved in high levels of management

overruled—ruled against by a subsequently higher court decision

parens patriae—the responsibility of the state as sovereign and guardian of persons with a legal disability

partnership—an association of two or more individuals to act as co-owners of a business venture

patent defect—a malfunction easily discovered upon examination of a product

paternalism—providing for people's needs but giving them no responsibility

peer review—a review by persons with similar professional qualifications

per capita payment—pay equally according to the number of individuals

perjury—a false statement under oath

personality traits—distinctive individual qualities of a person

pharmacopoeia—a book officially listing medical drugs along with information about their preparation and use; a stock of drugs in a pharmacy

philosophy—a basic viewpoint of the system of values of an individual or society

piecework—work paid for according to the quantity of production

plaintiff—one who brings a court action against another

pluralistic—pertaining to the belief that there is no single explanation for all the extraordinary aspects of life, particularly in a society of numerous distinct cultures

politics—the methods used to administer public affairs, particularly those of a government

premises—preliminary explanatory statements made as a basis for a legal argument

preponderance of evidence—evidence that is more convincing than that offered by the opposition

pretrial conference—the first court conference of parties involved in a dispute

preventive medicine—medical practices and precautions designed to ward off litigation

principal—the employer, or source of authority, of the agent, or employee

privileged communication—a confidential communication that a person on the witness stand cannot be forced to disclose

probable cause (reasonable cause)—having more evidence for than against

probation—a sentence releasing a defendant into the community with court supervision

procedural—that law which prescribes a method of enforcing rights or obtaining redress for their invasion

procedures manual—a reference handbook explaining the procedures by which a legal right may be enforced

product liability—a tort making a manufacturer liable for compensation to anyone using his or her product if damages or injuries occur from defects in that product

profits—the gains accrued from business or investments after the payment of expenses

property right—the right of ownership

prospective—likely to come about; looking forward to the future

proximate cause—that which, in any natural and continuous sequence, unbroken by any intervening cause, produces injury

psychological—influencing mental or emotional behavior

psychosomatic—characterized by both physiological and psychological illness

purist—one who practices absolute correctness

quality assurance—responsibility to uphold the quality of care of patients in treatment situations

random—without a definite systematic method

rape—unlawful sexual intercourse with a female against her will

reasonable care—acceptable degree of care under certain circumstances

reasonable person—a prudent person, whose behavior would be considered appropriate under the circumstances

reformation—the rehabilitation of a criminal; changed behavior

remedies—legal ways to correct or prevent a wrong or to enforce a right

res ipsa loquitur ("the thing speaks for itself")—the rule or evidence showing that negligence by the accused person may be reasonably inferred from the nature of the injury occurring to the plaintiff

respectable minority—a minority acceptable to its peer group

respondeat superior ("Let the master answer")—an employer is vicariously liable for the behavior of an employee working within his or her scope of employment

restraint—restriction of liberty

retirement benefits—benefits paid to an employee for a prior term of service after he or she discontinues work for that employer

retribution—something given or demanded in payment or as a punishment for criminal wrongdoing

revoke—to make void by taking back

Richardson Commission—a commission appointed by the United States Government

risk management—minimizing the danger or hazard

robbery—the forcible stealing of the personal property of another either from his or her person or in the immediate presence of the victim

sample—a representative segment or portion

sanction—a penalty imposed for violating a law or accepted procedure

sanctity—the condition of being inviolable

scientific investigation—an investigation using scientific rules and concepts to reach a valid conclusion

search warrant—a written legal order giving authority for a search

self-defense—the right to protect oneself reasonably from acts of violence or threatened violence

sentence—the judicial pronouncement of the penalty for the party found guilty

settlement—an adjustment or agreement settling matters is dispute

sexual harassment—sex discrimination caused by unwanted attention from peers, coworkers, supervisors, customers, clients, or anyone with whom the victim is obliged to work

shares—units of stock giving the possessor part ownership in a corporation

shibboleth—any phrase or custom peculiar to a certain class or faction

slander—the utterance of a false charge that damages another's reputation

sociological—pertaining to human social behavior

sodomy—unnatural copulation of human beings with each other or with an animal

sole proprietorship—ownership of a business by one person

specific performance—the remedy of carrying out a contract as specified

standard of care—the degree of care that a reasonably prudent person should exercise under the same or similar circumstances

statute of frauds—the provision that no suit or action shall be maintained concerning a particular type of contract unless there is a memorandum of that contract signed by the person to be charged or by his or her authorized agent

statute of limitations—the law setting a time limit within which one person can sue another

statutes—laws passed by state legislatures

statutory—pertaining to a law

stockholders—those who hold an interest (stock) in a corporation

strict liability—responsibility of a seller or manufacturer for any defective product unduly threatening a consumer's personal safety

strict tort—responsibility of all members of a corporation or association involved in the manufacture and sales of a defective product

subpoena—a command to appear at a specified time and place to testify

subpoena duces tecum—the court command to a witness to produce at trial a certain pertinent document he or she holds

subscribers—one who agrees to buy or belong for a period of time

substantive law—the part of law that creates, defines, and regulates rights

substitute judgment—one who makes a decision for another

suit-prone—apt to start a suit or to be the object of a suit

superior court—a court of general jurisdiction to which a case is removed for review or appeal

survival action—any technique used to help someone to survive

technology—methods and materials used to achieve commercial or industrial objectives. The application of scientific methods to achieve a certain objective

teleological—ethical theory concerned with outcome, whether an action produces greater good in the world

tendered—an offer of money from one person to another

terminally ill—fatally ill with a condition for which there is no reliable cure

testimony—evidence given by a competent witness

theft—stealing property without consent of the owner

tolling—a temporary suspension of the statute while the defendant is absent from the jurisdiction or while the plaintiff is a minor

tort—a private wrong or injury, other than breach of contract, for which the court will provide a remedy

tracked—detectable evidence that something has passed

trespasser—someone who enters a property illegally

undue influence—any improper persuasion to make someone act differently from his or her own will

union—an organization founded to promote the interests and rights of the group of workers it represents

utilization review—a process by which hospitals review patient progress in order to efficiently allocate scarce medical resources

values—principles considered desirable

venue—the particular county or geographical area where a court may try a case

verdict—decision or judgment

vicariously liable—legally obligated in place of someone else

virtue—goodness conforming to the standard of moral excellence

waiver—document by which one voluntarily gives up a right, privilege, or claim

waives—to surrender a claim, privilege, or right

wanton—done with reckless disregard of another's rights or needs

warranty—a promise that certain facts are truly represented

witness—a person testifying under oath to what he or she has heard or noticed

writ of certiorari—a device used by the United States Supreme Court to choose the cases in wishes to hear

wrongful death—death caused by negligence

zone of privacy—right of privacy lies within an area where the government cannot interfere

Bibliography

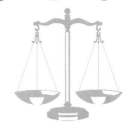

CASES

Adams v. State of Indiana, 229 N.E.2d 834 (Ind. 1973).

In re Adoption of Anonymous, 74 Misc. 2d 99, 345 N.Y.S.2d 430 (1973).

Alberts v. Devine, 395 Mass. 59 (1985).

Amadio v. Levin, 501 A.2d 1085 (Pa. 1985).

Anderson v. Somberg, 67 N.H. 291, 338 A.2d 1 *cert. denied,* 423 U.S. 929, S. Ct. 279 (1975).

Applebaum v. Board of Directors of Barton Memorial Hospital, 104 Cal. App. 3d 648, 163 Cal. Rptr. 831 (1980).

Armstrong v. Svoboda, 49 Cal. Rptr. 701 (1966).

Ascher v. Gutierre, 175 U.S. App. D.C. 900, 533 F.2d 1235 (1976).

August v. Offices Unlimited, Inc., 981 F.2d 576 (1st Cir. 1992).

Avery v. Maryland, 292 A.2d 728 (Md. 1972).

Backus v. Baptist Medical Center, 510 F. Supp. 1191 (1980).

Barnette v. Potenza, 79 Misc. 2d 51, 359 N.Y.S. 432 (1974).

Beadles v. Megayka, 311 P.2d 711 (Colo. 1957).

Becker v. Janiski, 15 N.Y.S. 675 (1891).

Becker v. Schwartz, 46 N.Y.2d 401, 413 N.Y.S. 895, 386 N.E.2d 807 (1978).

Bence v. Denbo, 183 N.E. 326 (Ind. Ct. App. 1932).

Berg v. New York Society for the Relief of the Ruptured & Crippled, 136 N.E.2d 513 (N.Y. 1956).

Estate of Berthiaume v. Pratt, 365 A.2d 792 (Me. 1976).

Bishop v. Byrne, 265 F. Supp. 460 (W. Va. 1967).

Bonner v. Moran, 75 U.S. App. D.C. 156, 126 F.2d 121 (1941).

Bouvia v. Superior Court of Los Angeles County, 179 Cal. App. 3d 1172, 225 Cal. Rptr. 297 (Ct. App. 1986).

Brophy v. New England Sinai Hospital, 398 Mass. 417 (1986).

Burton v. Leftwich, 123 So. 2d 766 (La. 1960).

Butler v. Louisiana State Board of Education, 331 So. 2d 192 (La. 1976).

Butterworth v. Swint, 186 S.E. 770 (Ga. 1936).

C.M. v. C.C. 152 N.J. Super. 160, 377 A.2d 821 (1977).

Campbell v. Wainright, 416 F.2d 949 (1969).

Cannell v. Medical & Surgical Clinic, 315 N.E.2d 278 (Ill. 1974).

Carey v. Mercer, 132 N.E. 353 (Mass. 1921).

Carr v. St. Paul Fire & Marine Insurance Co., 384 F. Supp. 821 (Ark. 1974).

Carr v. Shippolette, 82 F.2d 874 (D.C. Cir. 1936).

Carter v. Cangello, 164 Cal. Rptr. 361 (1980).

Christy v. Saliterman, 179 N.W.2d 288 (Minn. 1970).

Cobbs v. Grant, 8 Cal. Rptr. 505, 502 P.2d 1 (1972).

Cochran v. Sears Roebuck, 34 S.E.2d 296 (Ga. 1945).

Commissioner of Correction v. Myers, SJC Mass. (1979).

Commonwealth v. Edelin, 3 Mass. Adv. 2795, 359 N.E.2d 4 (1976).

Commonwealth v. Golston, 366 N.E.2d 744 (1977).

Connell v. Medical & Surgical Clinic, 315 N.E.2d 278 (Ill. 1974).

In re Conroy, 98 N.J. 321, 486 A.2d 1209 (1985).

Cook v. Rhode Island, 10 F.3d 17 (1st Cir. 1993).

Cooper v. Sisters of Charity, 272 N.E.2d 97 (Ohio 1971).

Corne & De Vane v. Bausch & Lomb, 390 F. Supp. 161 (1975).

Cox v. Stanton, 529 F.2d 247 (1975).

Crawford v. McDonald, 187 S.E.2d 542 (Ga. 1972).

Crow v. McBride, 153 P.2d 727 (Cal. 1944).

Crowe v. Provost, 374 S.W.2d 645 (Tenn. 1963).

Cruzan v. Director, Missouri Department of Health, 110 S. Ct. 2841
    (Mo. 1990).

In re Culbertson's Will, 292 N.Y.S.2d 806 (1968).

Delaney v. Rosenthal, 196 N.E.2d 878 (Mass. 1964).

DeMay v. Roberts, 9 N.W. 146 (Mich. 1881).

Doe v. Southeastern Pennsylvania Transportation, No. 93-5988 (U.S. Dist.
    Ct., E.D. Pa., December 5, 1994), 95 LWUSA 96, p. 8.

Donaldson v. O'Connor, 493 F.2d 507 (1974).

East Chicago Rehabilitation Center, Inc. v. NLRB, 710 F.2d 397 (1983).

Gashgai v. Maine Medical Association, 350 A.2d 511 (1976).

Geddes v. Daughters of Charity, 348 F.2d 144 (1965).

Gelder Medical Group v. Webber, 363 N.E.2d 573 (N.Y. 1977).

Gillanza v. Sands, 316 So. 2d 77 (Fla. 1975).

Gillette v. Tucker, 65 N.E. 865 (Ohio 1902).

Goldman v. Kossove, 117 S.E.2d 35 (N.C. 1960).

Gotkin v. Miller, 379 F. Supp. 859 (E.D.N.Y. 1974), *aff'd* 514 F.2d 125
    (2d Cir. 1975).

Gray v. Grunnagle, 23 A.2d 663 (Pa. 1966).

Greaves v. State, 528 P.2d 805 (1974).

Griece Mills v. Derwinski, 967 F.2d 794 (2d Cir. 1992).

Griffin v. Medical Society of New York, 11 N.Y.S.2d 109 (1939).

Griggs v. Duke Power, 401 U.S. 424 (1971).

Griswold v. Connecticut, 381 U.S. 479, 85 S. Ct. 1678 (1965).

Guilmet v. Campbell, 385 Mich. 57, 188 N.W.2d 601 (1971).

Hawker v. New York, 170 U.S. 189 (1898).

Hawkins v. McGee, 146 A. 611 (N.H. 1929).

Helling v. Carey, 83 Wash. 2d 514, 519 P.2d 981 (1974).

Helms v. St. Paul Fire & Marine Insurance Co., 289 So. 2d 288 (La. 1974).

Hiatt v. Grace, 523 P.2d 320 (Kan. 1974).

Hicks v. Arkansas State Medical Board, 260 Ark. 31, 537 S.W.2d 794
    (Ark. 1976).
Hood v. Phillips, 554 S.W.2d 160 (Tex. 1977).
Horne v. Patton, 287 So. 2d 824 (1973).
Horton v. Niagara Falls Memorial Medical Center, 380 N.Y.S. 116 (1976).
Howard v. Lecher, 42 N.Y.2d 109, 397 N.Y.S.2d 363 (1977).
Humphrey v. First Interstate Bank of Oregon, 696 P.2d 527 (1985).
Hurley v. Eddingfield, 156 Ind. 416, 59 N.E. 1058 (1901).

Jacobs v. Theimer, 519 S.W.2d 846 (Tex. 1975).
James v. Spear, 338 P.2d 22 (Cal. 1959).
Jefferson v. United States, 77 F. Supp. 706 (Md. 1948).
Jeswald v. Hutt, 239 N.E.2d 37 (Ohio 1968).
Johnson v. Woman's Hospital, 527 S.W.2d 133 (Tenn. 1975).
Johnston v. Black Co., 91 P.2d 921 (Cal. 1939).
Jones v. Fakehany, 67 Cal. Rptr. 810 (1968).

Katko v. Briney, 183 N.W.2d 657 (Iowa 1971).
Kennedy v. Parrott, 243 N.C. 355, 90 S.E.2d 754 (1956).
J. F. Kennedy Hospital v. Heston, 58 N.J. 576, 279 A.2d 670 (1971).
Kirk v. Michael Reese Hospital, No. 81-2408 (Ill. App. Ct.
    August 28, 1995).

Laperi Administrator v. Sears Roebuck Co., Mass. Lawyers Weekly
    No. A 92-24.

Mahavier v. Beverly Enterprises, 540 S.W.2d 813 (Tex. 1976).
Markus v. Frankford Hospital, 283 A.2d 69 (Pa. 1971).
Mattocks v. Bell, 194 A.2d 307 (D.C. 1963).
Mazer v. Lipschutz, 327 F.2d 42 (1963).
McCormack v. Mt. Sinai Hospital, 44 N.Y.S.2d 702 (1981).
McCormick v. Haley, 307 N.E.2d 34 (Ohio 1973).
McCune v. Neitzel, No. 88-552 (Neb. Sup. Ct. Lawyer's Alert No. 215-23,
    July 13, 1990).
McGulpin v. Bessmer, 43 N.W.2d 121 (Iowa 1950).
McLaughlin v. Mine Safety Appliances Co., 11 N.Y.2d 62, 226 N.Y.S.2d
    407, 181 N.E.2d 430 (1962).
McNamara v. Emmons, 97 P.2d 503 (Cal. 1939).
Miles v. Hoffman, 221 P. 316 (Wash. 1923).
Millsaps v. Bankers Life Co., 35 Ill. App. 3d 735, 342 N.E.2d 329 (1976).
Mone v. Greyhound Lines, 368 Mass. 358, 331 N.E.2d 916 (1976).
Mullins v. Duvall, 104 S.E. 513 (Ga. 1920).

Nolan v. Kechibrigian, 64 A.2d 866 (R.I. 1949).

O'Neill v. Montefiore Hospital, 202 N.Y.S.2d 436 (1960).

Orthopedic Clinic v. Hanson, 415 P.2d 991 (Okla. 1966).
In re Osborne, 294 A.2d 372 (1972).

Park v. Chassin, 80 App. Div. 2d 60, 400 N.Y.S. 110 (1977).
Pearch v. Canady, 52 Tenn. 343, 373 S.W.2d 617 (1963).
People v. Brown, 88 Cal. App. 3d 283, 151 Cal. Rptr. 749 (1979).
People v. Sorenson, 68 Cal. 2d 680, 66 Cal. Rptr. 7, 437 P.2d 495 (1968).
People v. Yukl, 83 Misc. 2d 364, 372 N.Y.S. 2d 313 (1975).
Pinkus v. MacMahon, 129 N.J. 367, 29 A.2d 885 (1943).
Plutshack v. University of Minnesota Hospital, 316 N.W.2d 1 (Minn. 1982).
Price v. Sheppard, 239 N.W.2d 905 (Minn. 1976).

In re Quinlan, 70 N.J. 10, 355 A.2d 647 (1976).

Redder v. Hanson, 338 F.2d 244 (1964).
Reeder v. City of New York, 197 N.Y.S.2d 572 (1960).
Estate of Reiner, 383 N.Y.S.2d 504 (1976).
Renslow v. Mennonite Hospital, 67 Ill. 348, 10 Ill. Dec. 484 (1977).
Reyes v. Wyeth Laboratories, 498 F.2d 1264, *cert. denied,* 419 U.S. 1096 (1974).
Reynolds v. McNichols, 488 F.2d 1378 (1973).
Riff v. Morgan Pharmacy, 508 A.2d 1247 (Pa. 1986).
Robins v. California, 370 U.S. 660, 82 S. Ct. 1417 (1962).
Rochester v. Katalan, 320 A.2d 704 (Del. 1974).
Rockhill v. Pollard, 259 Or. 54, 485 P.2d 28 (1971).
Roe v. Wade, 410 U.S. 113, 93 S. Ct. 705, 35 L. Ed. 2d 147 (1973).
Rogers v. Lawson, 170 F.2d 157 (D.C. Cir. 1948).
Rudick v. Prineville Memorial Hospital, 319 F.2d 764 (1963).
Rule v. Cheeseman, 317 P.2d 472 (Kan. 1957).

In re Sampson, 317 N.Y.S.2d 241 (1970).
Schachter v. Whalen, 581 F.2d 35 (1978).
Schlesser v. Keck, 271 P.2d 588 (Cal. 1954).
Sherlock v. Stillwater Clinic, 260 N.W.2d 269 (1977).
Shoemaker v. Friedberg, 183 P.2d 318 (Cal. 1947).
Simonsen v. Swenson, 177 N.W. 831 (Neb. 1920).
Skodje v. Hardy, 288 P.2d 471 (Wash. 1955).
Smalley v. Baker, 262 Cal. App. 2d 824, 69 Cal. Rptr. 521 (1968).
In re Smith, 295 A.2d 238 (Md. 1972).
Smith v. Sibley, 431 P.2d 719 (Wash. 1967).
Snyder v. Holy Cross Hospital, 30 Md. App. 317 (1976).
In re Spring, 380 Mass. 629, 405 N.E.2d 115 (1978).
Stahlin v. Hilton Hotels Corp., 484 F.2d 580 (1973).
State Board of Medical Examiners v. Finch, 514 S.W.2d 608 (Mo. 1974).
Stowers v. Wolodzko, 191 N.W.2d 355 (1971).
Strunk v. Strunk, 445 S.W.2d 145 (1969).

Sullivan v. O'Connor, 363 Mass. 579, 296 N.E.2d 183 (1973).
Superintendent Belchertown v. Saikwicz, 370 N.E.2d 417 (1977).

Tarasoff v. Regents of University of California, 118 Cal. Rptr. 129 (1974).
Tarasoff v. Regents of University of California, 17 Cal. 3d 342, 131 Cal.
    Rptr. 14 (1976).
Thomas v. St. Joseph Hospital, 618 S.W.2d 791 (Tex. Civ. App. 1981).

United States v. Krizek, 859 F. Supp. 5 (D.D.C. 1994).
United States v. Morvant, 843 F. Supp. 1092 (E.D. La. 1994).
United States v. Wilson, 361 F. Supp. 510 (Md. 1973).

Venner v. State, 30 Md. App. 599, 354 A.2d 483 (1976).
Vigil v. Rice, 397 P.2d 719 (N.M. 1964).

Whalen v. Roe, 429 U.S. 589, 97 S. Ct. 869 (1977).
Wickline v. State of California, No. B 10156 (Cal. Ct. App. 2d Dist.,
    July 1, 1986).
Winters v. Miller, 446 F.2d 65, *cert. denied,* 404 U.S. 985 (1971).

PERIODICALS

AIDS patients' names mailed to Florida paper. (1996, September 20). *The
    Boston Globe.*
AMA opposes taking organs from brain-malformed babies. (1996, January
    7). *New York Times,* p. 22.
American Bar Association Journal, 83. (1993, January).
Anderson, M.T. (1985, April). Reporting elder abuse: It's the law. *AJN,* 371.
Annas, George J. (1986, September). Made in the U.S.A.: Legal and ethical
    issues in artificial heart experimentation. *Law, Medicine and Health
    Care, 14*(3–4).
Appleman, John Alan. (1976, November/December). Malpractice insurance
    rates—What's the answer? *Journal of Legal Medicine,* 37.
Barnicle, Mike. (1995, July 16). Father battles insane system. *The Boston
    Globe.*
Bass, Alison. (1995, February 22). Computerized medical data put privacy
    on the line. *The Boston Globe,* p. 5.
Bass, Alison. (1995, May 12). Children's mental health coverage often
    falling short. *The Boston Globe,* p. 1.
Beck, Leif C. (1972, April 15). Patient information: When—and when not to
    divulge. *Patient Care, 72,* 60.
Bergerson, Stephen R. (1984). Charting with a jury in mind. *Nursing,* 5.
Besharov, Douglas J. (1988, Spring). Child abuse and neglect . . . *Family
    Law Quarterly, XXII*(1), 8.
Bishop, Jerry E. (1981, December 16). Physical isn't needed yearly. *The
    Wall Street Journal,* p. 1.

The Boston Globe. (1980, October 31).

The Boston Globe. (1985, October 31).

The Boston Globe, p. 5 (1995, February 22).

The Boston Globe, p. 1 (1995, May 12).

Brant, Jonathan. Medical malpractice insurance. *Valparaiso University Law Review,* 6, 152, n. 41, 157, n. 31.

Brelis, Matthew. (1995, April 11). Patients' files allegedly used for obscene calls. *The Boston Globe,* p. 1.

Brittain, Robert S. (1978). Physician defines role of medical profession in claims prevention. *Lawyers Medical Journal* 7, 203–205.

Brooke, James W. (1970). *Willamette Law Review,* 6, 225, 232.

California judge dismisses fetal abuse charges. (1987, February 28). Associated Press, San Diego, *The Boston Globe.*

Capeci, Jerry. (1985, March 8). Docs nabbed in abortion scheme. *The Boston Herald.*

Caplan, Arthur L. (1992, November–December). When evil intrudes. *Hastings Center Report,* 29.

Case conference: Fain would I change that note. (1978). *Journal of Medical Ethics,* 4, 207–209.

Cepelewicz, Barry B. (1996, July). Telemedicine: A virtual reality, but many issues need resolving. *Medical Malpractice Law and Strategy, XIII*(9). Leader Publications: Division of New York Law Publishing Company.

Chase, Marilyn. (1994, December 5). Can a doctor who's a gatekeeper give enough care? *New York Times,* p. B1.

A clinic stopover for smugglers of drugs is found after arrest. *New York Times.*

Connecticut boy's transplant bill is settled. (1995, October 10). *The Boston Globe,* p. A21.

Coverup seen in death at rest home. (1995, February 5). *New York Times,* p. 33.

Cox, Thomas. A risk management approach to computerizing a physician's office. *Forum,* Harvard Risk Management Foundation.

Crane, Mark. (1989, March 20). Why did it take so long to nail this crooked doctor? *Medical Economics,* 54–64.

Davis, Maia. (1996, August 1). An empty feeling. *The Patriot Ledger,* p. 15.

Davis, Robert. (1995, March 22). On line medical records raise privacy fears. *USA Today,* p. 1A.

Dentzer, Susan, et al. (1986, May 5). Can you pass the job test? *Newsweek,* 46.

Dixon, Jennifer. (1995, July 29). Agency remains firm in refusal of benefits in frozen-sperm birth. *The Patriot Ledger.*

Doctor accused of trying to murder ex-boss. (1996, September 3). *New York Times,* p. 28.

Doctor tries to sidestep child abuse reporting laws. (1990, January/February). *National District Attorneys Association Bulletin,* 9(1).

Doctors' union pres looking to enlist members. (1987, January 14). *The Patriot Ledger.*

Doris Duke's nurse enters a guilty plea. (1995, October 15). *New York Times,* p. 40.

Dumanoski, Dianne. (1982, March 22). The von Bulow case: Trek through medical records. *The Boston Globe,* p. 1.

Editorial. (1987, June 6). *The Baltimore Sun.*

Estabrook, Gregg. (1987, January 26). The revolution in medicine. *Newsweek,* 40.

Ethical issues in managed care. (1995, January 25). *JAMA,* 330–335.

Failure to report abuse charge leads to 5-year exclusion. (1991, May). *Civil Money Penalties Reporter, Medicare/Medicaid Fraud & Abuse,* 5(1), 1.

Family leave: A government survey. (1996, March 26). *The Wall Street Journal,* p. 1.

Florida man 75 gets life for mercy killing of ailing wife. (1985, May 10). *The Boston Globe.*

Four at a clinic are accused of Medicaid fraud. (1995, February 8). *New York Times,* p. B2.

Freudenheim, M. (1991, January 1). Guarding medical confidentiality. *New York Times.*

Gage, S.M. (1981, Spring). Alteration, falsification and fabrication of medical records in medical malpractice actions. *Medical Trial Quarterly,* 27, 476.

Gaylin, Willard. (1994, June 12). Faulty diagnosis. *New York Times,* sec. 4A, p. 1.

Gaylin, William. (1980, August). XYY controversy: Researching violence and genetics. *The Hastings Center Special Supplement.*

Gilbert, Susan. (1996, August 21). Life saving medical history. *New York Times,* p. 1.

Girl accused of making false AIDS calls. (1995, March 1). *New York Times.*

Graedon, J. (1980). *The People's Pharmacy,* 2.

Greenhouse, Linda. (1996, June 14). [*Jaffee v. Redmond,* No. 95-266]. Justices uphold psychotherapy privacy rights. *New York Times,* p. A1.

Greve, Paul A. (1990, December). Keep quiet or speak up? Issues in patient confidentiality. *RN,* 53.

Groups spar over outcome of Kentucky medical record law. (1995, January 23/30). *American Medical News,* 29.

Haralambie, Ann M. (1988, Winter). Special problems in custody and abuse cases. *Family Advocate,* 10(3), 15.

Harvard Health Letter, 20(11), 1. (1995, September).

Headlines. (1992, August). *American Journal of Nursing,* 9.

Health care facility records: Confidentiality, computerization and security. (1995, July). *Forum on Health Law,* 13. The American Bar Association.

Hearn, Wayne. (1996, October 21). When the president is the patient. *American Medical News,* 13.

Herbert, Joe. (1994, September 11). Profits before patients. *New York Times,* p. E19.

Hirsch, H.L. (1978, Spring). Tampering with medical records. *Medical Trial Quarterly,* 450.

Holthaus, David. (1989, October). Employer's power to fight drug use. *Trustee,* 20.

Horsley, Jack E. (1990, January). Legally speaking: Don't tolerate sexual harassment at work. *RN,* 69.

Hospital Ethics. American Hospital Association, Advertising Publication.

Hyer, Marjorie. (1987, March 12). *St. Petersburg Times,* p. 21A, col. 1.

Isler, Charlotte. (1979, February). Six mistakes that could land you in jail. *RN,* 66–67.

Issue: Facsimile transmission of health information. (1994, May). American Health Information Management Association (AHIMA) Position Statement.

Jacobs, Margaret A. (1996, June 12). Women seek infertility benefits under disabilities law. *The Wall Street Journal,* p. B7.

Jones, Laurie. (1995, March 13). HIV tests urged for pregnant women. *AMNEWS,* 5.

Jonsen, Albert R. (1986, September). Bentham in a box: Technology, assessment and health-care allocation. *Law, Medicine and Health Care,* 14(3–4), 174.

Judge rule favors mother. (1995, January 10). *New York Times,* p. B5.

Kearney, Kerry A. (1996). Legal liability and risk considerations for a medical call center. *The Health Lawyer,* 9(3), 20.

Kelasa, Eileen V. (1993, January). HIV vs. a nurse's right to work. *RN,* 63.

Kennedy, Randy. (1995, September 14). 20 arrested in drug dealing in Brooklyn VA hospital. *New York Times,* p. B3.

Klein, Catherine F. (1995, Summer). Full faith and credit interstate enforcement of protection orders under the Violence Against Women Act of 1994. *Family Law Quarterly,* 29(2), 253–272.

Kolata, Gina. (1991, June 4). More babies being born to be donors of tissue. *New York Times,* p. 1.

Krupat, Edward. (1986, November). A delicate imbalance. *Psychology Today,* 22.

Kurkjian, Stephen. (1996, May 2). Gloves are coming off. *The Boston Globe,* p. 1.

Ladd, John. (1982). The concepts of health and disease and their ethical implications. In Gruzalski & Nelson (Eds.), *Value conflicts in health-care delivery,* p. 23. Ballinger Publishing Company.

The Lakeberg Siamese twins: Were risks, costs of separation justified? *Medical Ethics Advisor,* 9(10), 121.

Lambert, Lane. (1996, March 4). Mental health survey criticized. *The Patriot Ledger,* p. 1.

Landers, Ann. (1982, March 19). The inhumanity of some doctors. *The Boston Globe,* p. 33.

Landers, Louise. (1978, July). Why some people seek revenge against doctors. *Psychology Today,* 94.

Lee, Felicia R. (1993, March 6). Difficult custody decisions being complicated by AIDS. *New York Times,* p. 22.

Legal lines. (1986, August). *Professional Medical Assistant,* 16.

Letters to the editor. (1987, June 6). *The Baltimore Sun.*

Leung, Shirley. (1996, August 10). Father of shooting victim sues owner of clinic site. *The Boston Globe,* p. B8.

Levine, Joseph. (1986, September 29). A ray of hope in the fight against AIDS. *Time,* 60.

Levine, Robert. (1987, April). Waiting is a power game. *Psychology Today,* 24–33.

Lewin, Tamar. (1991, May 31). As elderly population grows, so does the need for doctors. *New York Times,* pp. 1, A16.

Lewin, Tamar. (1996, January 1). Blood banks starting to harvest umbilical cords. *New York Times,* p. 12.

Marshall, Ruth. (1987, March 30). AIDS: The search for a vaccine. *Newsweek,* 79.

Marwick, Charles. (1996, January 10). Childhood aggression needs definition, therapy. *JAMA, 275*(2), 90.

McGinley, Laurie. (1992, April 21). Fitness exams help to measure worker acuity. *The Wall Street Journal,* pp. B1, B9.

Medical records. (1996). *The Wall Street Journal.*

Medical World News, 7, 116 (1966, May).

Mills, David. (1984). Insurers use police tactics to snare doctors who file false claims. *The Wall Street Journal.*

Mittleman, Michael. (1980, February). What are the chances when malignancy leads to a malpractice suit? *Legal Aspects of Medical Practice,* 42.

Mooney, Brian C. (1990, September 5). *The Boston Globe,* p. 23.

Mycek, Shari. (1991, May). Domestic violence goes public. *Trustee, 49*(5), 18.

Nossiter, Adam. (1995, March 16). A mistake, a rare prosecution, and a doctor is headed for jail. *New York Times,* p. A1.

O'Rourke, Kevin. (1986, November 22). Tube feeding—A Catholic view. *America.*

Palinecsar & Cobb. (1982). The physician's role in detecting and reporting elder abuse. *Journal of Legal Medicine, 3,* 413–441.

Pappano, Laura. (1987, April 30). Tormented by fear of rejection. *The Patriot Ledger.*

Paris, John H. (1980). Court intervention and the diminution of patients' rights. The case of Brother Joseph Fox. *New England Journal of Medicine, 303,* 876.

Parker, Brant, & Hart, Johnny. (1982, March 14). The wizard of id. *The Boston Globe.*

The Patriot Ledger, p. 4. (1985, August 19).

The Patriot Ledger. (1986, June 25).

The Patriot Ledger, p. 26. (1988, March 30).

The Patriot Ledger. (1990, June 6).

Pave, Marvin. (1985, May 10). *The Boston Globe.*

Paxton, Harry T. (1988, February 1). Today's guidelines for patient confidentiality. *Medical Economics,* 198.

Peratta, Ed. (1996, June 6). Wellesley doctor settles complaint stemming from patient's HIV test. *Wellesley Townsman,* p. 1.

Personal comments in medical records may cause trouble. (1976, January 12). *Medical World News,* 125.

Poole, Derrick. (1986, June 25). *The Patriot Ledger.*

Poulos, C. Jean. (1987, May/June). A case of fraud. *The Professional Medical Assistant,* 14.

Preiser, S.E. (1976, October 4). The high cost of tampering with medical records. *Medical Economics,* 85.

Purtile, Ruth, & Sorrell, James. (1986, August). The ethical dilemmas of a rural physician. *The Hastings Report,* 25.

Rakowsky, Judy. (1995, August 3). Newton psychiatrist found guilty of fraud. *The Boston Globe,* p. 24.

Reese, Michael. (1985, May 6). A tragedy in Santa Monica. *Newsweek,* 10.

Report of the Ad Hoc Committee of the Harvard Medical School to examine the definition of brain death. (1968, August). *JAMA, 205,* 85.

Retrial begins in murder case tied to confession to an A.A. group. (1994, November 3). *New York Times METRO,* p. B7.

Ristuben, Karen R. (1996, June). Implications of managed care on patient care. *Health Law Section Newsletter,* Massachusetts Bar Association.

Robbery. *The Patriot Ledger.*

Robinson, Donald. (1989, May 28). Who should receive medical aid? *Parade Magazine,* 4.

Rosenthal, Elisabeth. (1995, November 11). Public advocate says HMO's often mislead poor and elderly. *New York Times,* p. B4.

Roth, Neal. (1977). The medical malpractice insurance crisis. *Insurance Counsel Journal, 41,* 469–473.

Rovner, Jack. (1996). Analysis of the provisions of the Health Insurance Portability and Accountability Act of 1996. *The Health Lawyer, 9*(3), 1.

Rubin, Paula N. & Dunne, Toni. (1995, February). The ADA: Emergency response systems and TDD's. pp. 1–7. National Institute of Justice: Research in Action.

Ryan, John. Dispelling common myths about documentation: Advice from a defense attorney. *Forum,* Harvard Risk Management Foundation.

Safeguarding the privacy of computer records. (1996, November 22). [*Knoxville News-Sentinel*]. *The Patriot Ledger,* p. 13.

Salcido, Robert. (1996, Mid-Winter). Application of the False Claims Act "knowledge" standard: What one must "know" to be held liable under the act. *The ABA Forum on Health Law, 8*(6), 1, 6.

Schulz, Ellen E. (1995, June 29). Fudging medical claims can backfire. *The Wall Street Journal,* p. C1.

Shao, Maria. Hospitals, patients settle suit on photocopy charges. *The Boston Globe.*

Snarey, John. (1987, June). A question of morality. *Psychology Today,* 6.

Stevens, William K. (1982, March 28). High medical costs. *New York Times,* pp. 1, 50.

Sullivan, Ronald. (1984, March 24). Queens hospital accused of denial of care. *New York Times,* p. 17.

Tammelleo, A. David. (1990, October). Who's to blame for faulty equipment? *RN,* 67.

Therapist punished for Simpson revelations. (1995, November 24). *The Boston Globe,* p. 19.

Thobaben, M., & Anderson, L. (1985). Reporting elder abuse: It's the law. *American Journal of Nursing, 85*(4), 371–374.

Tort law's victims. (1985, April 2). *The Wall Street Journal.*

US warns doctors, labs about kickbacks. (1994, October 14). *The Patriot Ledger,* p. 3.

Valente, Roberta L. (1985, Summer). Addressing domestic violence: The role of the family law practitioner. *Family Law Quarterly, 29*(1), 187–196.

Wagg, Dorothy. (1995, August 24). Medical records basic. p. 17. Massachusetts Hospital Association.

The Wall Street Journal, p. 1. (1982, July).

The Wall Street Journal, p. 1. (1990, February 13).

The Wall Street Journal, p. 83. (1993, January).

When dad's a sperm donor. (1993, January 15–17). *USA Weekend.*

Wilson, Paul T. Anesthesiology and malpractice lawsuits. *Medical Trial Technical Quarterly, 76,* 68–76, at 73.

Winslow, George & Ron. (1995, March 30). The HMO trend: Big, bigger, biggest. *The Wall Street Journal,* pp. B1, B4.

Winslow, Ron. (1995, April 26). Drug-industry sales pitches to doctors are inaccurate 11% of the time, study says. *The Wall Street Journal,* p. B6.

BOOKS

American College of Legal Medicine. (1988). *Legal medicine: Legal dynamics of medical encounter.*

Belli, Melvin M. (1986). *For your malpractice defense.* Medical Economics Books.

Biomedical safety and standards. (1985). Brea, CA: Quest Publishing Co.

Koop, Everett C. (1976). *The right to live; the right to die.* Wheaton, IL: Tyndale House Publishers.

Ladd, John. (1982). *Value conflicts in health care delivery.* Gruzalski Ballinger Publishing Co.

Landers, Louise. (1978). *Defective Medicine.*

Medico-legal forms with legal analysis. (1982). Chicago, IL: American Medical Association.

Nozick, Robert. (1974). *Anarchy, state and utopia.* NY: Basic Books.

Pfeiffer, J. W. (1974). *Nonrental communications: A collection of structured experiences for human relations training* (Vol. 2). La Jolla, CA: Univ. Assoc.

Provost, Gary. (1986). *Fatal dosage.* Bantam Books.

Scott, Russell, (1981). *The body as property.* NY: The Viking Press.

Trials of war criminals before the Nuremberg military tribunals under control council law (No. 10, Vol. 11). (October 1946–April 1949). Nuremberg.

MISCELLANEOUS

American Association of Medical Assistants, "Creed," 20 North Wacker Drive, Suite 1575, Chicago, IL 60606.

American Medical Association, "Principles of Medical Ethics," 535 North Dearborn Street, Chicago, IL 60610.

The Belmont Report: Ethical Principles and Guidelines for the Protection of Human Subjects of Research, Appendix I, DHEW Publications (OS) 78-0013. Washington, DC: Government Printing Office.

Child Abuse and Neglect Program, MCLE/NELI (October 25, 1984), Boston College, Massachusetts Continuing Legal Education, Inc., 20 West Street, Boston, MA 02111.

Excerpt from the decision at 331 F.2d 100 (D.C. Cir.), *cert. denied,* 377 U.S. 978 (1964). Reprinted as it appears in J. Katz (Ed.), *Experimentation with human beings,* pp. 551–552. (1972). NY: Russell Sage Foundation.

Gillespie, Karen. (June 1996). *Perspectives: Malpractice law evolves under managed care.* Princeton, NJ: The Robert Wood Johnson Foundation.

Medicare Part B Intermediary Letter No. 84-9: Payments to Respiratory Therapists by Durable Medical Equipment Suppliers and the Illegal Remuneration Provisions of the Social Security Act. (September 1984).

Medico-Legal Seminar, Roche Laboratories, Los Angeles, CA.

Presidents Commission. (1983). *Deciding for forego life-sustaining treatment,* p. 127.

Sexual Harrassment Survey, Massachusetts Department of Education, 1385 Hancock Street, Quincy, MA 02169.

Index

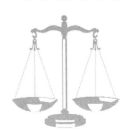